CHILDHOOD GLAUCOMA

Editors

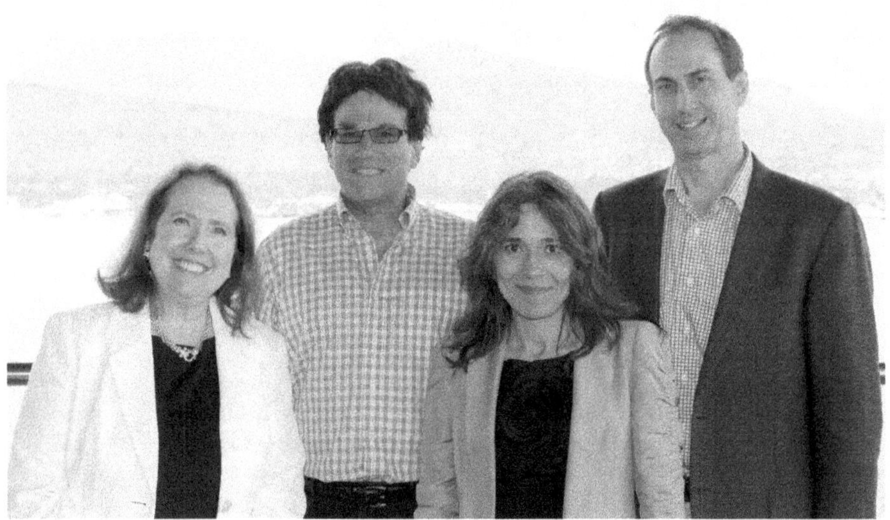

Alana L. Grajewski, Robert N. Weinreb, Maria Papadopoulos and John Grigg (L-R)

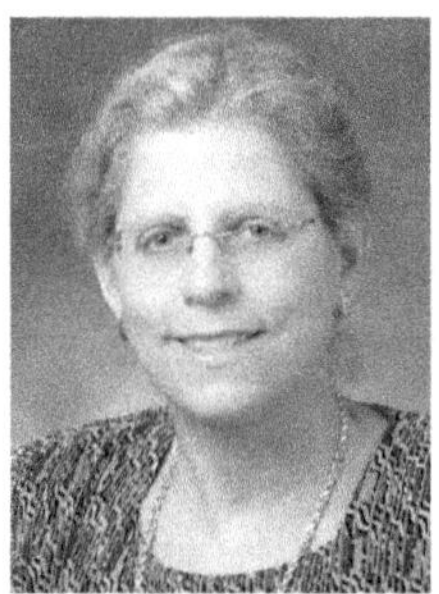

Sharon Freedman

CHILDHOOD GLAUCOMA

The 9th Consensus Report of the
World Glaucoma Association

Editors

Robert N. Weinreb
Alana L. Grajewski
Maria Papadopoulos
John Grigg
Sharon Freedman

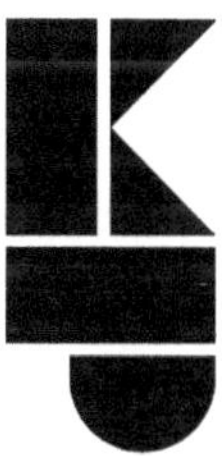

Kugler Publications/Amsterdam/The Netherlands

ISBN 13:978-90-6299-320-8

Standard soft cover print-on-demand edition. See our website for premium editions of our books.

Kugler Publications
P.O. Box 20538
1001 NM Amsterdam, The Netherlands
www.kuglerpublications.com

This publication is the ninth
of a series on
Consensus reports on Glaucoma
under the auspices of the
World Glaucoma Association

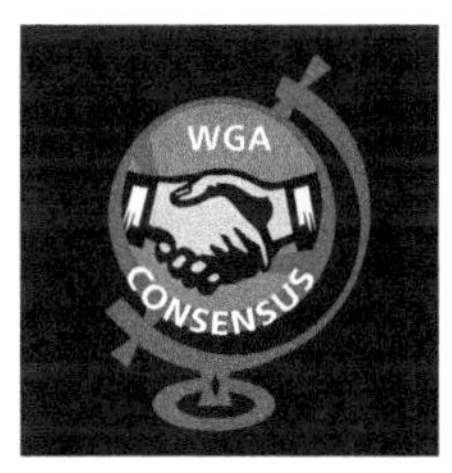

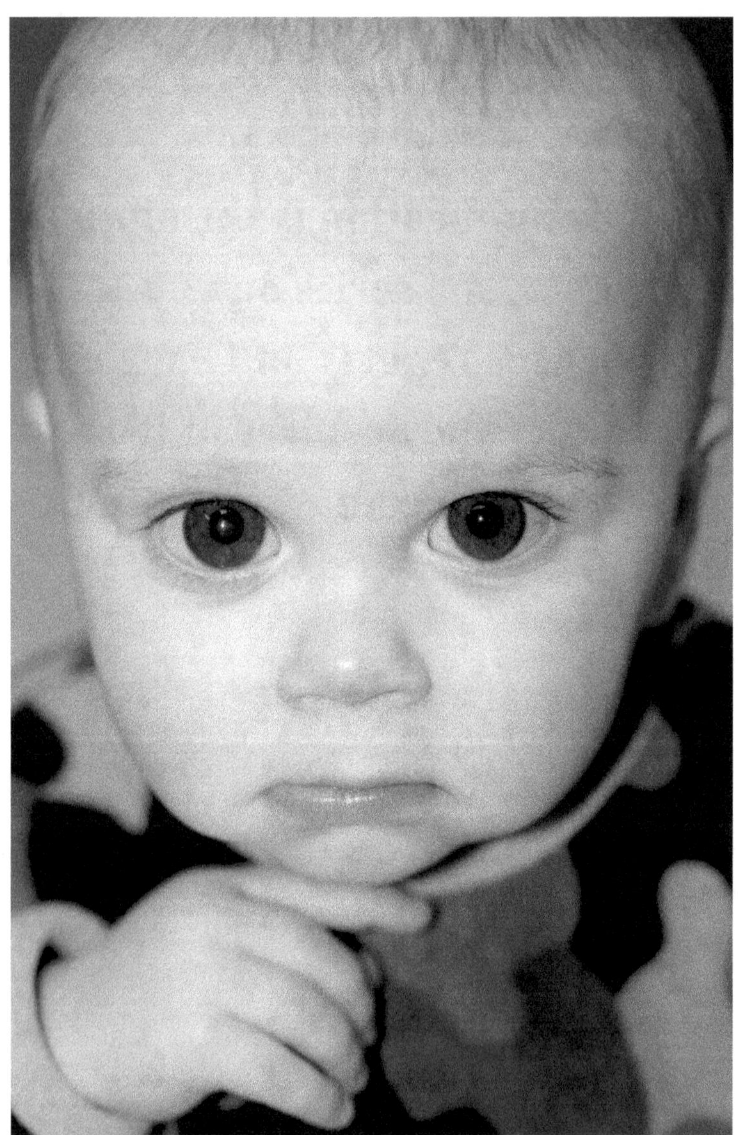

Photo provided by James D. Brandt

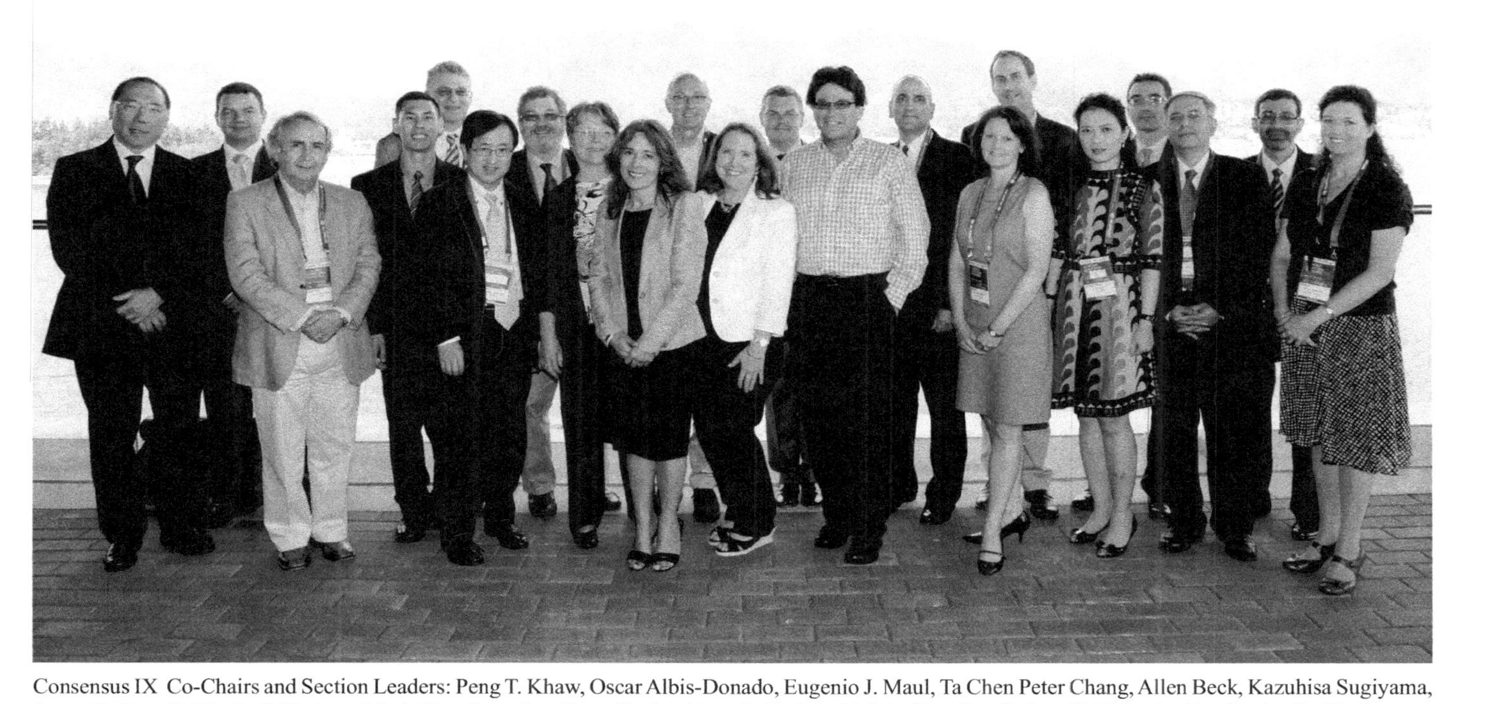

Consensus IX Co-Chairs and Section Leaders: Peng T. Khaw, Oscar Albis-Donado, Eugenio J. Maul, Ta Chen Peter Chang, Allen Beck, Kazuhisa Sugiyama, James D. Brandt, Elizabeth Hodapp, Maria Papadopoulos, Franz Grehn, Alana L. Grajewski, John Brookes, Robert N. Weinreb, Alex Levin, Cecilia Fenerty, John Grigg, Ching Lin Ho, Julian Garcia Feijoo, Tanuj Dada, Anil Mandal, Beth Edmunds (L-R)

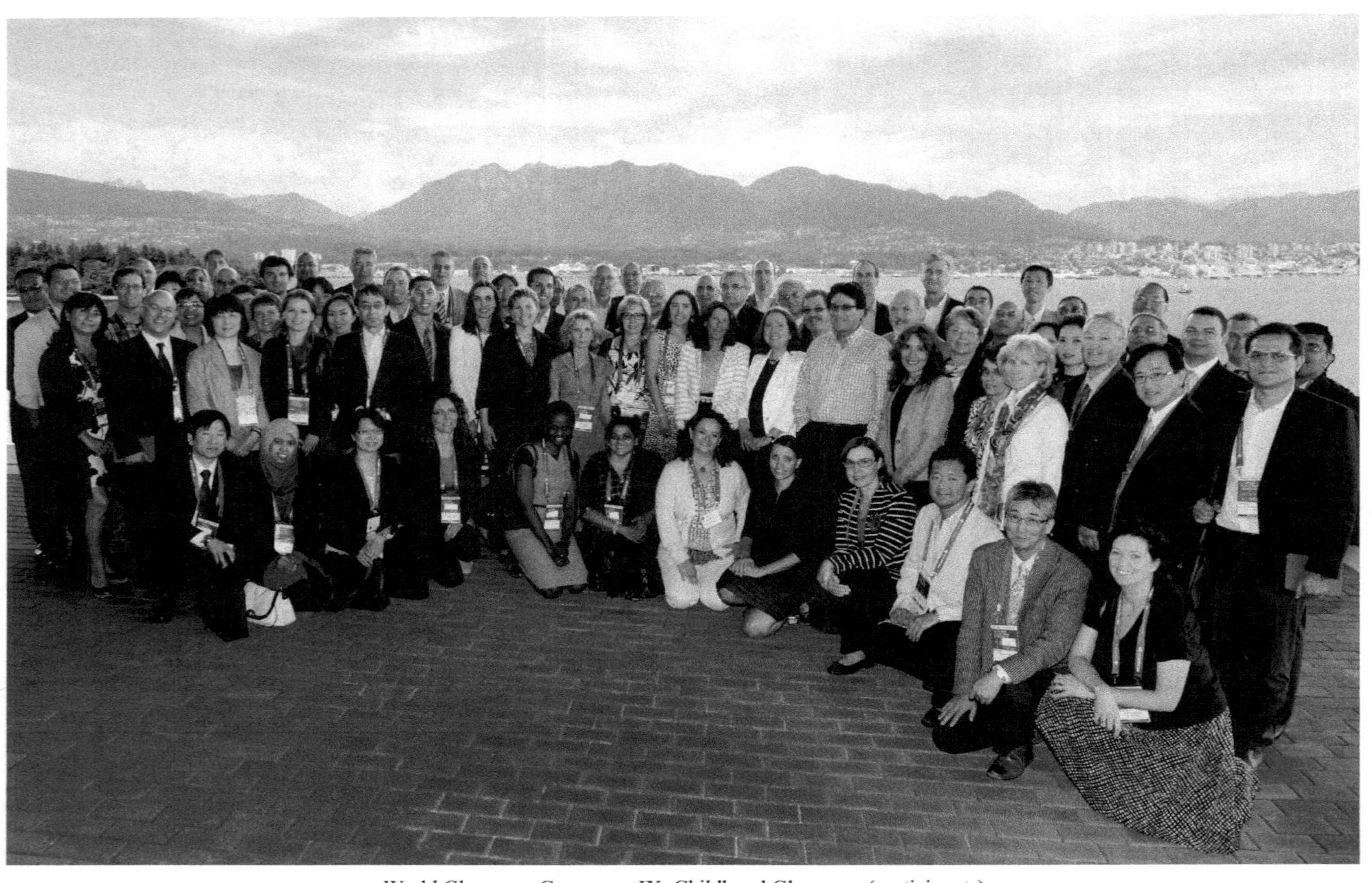

World Glaucoma Consensus IX: Childhood Glaucoma (participants)

FACULTY

Consensus Initiative Chair
Robert N. Weinreb, USA

Co-Chairs and Section Leaders
Sharon Freedman, USA
Alana L. Grajewski, USA
John Grigg, Australia
Maria Papadopoulos, UK

Co-Leaders
Oscar Albis, Mexico
Allen Beck, USA
Jamie Brandt, USA
John Brookes, UK
Valeria Coviltir, Romania
Tanuj Dada, India
Beth Edmunds, USA
Julián Garcia Feijoo, Spain
Cecilia Fenerty, UK
Nicola Freeman, South Africa
Franz Grehn, Germany
Viney Gupta, India
Ching Lin Ho, Singapore
Elizabeth Hodapp, USA
Peng Khaw, UK
Alex Levin, USA
David Mackey, Australia
Anil Mandal, India
Eugenio Maul, Chili
Ken Nischal, USA
Doug Rhee, USA
Kazuhisa Sugiyama, Japan

Participants
Joseph Abbott, UK
Ahmed Abdelrahman, Egypt
Manju Anilkumar, India
Michael Banitt, USA
Alberto Betinjane, Brazil
Susmito Biswas, UK
Elena Bitrian, Spain
Maria Cristina Brito, Portugal
Roberto Caputo, Italy

Kara Cavuoto, USA
Ta Chen Peter Chang, USA
Teresa Chen, USA
Mark Chiang, UK
Jocelyn Chua, Singapore
Anne Coleman, USA
Jamie Craig, Australia
Barbara Cvenkel, Slovenia
Tam Dang, Vietnam
Thomas Dietlein, Germany
Vera Essuman, Ghana
Robert Feldman, USA
John Fingert, USA
Simone Finzi, Brazil
Fede Fortunato, Italy
Tamiesha Frempong, USA
Stefano Gandolfi, Italy
Orna Geyer, Israel
Faisal Ghadhfan, Kuwait
Dawn Grovesnor, Barbedos
Patrick Hamel, Canada
Dale Heuer, USA
Tomomi Higashide, Japan
Gwen Hofman, Gabon
Hernán Iturriaga-Valenzuela, Chili
Farrah Ja'afar, Japan
Mohamad Jaafar, USA
Jan Erik Jakobsen, Norway
Robyn Jamieson, Australia
Karen Joos, USA
Shumita Kaushik, India
Ramesh Kekunnaya, India
Arif Khan, Saudi Arabia
Albert Khouri, USA
Yoshiaki Kiuchi, Japan
Thomas Klink, Germany
S.R. Krishnadas, India
Simon Law, USA
Ming Lee, Malaysia
Chris Lloyd, UK
Chris Lyons, Canada
Giorgio Marchini, Italy
Sheila Marco, Kenya

Carmen Méndez Hernández, Spain
Kimberley Miller, USA
Tony Moore, UK
Sy Moroi, USA
Akira Negi, Japan
Carlo Nucci, Italy
Michael O'Keefe, Ireland
Sola Olawoye, Nigeria
Mohammad Pakravan, Iran
Ki Ho Park, South Korea
Manoj Parulekar, UK
Norbert Pfeiffer, Germany
David Plager, USA
Pradeep Ramula, USA
Shira Robbins, USA
Christiane Rolim de Moura, Brazil
Jonathan Ruddle, Australia
Mansoor Sarfarazi, USA
Gabor Scharioth, Germany
Robert Schertzer, Canada
Lisa Schimmenti, USA
Sirisha Senthil, India
Janet Serle, USA
Alicia Serra-Castanera, Spain
Mark Sherwood, USA
Luis Silva, Venezuela
Scott Smith, United Arab Emirates

Nick Strouthidis, UK
Velota Sung, UK
Fatemeh Suri, Iran
Suman Thapa, Nepal
John Thygesen, Denmark
Carlo Traverso, Italy
Anya Trumler, USA
Deborah Vanderveen, USA
Ed Wilson, USA
Geoffrey Woodruff, UK
Chan Yun Kim, South Korea

Consensus Development Panel
Allen Beck, USA
Tanuj Dada, India
Sharon Freedman, USA
Alana L. Grajewski, USA
Franz Grehn, Germany
John Grigg, Australia
Jeff Liebmann, USA
Maria Papadopoulos, UK
Remo Susanna, Brasil
Robert N. Weinreb, USA

Recording Secretaries
Naama Hammel, USA
Kaweh Mansouri, USA

Glaucoma Societies/Sections of the following countries and regions have agreed to review the report:

Algeria, American Glaucoma Society, Argentina, Asia Pacific Glaucoma Society, Australian and New Zealand Glaucoma Interest Group, Austria, Azerbaijan, Bangladesh, Belgium, Bolivia, Brazil, Bulgaria, Canada, Chile, Chinese Glaucoma Society, Colombia, Costa Rica, Croatia, Czech, Denmark, Ecuador, Egypt, Estonia, European Glaucoma Society, Finland, France, Georgia, Germany, Glaucoma Society of India, Greece, Guatemala, Hungary, Iceland, Indonesia, International Society for Glaucoma Surgery, Iran, Ireland, Israel, Italy, Japan, Korea, Latin-American Glaucoma Society, Latvia, Lesotho, Lithuania, Mexico, Middle East African Glaucoma Society, Netherlands, Nigeria, Norway, Optometric Glaucoma Society, Pakistan, Pan American Glaucoma Society, Panama, Paraguay, Peru, Philippines, Poland, Portugal, Puerto Rico, Romania, Russia, Saudi Arabia, Serbia, Singapore, Slovakia, Slovenia, South Africa, Spain, Sweden, Switzerland, Taiwan, Thailand, Turkey, Ukraine, United Kingdom, Uruguay, Venezuela, Zambia

CONTENTS

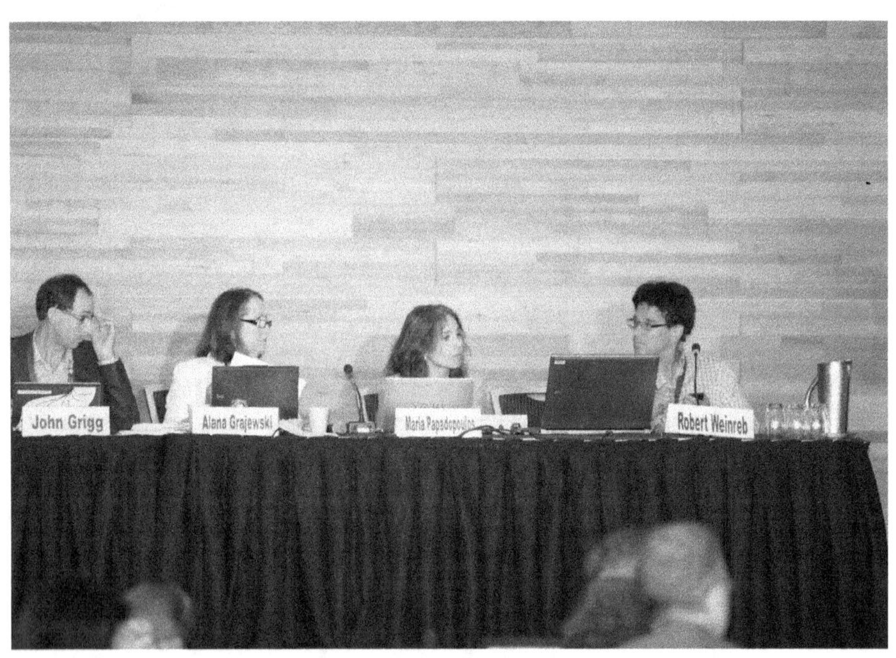

John Grigg, Alana L. Grajewski, Maria Papadopoulos, Robert N. Weinreb (L-R)

PREFACE

Childhood is the topic of the ninth World Glaucoma Association Consensus. There has been only sparse attention to the diagnosis and treatment of childhood glaucoma. Both pediatric ophthalmologists and glaucoma specialists provide care for such children. In some instances, they manage these individuals alone and, in others, the management is shared. For this consensus, the participation of both groups was solicited. The global faculty, consisting of leading authorities on the clinical and scientific aspects of childhood glaucoma, met in Vancouver on July 16, 2013, just prior to the World Glaucoma Congress, to discuss the reports and refine the consensus statements.

As with prior meetings, it was a daunting task to seek and obtain consensus on such a complicated and nuanced subject. It is unclear how each of us decides how we practice, and evidence to guide us often is sparse. It is remarkable how few high level studies have been conducted on the management of childhood glaucoma. Hence, this consensus, as with the others, is based not only on the published literature, but also on expert opinion. Although consensus does not replace and is not a surrogate for scientific investigation, it does provide considerable value, especially when the desired evidence is lacking.

The goal of this consensus was to provide a foundation for diagnosing and treating childhood glaucoma and how it can be best done in clinical practice. Identification of those areas for which we have little evidence and, therefore, the need for additional research also was a high priority. We hope that this consensus report will serve as a benchmark of our understanding. However, this consensus report, as with each of the others, is intended to be just a beginning. It is expected that it will be revised and improved with the emergence of new evidence.

Robert N. Weinreb, Chair

Co-Chairs:
Alana L. Grajewski
Maria Papadopoulous
Sharon Freedman
John Grigg

Consensus Secretaries

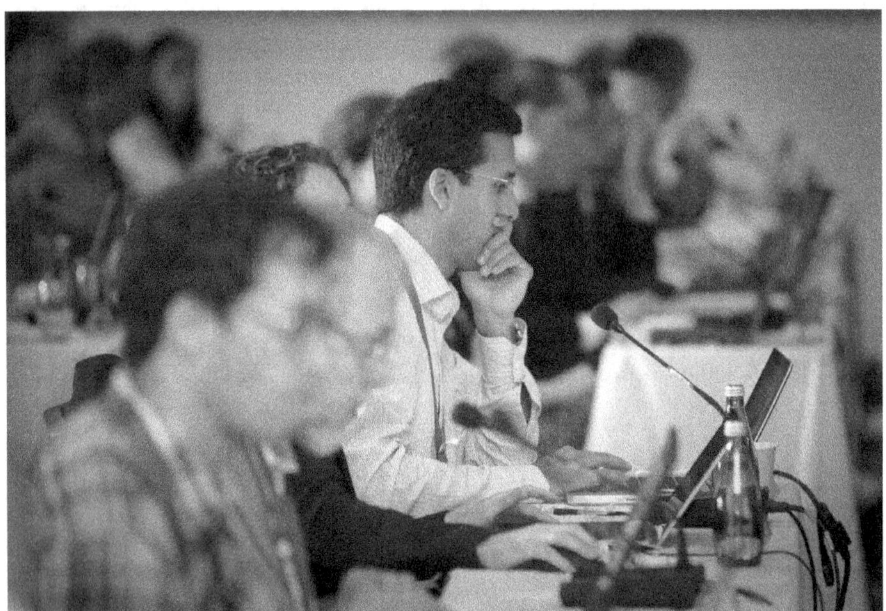

Kaweh Mansouri

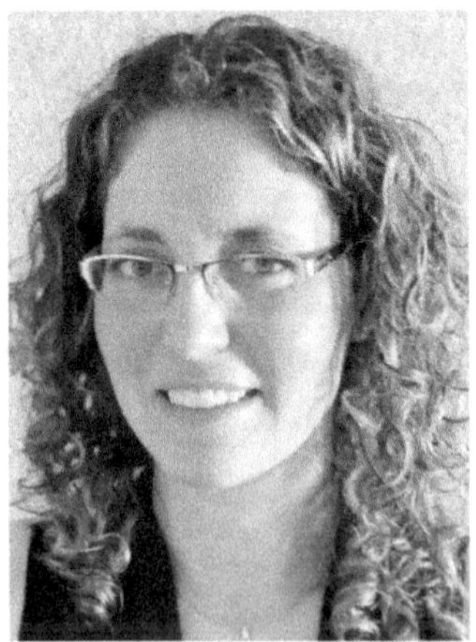

Naama Hammel

INTRODUCTION

One decade has passed since the first World Glaucoma Association Glaucoma Consensus was held in San Diego. The topic at that time was Glaucoma Diagnosis. Since then, a plethora of other topics in glaucoma have been addressed. For this Consensus, the ninth one, the topic is Childhood Glaucoma.

Global experts were invited and assembled by our international co-Chairs beginning in November, 2012, to participate in the Project Forum E-Room, a unique online forum that has facilitated discussion for each of the consensus meetings. The content was divided into ten sections and an important goal was to reach consensus on key issues that surround and permeate all aspects of childhood glaucoma. The results of these thoughtful discussions then were summarized by each of the sections with preliminary consensus statements. The Draft of the Consensus Report, including the preliminary consensus statements, was distributed to the Societies and Partners for review and comments prior to the Consensus Meeting that took place in Vancouver on Tuesday, July 16, 2013.

On this day, relevant stakeholders engaged in a stimulating, educational, and thought-provoking session that highlighted the review and revision of the consensus statements. The first presentation of the Report and the statements took place in a dedicated symposium during the fifth World Glaucoma Congress that followed the Consensus Meeting. The Consensus Report then was finalized by Consensus co-Chairs and Editors.

Robert N. Weinreb, Editor
La Jolla, California, USA

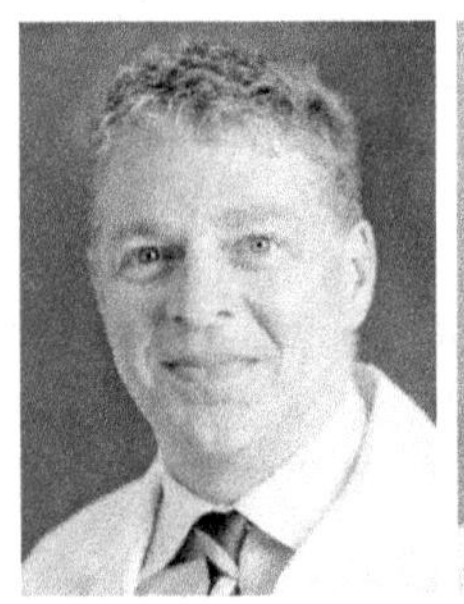

Allan Beck

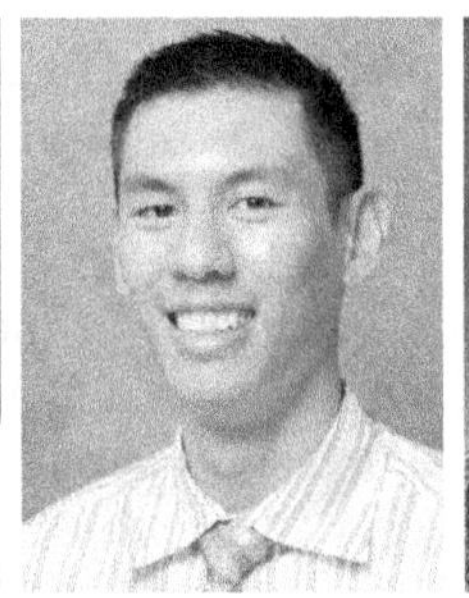

Ta Chen Peter Chang

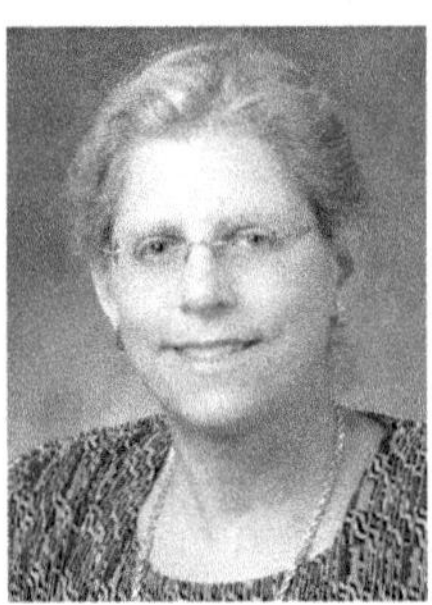

Sharon Freedman

1. DEFINITION, CLASSIFICATION, DIFFERENTIAL DIAGNOSIS

Allen Beck, Ta Chen Peter Chang, Sharon Freedman

Section leaders: Sharon Freedman, Allen Beck, Franz Grehn
Contributors: Maria Cristina Brito, Alberto Bentinjane, Thomas Dietlein

Consensus statements

1. Childhood glaucoma is intraocular pressure (IOP) related damage to the eye.
   Comment: In addition to the IOP, optic disc appearance and visual fields, the definition of glaucoma also reflects the effect of IOP on other ocular structures in infancy.
2. The interpretation of IOP measurement in infants and young children, especially during examination under anesthesia, can potentially be affected by many factors.
   Comment: Other signs of glaucoma in infants and young children, such as ocular enlargement, Haab striae and increased cup-to-disc ratio, may be more important than the IOP value in the assessment.
3. Childhood glaucoma is classified as primary or secondary. Secondary childhood glaucoma is further classified according to whether the condition is acquired after birth or is present at birth (non-acquired). Non-acquired childhood glaucoma is categorized according to whether the signs are mainly ocular or systemic.
   Comment: Terms such as 'developmental', 'congenital' or 'infantile' glaucoma lack clear definition and their use is to be discouraged.
4. A child should not be labeled as having glaucoma or subjected to surgical treatment unless one is reasonably sure of the diagnosis and has excluded other conditions that may mimic glaucoma.

Introductory / summary issues (main aims of this section)

General agreement with the definition of childhood glaucoma (with the use of clinical cases to validate in the development phase)

All responding participants have agreed with the definitions for childhood glaucoma and glaucoma suspect. There was some discussion on the impact of central

Childhood Glaucoma, pp. 3-10
Edited by Robert N. Weinreb, Alana L. Grajewski, Maria Papadopoulos, John Grigg,
and Sharon Freedman
2013 © Kugler Publications, Amsterdam, The Netherlands

corneal thickness (CCT) on IOP assessment, but the consensus was that more study is needed on this topic. The use of nomograms that 'adjust IOP' based on CCT is discouraged. The normal values for IOP during infancy were also discussed as being lower than adult normative values, and the impact of anesthesia on measuring IOP was acknowledged. For that reason, the recommendation was made that other signs of glaucoma (ocular enlargement, corneal signs such as Haab striae, and increased cup-to-disc ratio) may be more important than the IOP value during the examination under anesthesia of an infant with glaucoma or with suspected glaucoma.

General agreement with the classification, with the use of clinical cases to validate. (There will certainly continue to be disagreement since there are many classifications of childhood glaucoma and the disease itself comprises a heterogeneous group of disorders)

The responding participants used the new classification system to correctly classify all seven test cases, designed to represent each of the seven categories of the new system (Glaucoma Suspect plus the six groups of childhood glaucoma). This step provides some validation for the new classification system as both easy to use and applicable to common childhood glaucoma scenarios. The use of the term Childhood versus Pediatric was discussed, as well as the UNICEF definition of a child (younger than 16 years of age). The differential features of primary congenital glaucoma (PCG) as compared to juvenile open-angle glaucoma (JOAG) were addressed, namely the lack of ocular enlargement with JOAG and the normal angle findings in JOAG versus the described angle anomalies in PCG. It was decided that a complete description of the angle anomalies associated with PCG was beyond the scope of the classification system (*see* Section 2).

The classification of a case with cataract and signs of persistent fetal vasculature created the most controversy. Arguments for inclusion in the 'glaucoma-associated with non-acquired ocular anomalies' category versus inclusion in the 'glaucoma following congenital cataract surgery' category were offered and considered. A decision was made to modify the title of the latter category to: 'glaucoma following cataract surgery' with three sub-categories: (1) congenital idiopathic cataract; (2) congenital cataract associated with non-acquired ocular anomalies or systemic diseases; and (3) acquired cataract. This approach removes the dilemma of which category is most appropriate for a child with cataract who then develops glaucoma after surgery, yet captures important details about associated conditions which may play a role in the development of glaucoma.

The classification of glaucoma associated with congenital rubella syndrome created a similar dilemma of two potential classification scenarios. Compelling arguments were made to put congenital rubella in the 'glaucoma associated with non-acquired systemic disease/syndrome' category (based on ocular and systemic abnormalities present at birth) versus the 'glaucoma associated with acquired conditions' category (since rubella is an acquired infection transmitted from the mother to the fetus *in utero*). It was decided to place congenital rubella syndrome in the 'glaucoma associated with non-acquired systemic disease/syndrome' category, based on the presence of abnormalities at birth, and to clarify that the 'glaucoma associated with acquired condition' category is for conditions acquired after birth. This step simplifies the classification process for these two categories.

Keep classification as simple and logical as possible, resisting temptation to increase complexity until truly value-added

The aim is not to populate the classification with every cause of childhood glaucoma described or reported but instead with the most common conditions, and to provide guidance on categorization so that most people can logically ascertain where in the classification a given condition should be placed.

A discussion of the term 'developmental glaucoma' instead of 'non-acquired ocular anomalies' led to the decision to use the newer terminology, 'non-acquired ocular anomalies', due to its unambiguous meaning. Developmental glaucoma has been used in the past but lacks a clear definition and has become a 'wastebasket' category.

A discussion of the inclusion of Zellweger syndrome led to the decision to exclude it from the list of systemic syndromes due to rarity and extremely poor prognosis. Cutis marmorata telangiectiasia was eliminated for the same reason. The classification system allows rare syndromes to be included in the 'glaucoma associated with non-acquired systemic disease/syndrome' category without an exhaustive listing of all the rare diseases and syndromes that have been associated with childhood glaucoma. A suggested algorithm for using the new classification is detailed in Figure 1.

Emphasize features of clinical examination which help differentiate glaucoma from other conditions

No discussion ensued on the topic of differential diagnosis. The diagnostic features that distinguish PCG from other disorders that affect corneal clarity (Table 4) are part of the definition of childhood glaucoma. PCG can be distinguished from glaucoma associated with non-acquired ocular or systemic conditions by the presence or absence of associated ocular or systemic findings (Tables 1 and 2). PCG can be distinguished from conditions that cause epiphora or optic nerve findings such as a large cup-disc ratio by the absence of supportive findings such as ocular enlargement and elevated IOP (Table 4). A more detailed approach to the differential diagnosis is addressed in Section 2.

Definitions (Childhood Glaucoma Research Network (CGRN))

Definition of childhood

Based on national criteria: < 18 years of age (USA); ≤ 16 years of age (UK, Europe, UNICEF).

Definition of glaucoma – two or more required

- IOP > 21 mmHg (investigator discretion if examination under anesthesia data alone due to the variable effects of anesthesia on all methods of IOP assessment);
- Optic disc cupping (neuroretinal rim narrowing): a progressive increase in cup-disc ratio (diffuse rim narrowing), cup-disc asymmetry of ≥ 0.2 when the optic discs are of similar size, or focal rim narrowing;
- Corneal findings: Haab striae, corneal edema or diameter ≥ 11 mm in newborn, > 12 mm in child < 1 year of age, > 13 mm any age;
- Progressive myopia or myopic shift coupled with an increase in ocular dimensions out of keeping with normal growth;
- A reproducible visual field defect that is consistent with glaucomatous optic neuropathy with no other observable reason for the visual field defect.

Definition of glaucoma suspect – at least one required

- IOP > 21mmHg on two separate occasions;
- Suspicious optic disc appearance for glaucoma, *i.e.*, increased cup-disc ratio for size of optic disc;
- Suspicious visual field for glaucoma;
- Increased corneal diameter or axial length in setting of normal IOP.

Classification of Childhood Glaucoma (CGRN)

Primary childhood glaucoma

- Primary congenital glaucoma (PCG);
- Juvenile open-angle glaucoma (JOAG).

Secondary childhood glaucoma

- Glaucoma associated with non-acquired ocular anomalies;
- Glaucoma associated with non-acquired systemic disease or syndrome;
- Glaucoma associated with acquired condition;
- Glaucoma following cataract surgery.

Primary congenital glaucoma (PCG)

- Isolated angle anomalies ($\pm$ mild congenital iris anomalies);
- Meets glaucoma definition (usually with ocular enlargement);
- Subcategories based on age of onset
    1. Neonatal or newborn onset (0-1 month);
    2. Infantile onset (> 1-24 months);
    3. Late onset or late-recognized (> 2 years);
- Cases with normal IOP and optic discs but typical signs of PCG (*e.g.*, buphthalmos and Haab striae) that are not progressive may be classified as spontaneously arrested PCG.

Juvenile open-angle glaucoma (JOAG)

- No ocular enlargement;
- No congenital ocular anomalies or syndromes;
- Open angle (normal appearance);
- Meets glaucoma definition.

Glaucoma associated with non-acquired ocular anomalies

- Includes conditions of predominantly ocular anomalies present at birth which may or may not be associated with systemic signs;
- Meets glaucoma definition;
- List common ocular anomalies (*see* Table 1).

Glaucoma associated with non-acquired systemic disease or syndrome

- Includes conditions predominantly of systemic disease present at birth which may be associated with ocular signs;
- Meets glaucoma definition;
- List common systemic syndrome or disease (*see* Table 2).

Glaucoma associated with acquired condition

- Meets glaucoma definition after the acquired condition is recognized. An acquired condition is one that is not inherited or present at birth but which develops after birth;
- Glaucoma developing after cataract surgery is excluded from this category to highlight its frequency and differences from other conditions in the acquired condition category;
- List common acquired conditions (*see* Table 3);
- Based on gonioscopy results:
    1. Open-angle glaucoma ($\geq$ 50% open);
    2. Angle-closure glaucoma (< 50% open or acute angle closure).

Glaucoma following cataract surgery

- Meets glaucoma definition after cataract surgery is performed and is sub-divided into three categories based upon cataract type:
    1. Congenital idiopathic cataract;
    2. Congenital cataract associated with ocular anomalies / systemic disease (no previous glaucoma);
    3. Acquired cataract (no previous glaucoma).
- Based on gonioscopy results:
    1. Open-angle glaucoma ($\geq$ 50% open) or
    2. Angle-closure glaucoma (< 50% open or acute angle closure)

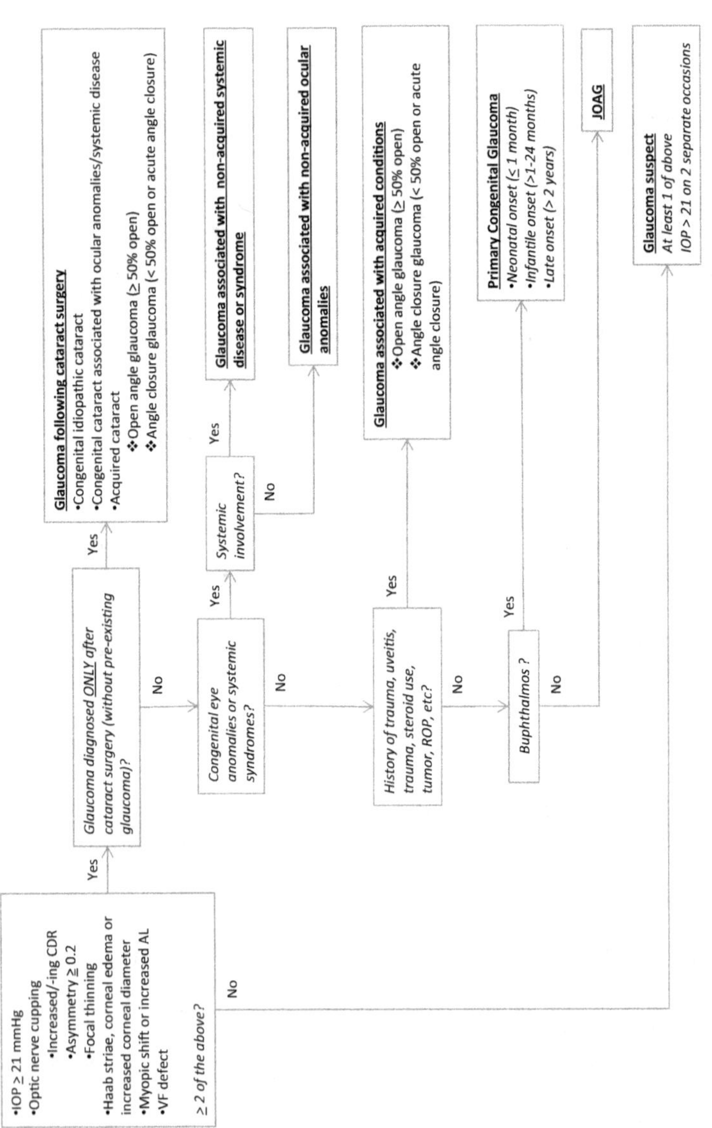

Fig. 1. Childhood glaucoma classification algorithm. The flow is from left to right, beginning with required factors for the definition of glaucoma and glaucoma suspect to final classification.

Table 1. Glaucoma associated with non-acquired ocular anomalies

Conditions with predominantly ocular anomalies **present at birth** which may or may not be associated with systemic signs

Axenfeld Rieger anomaly (syndrome if systemic associations)
Peters anomaly (syndrome if systemic associations)
Congenital ectropion uveae
Congenital iris hypoplasia
Aniridia
Persistent fetal vasculature (if glaucoma present before cataract surgery)
Oculodermal melanocytosis (Nevus of Ota)
Posterior polymorphous dystrophy
Microphthalmos
Microcornea
Ectopia lentis
    Simple ectopia lentis (no systemic associations)
    Ectopia lentis et pupillae

Table 2. Glaucoma associated with non-acquired systemic disease or syndrome

Conditions predominantly with known syndromes, systemic anomalies or systemic disease present at birth which may be associated with ocular signs

Chromosomal disorders such as Trisomy 21 (Down syndrome)
Connective tissue disorders
    Marfan syndrome
    Weill-Marchesani syndrome
    Stickler syndrome
Metabolic disorders
    Homocystinuria
    Lowe syndrome
    Mucopolysaccharidoses
Phacomatoses
    Neurofibromatosis (NF-1, NF-2)
    Sturge-Weber syndrome
    Klippel-Trenaunay-Weber syndrome
Rubinstein-Taybi
Congenital rubella

Table 3. Glaucoma associated with acquired condition

Conditions which are not inherited or present at birth but which develop after birth

Uveitis
Trauma (hyphema, angle recession, ectopia lentis)
Steroid induced
Tumors (benign/malignant, ocular/orbital)
Retinopathy of Prematurity (ROP)
Post surgery other than cataract surgery

Table 4. Differential diagnosis of primary congenital glaucoma in infancy (for detailed discussion of the differential diagnosis refer to Section 2)

A. Glaucoma associated with non-acquired ocular anomalies or with non-acquired systemic disease or syndrome
B. Corneal / ocular enlargement
   1. X linked megalocornea
   2. Congenital high myopia
   3. Connective tissue disorders (*e.g.*, Marfan syndrome, osteogenesis imperfecta)
   4. LTBP2 mutations
C. Corneal haziness
   1. Obstetric trauma
   2. Corneal dystrophies (*e.g.*, PPMD, CHED)
   3. Metabolic disorders (*e.g.*, mucopolysaccharidoses, mucolipidoses, cystinosis)
   4. Infection (*e.g.*, congenital rubella without IOP increase or other signs of glaucoma)
   5. Peters anomaly / sclerocornea (without IOP increase or other signs of glaucoma)
D. Other causes of epiphora
   1. Nasolacrimal duct obstruction
   2. Conjunctivitis
   3. Corneal abrasion/keratitis
E. Congenital optic nerve cupping
   1. Physiologic cupping of large optic nerves
   2. Optic nerve hypoplasia with periventricular leukomalacia
   3. Optic nerve coloboma
   4. Optic nerve pit
   5. Other optic nerve abnormality

References

1. Yeung HH, Walton DS. Clinical classification of childhood glaucomas. Arch Ophthalmol 2010; 128: 680-684.
2. Hoskins HD Jr, Shaffer RN, Hetherington J. Anatomical classification of the developmental glaucomas. Arch Ophthalmol 1984; 102: 1331-1336.
3. Papadopoulos M, Cable N, Rahi J, Khaw PT; BIG Eye Study Investigators. The British Infantile and Childhood (BIG) Eye Study. Invest Ophthalmol Vis Sci 2007; 48: 4100-4106.
4. Beck AD, Freedman SF, Lynn MJ, Bothun E, Neely DE, Lambert SR; for the Infant Aphakia Treatment Study Group. Glaucoma-related adverse events in the Infant Aphakia Treatment Study: 1 year results. Arch Ophthalmol 2012; 130: 130-135.
5. Chen TC, Walton DS, Bhatia LS. Aphakic glaucoma after congenital cataract surgery. Arch Ophthalmol 2004; 122: 1819-1825.
6. Isenberg SJ. Physical and refractive characteristics of the eye at birth and during infancy. In: Isenberg SJ (Ed.), *The Eye in Infancy*. St. Louis: Mosby 1994.
7. Freedman S, Walton, DS. Glaucoma in infants and children. In: Nelson LB, Olitsky S (Eds.), Harley's Pediatric Ophthalmology. Philadelphia: W.B. Saunders Company 2005.
8. Khan AO. Conditions that can be mistaken as early childhood glaucoma. Ophthalmic Genet 2011; 32: 129-137.

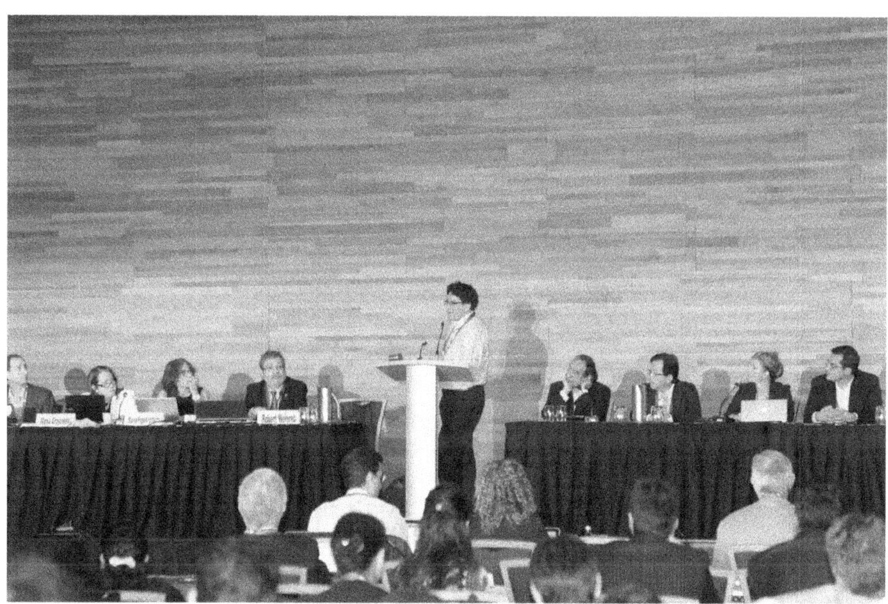

John Grigg, Alana L. Grajewski, Maria Papadopoulos and James D. Brandt, Robert N. Weinreb, Hernán Iturriaga-Valenzuela, Kazuhisa Sugiyama, Shira Robbins, Mohammad Pakravan (L-R)

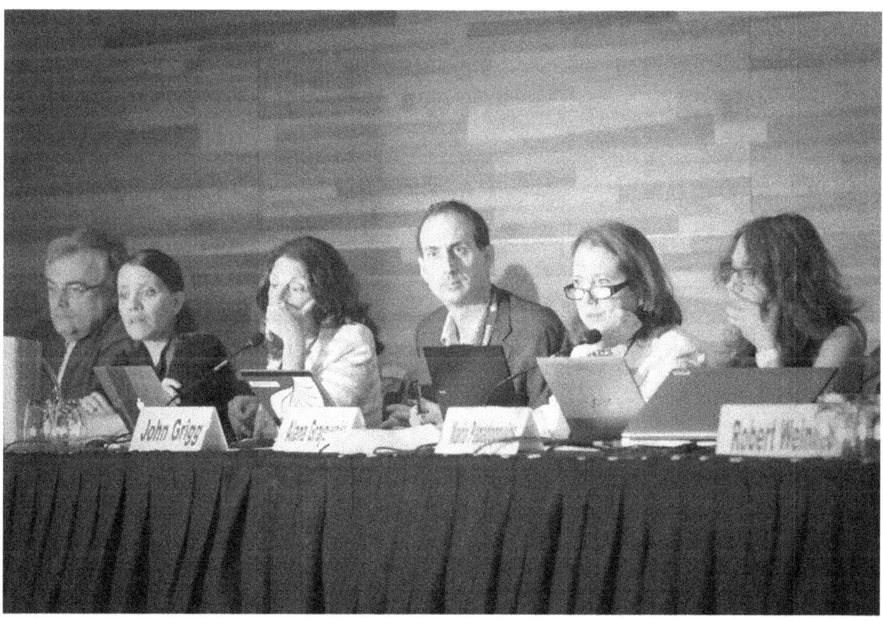

Stefano Gandolfi, Anya Trumler, Janet Serle, John Grigg, Alana L. Grajewski, Maria Papadopoulos (L-R)

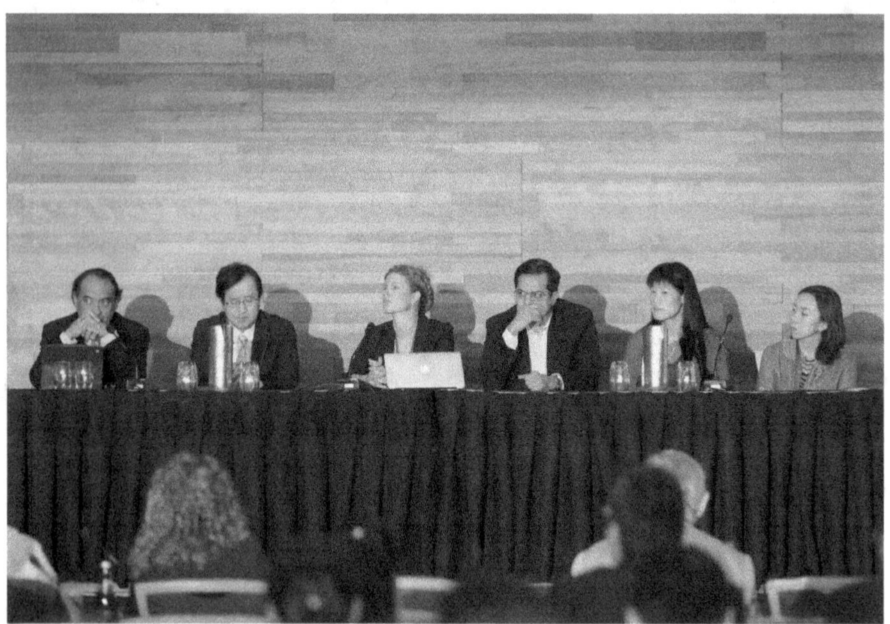

Hernán Iturriaga-Valenzuela, Kazuhisa Sugiyama, Shira Robbins, Mohammad Pakravan, Teresa Chen, Jocelyn Chua (L-R)

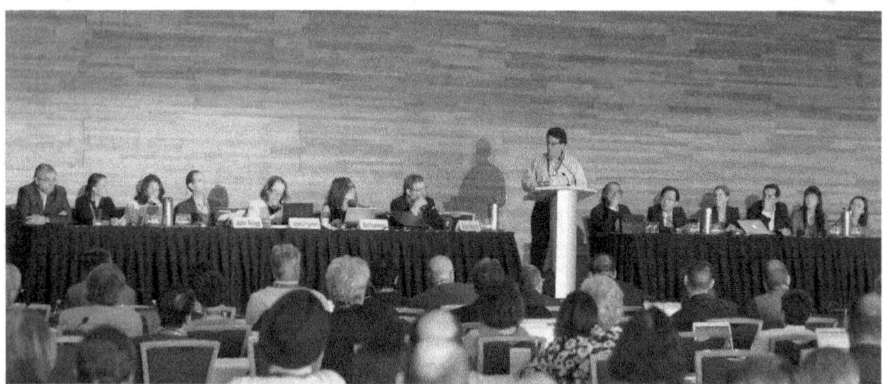

Stefano Gandolfi, Anya Trumler, Janet Serle, John Grigg, Alana L. Grajewski, Maria Papadopoulos, James D. Brandt, Robert N. Weinreb, Hernán Iturriaga-Valenzuela, Kazuhisa Sugiyama, Shira Robbins, Mohammad Pakravan, Teresa Chen, Jocelyn Chua (L-R)

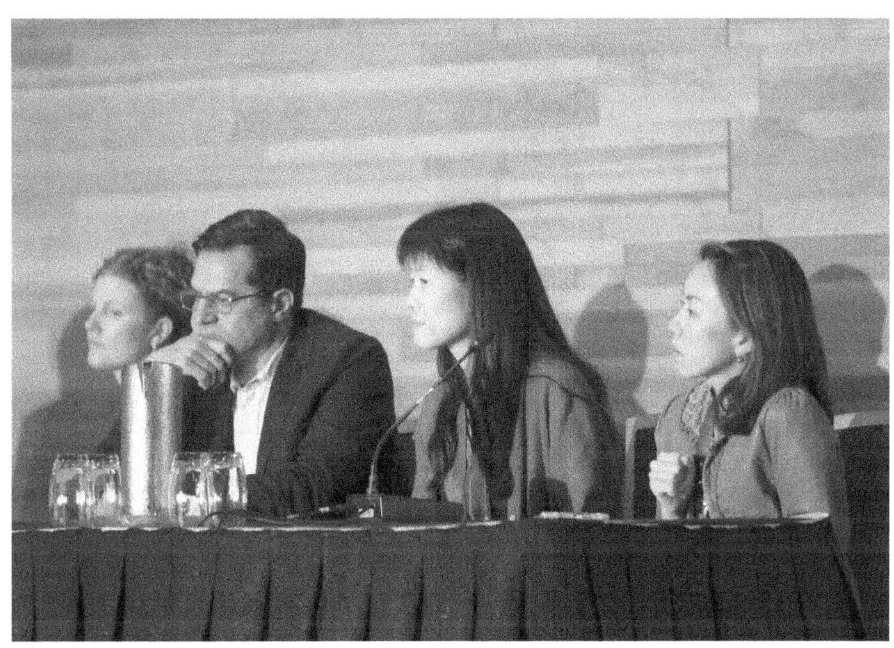

Shira Robbins, Mohammad Pakravan, Teresa Chen, Jocelyn Chua (L-R)

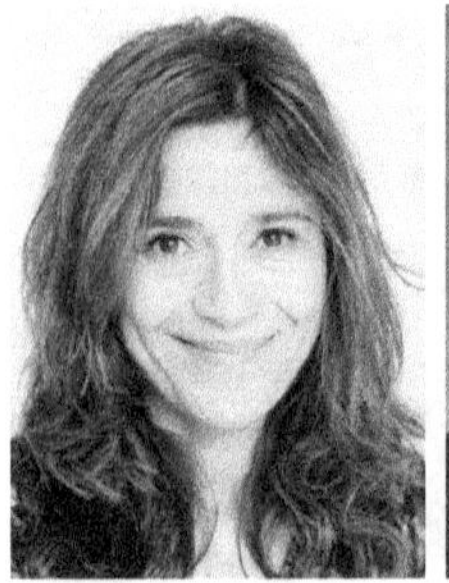

Maria Papadopoulos

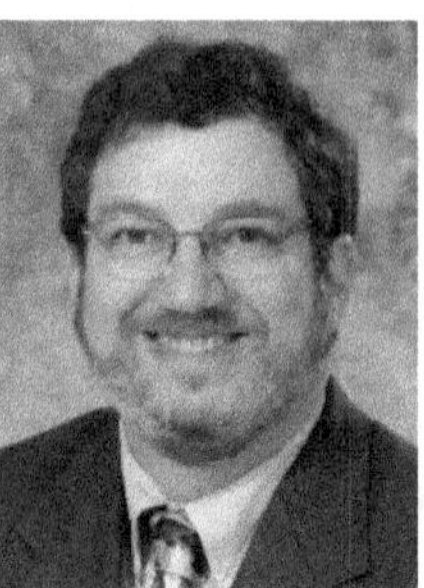

James D. Brandt

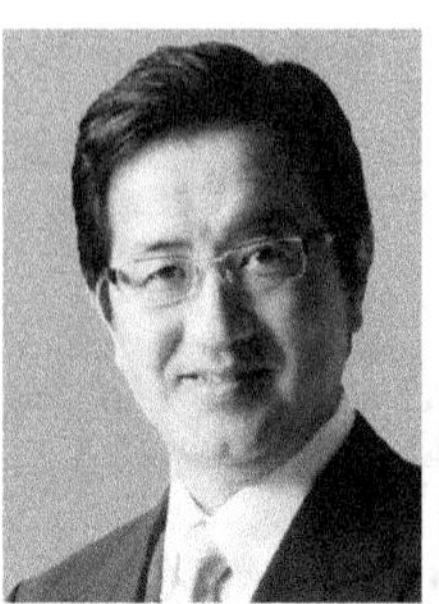

Kazuhisa Sugiyama

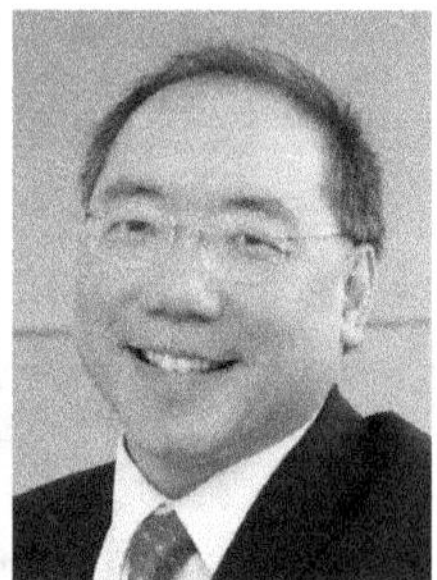

Peng T. Khaw

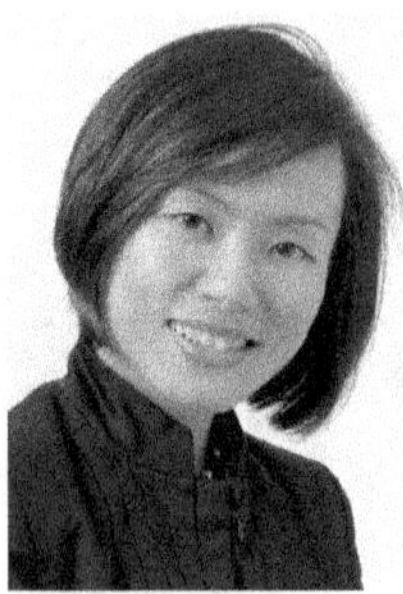

Jocelyn Chua

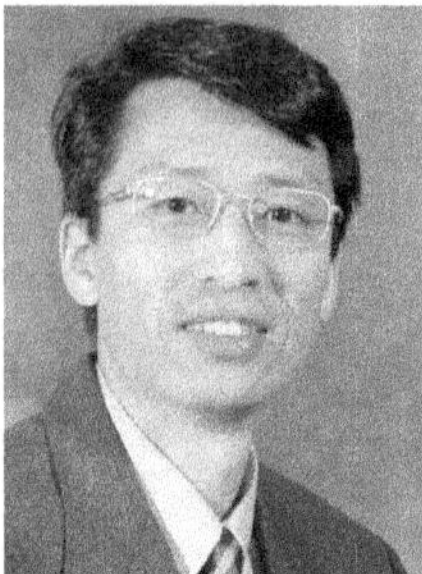

Simon Law

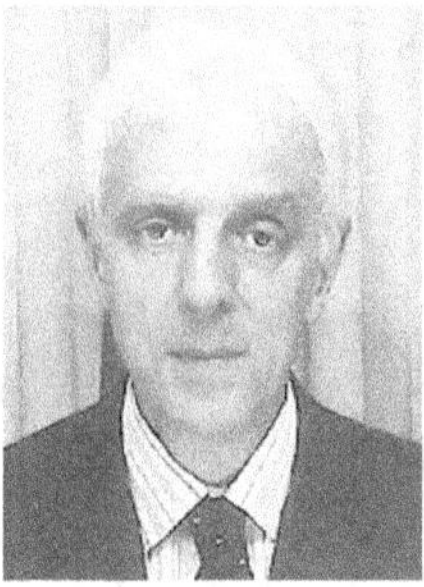

Alberto Betinjane

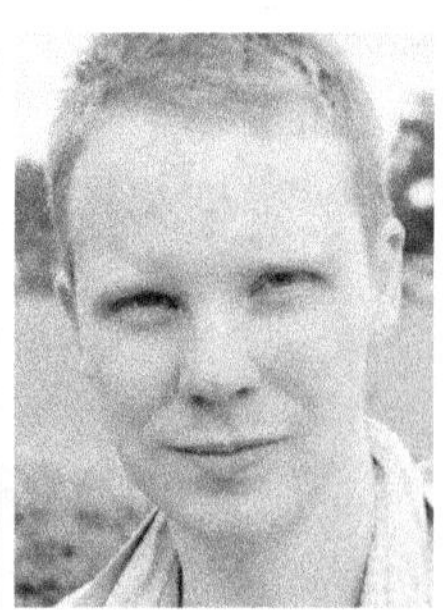

Joseph Abbott

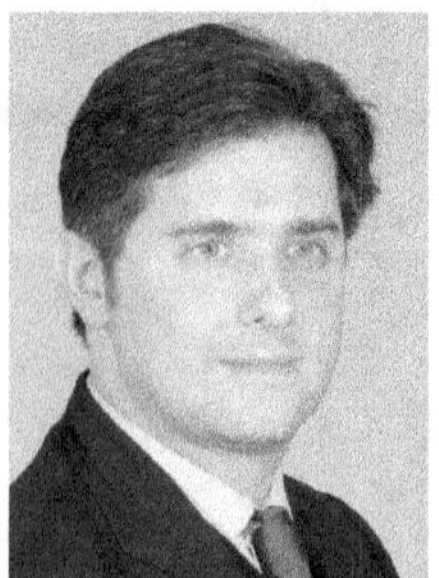

Nick Strouthidis

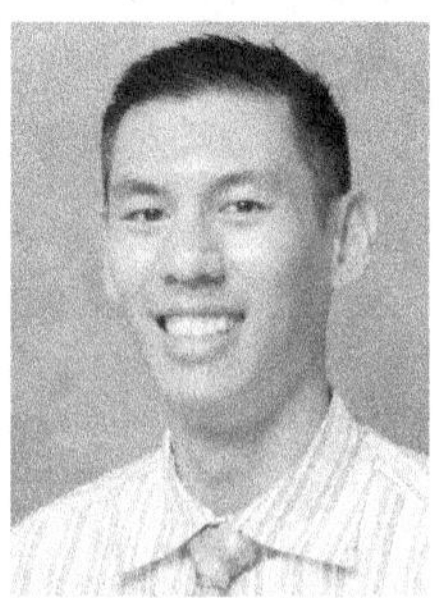

Ta Chen Peter Chang

2. ESTABLISHING THE DIAGNOSIS AND DETERMINING GLAUCOMA PROGRESSION

Maria Papadopoulos, James D. Brandt, Kazuhisa Sugiyama, Peng T. Khaw, Jocelyn Chua, Simon Law, Alberto Betinjane, Joseph Abbott, Nick Strouthidis, Ta Chen Peter Chang

Section Leaders: Maria Papadopoulos, James D. Brandt, Kazuhisa Sugiyama
Contributors: Arif Khan, Mohammad Pakravan, Anya Trumler, Alicia Serra-Castanera, Shira Robbins, Teresa Chen, Suman Thapa, Hernán Iturriaga-Valenzuela, Janet Serle, Albert Khouri, Farrah Ja'afar

Consensus statements

1. Prompt diagnosis of childhood glaucoma and appropriate prompt treatment can minimize the degree of visual impairment.
    Comment: Examination under anesthesia or sedation may be appropriate to make the diagnosis, perform surgery or plan further treatment.
2. A child should not be labeled as having glaucoma or subjected to surgical treatment unless one is reasonably sure of the diagnosis and has excluded other conditions that may mimic glaucoma.
    Comment: If doubt exists about the diagnosis or evidence of progression cannot be determined, then appropriately timed follow-up or examination under anesthesia or sedation is advisable.
    Comment: Children should be encouraged onto the slit lamp for more accurate evaluation [intraocular pressure (IOP) measurement and optic disc assessment] when it appears this may be possible.
3. Glaucoma in children is characterized by the presence of elevated IOP and characteristic optic disc cupping. In addition to these features, glaucoma in infancy is associated with ocular enlargement, *buphthalmos*.
    Comment: IOP measurement and optic disc appearance are fundamental features of the examination throughout the life of a child with glaucoma. In an infant whose eye is still vulnerable to other effects of elevated IOP, proxies of persistent elevated IOP (enlarging corneal diameter, increasing axial length and progressive myopia) also need to be taken into consideration and regularly assessed.

Childhood Glaucoma, pp. 15-41
Edited by Robert N. Weinreb, Alana L. Grajewski, Maria Papadopoulos, John Grigg,
and Sharon Freedman
2013 © Kugler Publications, Amsterdam, The Netherlands

Comment: In children, the conclusion with regard to the diagnosis or progression of glaucoma must be based on the overall clinical findings and investigation results.

4. IOP measurement *in infancy and early childhood* can be influenced by many factors so is often unreliable when used in diagnosis and management.

5. IOP response to anesthetic agents is unpredictable. All inhaled agents lower IOP, sometimes rapidly and profoundly.
   Comment: Chloral hydrate, ketamine and midazolam appear not to lower IOP.
   Comment: Use the same anesthetic for serial examinations.

6. Increasing corneal diameter is the hallmark of all forms of glaucoma in infancy and early childhood.
   Comment: Corneal enlargement due to elevated IOP usually occurs before three years of age. Serial corneal diameter measurements are useful in establishing the diagnosis and in the monitoring of progression of glaucoma up to the age of three years.
   Comment: Central corneal thickness (CCT) should not be used to adjust IOP measurements as its role in childhood tonometry remains to be determined.

7. Gonioscopy is crucial in making the correct diagnosis and for planning surgical treatment. It should be performed at least once when possible.

8. Optic disc appearance is an important and sensitive parameter for both diagnosis and determination of progression in childhood glaucoma.
   Comment: Optic nerve size, the cup-disc ratio, focal areas of rim loss, and nerve fiber layer defects should be documented, preferably through a large pupil.
   Comment: A magnified binocular view is preferable, so attempt to examine a child on the slit lamp as soon as they are cooperative.
   Comment: Documenting the appearance of the disc at baseline and follow-up is desirable in determining both diagnosis and response to treatment.
   Comment: Cupping reversal is common in successfully-treated childhood glaucoma.
   Comment: Automated optic nerve imaging (*e.g.*, OCT) is limited by the lack of normative data and portability of the devices.

9. Rapid changes in refractive status and axial length (AL) determination are helpful in both diagnosing the disease and determining response to treatment while the sclera remains vulnerable to the effects of elevated IOP.
   Comment: AL outside normal limits is strongly suggestive of glaucoma.
   Comment: Continued enlargement of AL beyond the normal range suggests inadequately-treated glaucoma.
   Comment: Progressive myopia is additional evidence of glaucoma progression.

10. Assessment of the visual field in children can be useful but is challenging.
    Comment: It may be helpful to use the shortest possible test (*e.g.*, program 24-2 Sita Fast).
    Comment: Repeat visual fields to confirm deficits. If repeated testing shows consistent findings, the measurements are probably valid.

Comment: Although there is no normative database for children, age correction of the mean deviation for standard automated perimetry is small (0.7 db/decade). Moreover, useful metrics, such as pattern standard deviation, glaucoma hemifield test and glaucoma change probability, are largely unaffected by age.

Introduction

Glaucoma in children is a uniquely disabling disease. Early diagnosis and appropriate treatment can minimize a lifetime of visual impairment. Therefore the suspicion of glaucoma in a child should always be treated seriously and with urgency. However, the assessment of a child with glaucoma or suspected glaucoma can be challenging. It requires examination in either the clinic, office or under anesthesia depending on the child's age and ability to cooperate. A neonate or infant who is feeding or sleeping can often be thoroughly examined in the clinic or office. However, most infants and young children require an examination under anesthesia (EUA) or sedation (EUS) until they can cooperate with all the components of an office exam, which often occurs by the age of four or five.

Glaucoma in children is characterized by the presence of elevated intraocular pressure (IOP) and characteristic optic disc cupping. In addition to these features, glaucoma in infancy is associated with ocular enlargement, *buphthalmos*, which results from the biomechanical effects of elevated IOP in an eye with immature connective tissues (primarily collagen). The age of glaucoma onset determines the relevant questions to ask during the history taking and the clinical findings to identify. Although IOP measurement and optic disc appearance are fundamental features of the examination throughout the life of a child with glaucoma, in an infant whose eye is still vulnerable to other effects of elevated IOP, proxies of persistent elevated IOP (enlarging corneal diameter, increasing axial length and progressive myopia) must also be taken into consideration and regularly assessed. In infants, the conclusion with regard to the diagnosis or progression of glaucoma must be based on the *overall* clinical findings and investigation results. As a child grows older, the cornea and sclera mature (become less elastic), so findings such as corneal diameter and axial length (AL) become less useful measurements. Improved cooperation with slit lamp examination allows more accurate evaluation of the anterior segment, assessment of IOP, and visualization of the optic disc and the nerve fiber layer with greater magnification. Hence, children should be encouraged onto the slit lamp for evaluation as soon as it appears this may be possible. Eventually, visual fields become feasible to assess functional vision, which are especially useful in advanced cases.

The initial consultation and assessment is an absolutely vital part of managing children with glaucoma as it is the beginning of what may become a lifetime relationship between the ophthalmologist, patient and his/her parents. The aim of the initial assessment is either to: (1) make a diagnosis of glaucoma and determine the type of glaucoma, primary or secondary (vital in determining management); or

(2) if glaucoma cannot be ruled out, to establish that enough evidence for glaucoma exists to justify further follow up or an EUA/S for a more complete examination and possible surgery. In established glaucoma cases, the aim is to determine the presence or absence of progression. In cases where doubt exists and a diagnosis or evidence of progression cannot be determined, then an EUA/S is advisable. A child should not be labeled as having glaucoma or subjected to surgery unless one is reasonably sure of the diagnosis.

Assessment

History

Children with glaucoma will present either: (1) with signs of glaucoma in infancy; (2) with a condition known to predispose them to glaucoma, *e.g.*, aniridia; (3) with a family history of childhood glaucoma, following screening; or (4) having failed routine school vision testing.

A detailed history must be obtained from family members, including the onset of clinical signs and symptoms, such as generalized irritability and discontent, as well as family and gestational history. Aspects of each of these can have a profound influence on the prognosis (*e.g.*, time of onset), treatment plan, genetic counseling and future child-bearing plans for the parents. It is important to determine:

(a) Signs and symptoms:
- Age of clinical onset for prognosis.
- In a neonate or infant, enquire about a history of epiphora (without discharge), photophobia (first symptom the child experiences), blepharospasm, corneal haze/opacification (usually first sign noticed by parents), change in ocular appearance with time or in response to treatment:
  o The classic triad of signs (epiphora without discharge, photophobia, blepharospasm) all relate to the effect of elevated IOP on the cornea and can result from any cause of glaucoma (primary or secondary).
  o Old photographs may help confirm a change in eye size.
  o With prompting, parents may recall an episode of a cloudy cornea that has since resolved.
  o Glaucoma may present as a 'red eye' mimicking conjunctivitis and is often misdiagnosed as such by general practioners, but as opposed to glaucoma, conjunctivitis is often associated with discharge. Similarly, nasolacrimal duct obstruction is associated with epiphora and discharge, but no photophobia. Corneal abrasions are common causes of acute ocular irritation with epiphora and photophobia but are often diagnosed from the history and examination. With all the above conditions there is no ocular enlargement and the optic nerve is normal.

(b) Gestational history:
- Problems during pregnancy (*e.g.*, maternal rubella).
- Delivery history (*e.g.*, use of forceps).

(c) Family history:
- Family history of childhood glaucoma (if present, siblings must be examined, especially if it is due to an autosomal dominant condition).
- History of parental consanguinity (if present, siblings must be examined).

(d) General pediatric & syndromic history:
- Is child meeting developmental milestones? Neurologically normal?
- Is child being worked up for cardiac or genito-urinary abnormalities or dysmorphic issues?
- If child has history of pediatric cataract, is cause known? (*e.g.*, congenital rubella, Lowe syndrome).
- Anesthetic or airway issues (*e.g.*, homocystinuria, Rubinstein-Taybi syndrome)?
- History of atopic disease (*e.g.*, asthma – enquire about systemic prednisolone use, inhaled steroids, eczema – facial steroid creams)?

(e) Ocular history:
- In older children, a history of ocular trauma, intraocular inflammation, ocular surgery or topical corticosteroid use may be relevant.

Examination

General appearance, visual behavior and visual acuity assessment

The examination of an infant or child suspected to have glaucoma should begin by assessing their overall appearance and visual behavior, including the signs of nystagmus or strabismus. Age-appropriate visual acuity assessment is important with regards amblyopia management and may be useful as a measure of progression in advanced cases. Ambient illumination can be reduced to allow a neonate or infant to open their eyes, permitting a more complete examination by penlight or portable slit lamp. Through observation alone it may be possible to assess the presence of corneal edema, lacrimation, photophobia, blepharospasm and the relative and actual size of both eyes. The examination of infants can be greatly aided if performed during breast/bottle-feeding or whilst sleeping and so parents should be advised to arrange the feeding or sleeping schedule to coincide with the office or outpatient visit. When indicated, it is important to examine the patient's parents as the presence of subtle signs of Axenfeld-Rieger anomaly in the parents may change the genetic advice given and alter the management of subsequent siblings.

Intraocular pressure (IOP)

IOP in normal neonates is thought to be lower than the adult mean[1] with it increasing to adult levels by teenage years.[2]

Measuring the IOP in children can be challenging as it is potentially influenced by many factors such as: type of tonometer, cooperation, eye movements, anesthesia (discussed in a later section), intubation, speculum use and the cornea [oedema, opacities, biomechanical properties and central corneal thickness (CCT)]. In light of the above, IOP is among the least accurate and most variable of all the parameters measured when assessing a child for glaucoma – therefore the diagnosis of childhood glaucoma should never be made on the basis of elevated IOP alone. Instead it should be based on the overall clinical findings and investigation results.

The reference standard for IOP measurement is Goldmann applanation tonometry (GAT) and the Perkins tonometer (a handheld version of GAT) for use during EUA, whenever possible. The TonoPen™ is a modified Mackay-Marg electronic tonometer and often used in pediatric patients. However, the Tonopen™ is known to overestimate the IOP in children compared to Perkins in both normal children and those with glaucoma.[3-5] The pneumatonometer is frequently useful in young children. Eisenberg and colleagues performed manometric evaluation of these three different tonometers[6] in a small group of normal adult and pediatric eyes. They found that the pneumatonometer was unaffected by age and recommended it for use in pediatric eyes. However, they also commented that pneumatonometry produced a significantly higher estimation of IOP compared to applanation tonometry.

A disadvantage of both GAT and Tonopen™ for neonates and infants in the office/clinic setting is the need for topical anesthesia. More recently, the iCare™ portable rebound tonometer has become available for IOP measurement without the installation of topical anaesthetic drops. It can be used in the upright position and is well tolerated.[7, 8] As such, it is gaining popularity for pediatric IOP assessment in the office/clinic setting. However, it is thought to have a similar reliability to TonoPen™ and a tendency to overestimate in known or suspected glaucoma cases compared to applanation tonometry.[9-13] Dahlmann-Noor and colleagues,[10] found the magnitude of disagreement in children with glaucoma to increase with the level of IOP and with higher CCT. However, measurements within the normal range were likely to be accurate. Therefore, a normal measurement of IOP by rebound tonometry could spare the child an unnecessary EUA. A high reading should alert the clinician to retest the IOP using applanation tonometry if possible and to consider the measurement within the context of other clinical and investigation findings. iCare™ can be used in a supine baby by rolling them into a lateral position allowing the barrel of the iCare to remain parallel to the ground. The iCare™ PRO (currently not available for commercial use in the US) can be used in the supine position without moving the patient. However, the iCare™ is physically more robust and the rebounding probe has a longer range which children seem to tolerate better. Another practical advantage is that the smaller tips of the iCare™ and the TonoPen (compared to the Goldmann prism) allow them to be applied to more 'normal' areas of cornea when scarring or other pathology (*e.g.*, Peters anomaly) is present.

Regardless of the technique for IOP measurement, certain principles should be considered. Ideally, the IOP should be taken with the eyes in the primary position and motionless in a relaxed child. Avoid measuring the IOP when using a lid speculum or when the child is crying or squeezing their lids as all of these may falsely elevate the IOP. IOP measurements must be obtained prior to pupil dilation as it can also affect the IOP. It is advisable to use the same type of tonometer for serial examinations, as the literature suggests that there is less than perfect agreement between the various tonometers. Consider Goldmann applanation tonometry at the slit lamp as soon as the child is able to cooperate. In an infant or young child, attempt measuring the IOP early during the visit, before they become tired and less cooperative. Fundamentally, it is essential to consider IOP *only* in the context of other clinical findings such as optic disc assessment and, where relevant, ocular dimensions (corneal diameter, axial length), refraction and corneal clarity, to determine whether glaucoma is present or whether it is progressing. If the IOP measurement is out of keeping with the other clinical findings, it may be inaccurate. In these cases, tactile estimation of IOP may reassure the clinician that the real IOP is in keeping with the rest of the exam.

In older childen with normal IOP, in whom a high index of suspicion of glaucoma is raised, consider the diurnal curve by acquiring multiple IOP measurements throughout the day.

Anterior segment examination

The anterior segment of a neonate or infant is best examined with a hand held slit lamp in the clinic/office or during EUA/S and later, using a table-mounted slit lamp once the child is old enough to cooperate. The anterior segment exam is a very important part of the initial evaluation not only with regard to the diagnosis of glaucoma but also in determining the type of glaucoma. Commencing medical glaucoma treatment in confirmed glaucoma cases prior to an EUA/S may help clear the cornea and improve visualization of anterior segment structures and angle features with gonioscopy. Persistent corneal edema may be a sign of poorly-controlled glaucoma.

The use of an oblique slit beam and magnification can help identify subtle corneal features. The cornea should be examined for the presence of posterior embryotoxon, corneal edema, opacities and splits in Descemet membrane (DM). The presence of corneal enlargement and DM splits (Haab striae) is indicative of previously elevated IOP during infancy. Haab striae occur when DM stretches and breaks when its limit of elasticity is exceed by corneal stretching from elevated IOP (Fig. 1). They are usually concentric to the limbus in the periphery and more typically horizontal centrally near or across the visual axis where associated opacification and resultant astigmatism can limit the visual potential. Rarely, birth trauma from forcep injury can result in DM splits and corneal edema. However, they are usually central, vertical, unilateral[14] and, most importantly, occur in the presence of a normal corneal diameter. Furthermore, in the neonate often there is associated periocular bruising indicative of the force applied by the forceps to the eye and adnexa.

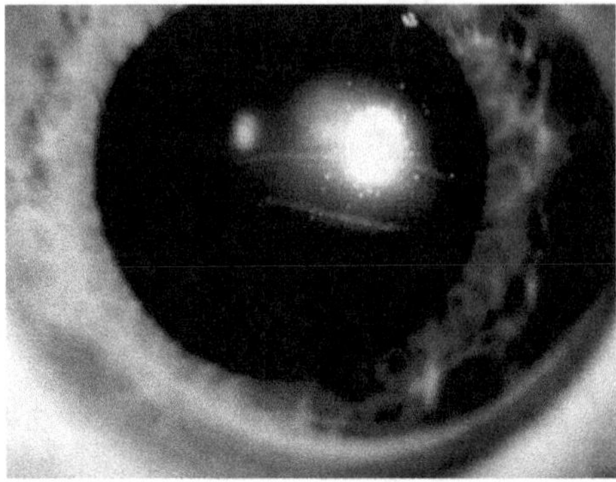

Fig. 1. Descemet membrane tears from elevated IOP Haab striae. (Courtesy of Dr Maria Papadopoulos).

Excluding primary corneal disease is important, and a useful distinguishing feature is the absence of corneal or ocular enlargement. For example, rarely congenital corneal dystrophies such as posterior polymorphous dystrophy (PPMD) can be diagnosed in neonates or young infants with corneal haze who are sometimes referred as glaucoma suspects. PPMD is usually asymptomatic and inherited as autosomal dominant condition so it is advisable to examine the parents for the condition. The signs are often asymmetrical and are found deep in the cornea at the level of DM as vesicular and band-like lesions best seen on retroillumination (Fig. 2). The bands in PPMD, due to localised excessive formation of aberrant DM, have an irregular, scalloped appearance,[15] whereas Haab striae represent the edges of the ruptured DM, appearing smooth and thickened due to the tendency of torn DM to curl and form a ridge. Photophobia and epiphora are unusual in corneal dystophies although in the recessive form of PPMD they can occur. These patients can develop glaucoma in the future due to abnormal cell migration across the angle and are best kept under observation.

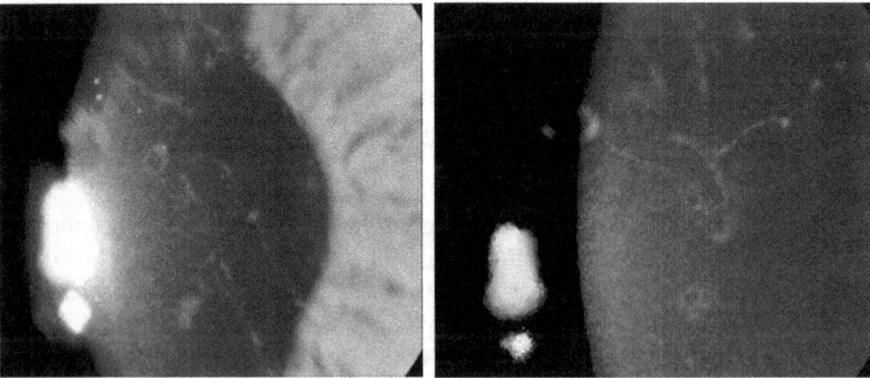

Fig. 2. Posterior polymorphous dystrophy characterized by vesicles and bands at the level of Descemet membrane. (Courtesy of Dr. Maria Papadopoulos)

Other corneal dystrophies tend to be symmetrical. Congenital hereditary endothelial dystrophy (CHED), which may be inherited as autosomal dominant or recessive, typically presents at birth or in the first few years of life and is characterized by bilateral, diffuse corneal edema with significant stromal thickening. The latter is not a feature of congenital hereditary stromal dystrophy (CHSD) which is very rare. Measured IOP may be falsely elevated with the corneal hereditary dystrophies making the differentiation from glaucoma difficult. However, normal corneal diameters and optic nerves (if visible) should raise the suspicion of corneal disease rather than glaucoma. Genetic testing may be helpful in confirming the diagnosis of CHED. However, the diagnosis remains clinical as a negative genetic result does not rule out the condition.[16] Some authors argue that CHED and glaucoma can co exist,[17] although others dispute this.[16,18]

Metabolic disorders, such as mucopolysaccharidoses (MPS) and cystinosis, can also produce corneal clouding mimicking the corneal edema of glaucoma. The corneal haze is typically bilateral and of late infantile, early childhood onset rather than congenital. The classic dysmorphic features can be helpful in identifying a young child with MPS. In MPS, the glycosaminoglycan depositions in the anterior segment can lead to secondary glaucoma. Furthermore, these deposits can increase corneal thickness and stiffness and thus influence the accuracy of IOP measurements. Transient or permanent corneal clouding with or without elevated IOP can result from intrauterine infection with rubella virus but there are often other systemic signs to suggest the diagnosis.

Normally neonates have shallow anterior chambers. When a deep anterior chamber in a neonate or young infant is associated with an enlarged cornea, glaucoma should be strongly suspected. For children not sufficiently cooperative in the office or clinic for a portable slit lamp exam, a 20-diopter lens with a light source can be used to provide a more limited exam of the anterior segment. In the operating room a detailed exam of the anterior segment can be obtained through a standard operating microscope or a portable slit lamp. Examining the iris and pupil for abnormalities is vital to determine the type of glaucoma, as they suggest a secondary cause of glaucoma. Iris abnormalities such as peripheral corneal adhesions may indicate the presence of Axenfeld-Rieger anomaly, especially in the setting of posterior embryotoxon. In primary congenital glaucoma (PCG) the iris may be normal or associated with stromal hypoplasia, loss of iris crypts, peripheral scalloping of posterior pigment iris layer and prominent iris vessels. Distinctive hypoplastic iris stroma, often in the context of a strong family history, is seen in congenital iris hypoplasia. Diffuse iris atrophy may indicate a subtle variant of aniridia, whereas inferior sectoral iris atrophy or distortion may indicate a colobomatous process.

Similarly, determining the coexistent presence of a congenital cataract and glaucoma may influence the diagnosis, in that you should consider secondary causes such as Lowe syndrome or congenital rubella syndrome. Furthermore, the presence of a cataract from any cause may affect the choice of glaucoma surgery. For example, you may be more likely to choose glaucoma drainage device surgery which may have a better chance of controlling IOP after lensectomy rather than a trabeculectomy. Furthermore, lens subluxation should be identified as it increases the likelihood of vitreous prolapse during intraocular surgery and worsens the prognosis.

Gonioscopy

Normal angle development is believed to occur by the posterior sliding of the ciliary body (CB) from Schwalbe line (fifth month) to the scleral spur (ninth month), and then to a location behind the scleral spur (postnatally) due to differential growth rates of the corneoscleral coat compared to the uveal tract.[19] Inhibited posterior migration of the uveal tract is thought to occur in PCG resulting in an anterior position of the CB and peripheral iris overlapping with the trabecular meshwork, similar to the late fetal position, and hence the appearance of an immature angle (Fig. 3). This arrest in maturation can occur at any stage leading to a wide variation in appearance of the PCG angle. Consequently, the angle appearance on gonioscopy is suggestive of PCG but not always diagnostic. By gonioscopy, it may be sometimes difficult to distinguish PCG from the normal infant angle, both of which differ from the adult angle (Fig. 3). The normal infant angle is thought to undergo continued development to become like an adult angle, unlike the angle in a PCG eye.[20]

In the normal newborn eye, the peripheral iris and ciliary body have usually recessed to at least the level of the scleral spur, often posterior to it. The trabecular meshwork is poorly pigmented and can be difficult to identify, but the scleral spur can be visualized as a whitish band. The iris insertion into the angle is flat, so the peripheral angle recess is usually absent in newborn eyes. In contrast, the iris insertion of eyes with PCG is higher than normal. The peripheral iris inserts to the

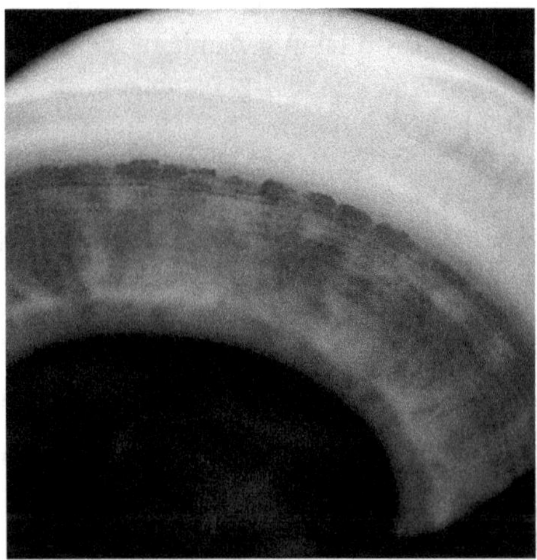

Fig. 3. The immature angle appearance of a primary congenital glaucoma. (Courtesy of Dr. James D. Brandt)

trabecular meshwork and the scleral spur is not visualized. The level of insertion may vary in different areas of the angle. In very immature angles, pale amorphous tissue may be present in the angle. Angle abnormalities are usually bilateral. Even in patients with 'unilateral' glaucoma, the fellow eyes often have enlarged corneal diameters but the optic discs are normal. In these eyes, it is thought that with continued postnatal angle maturation, sufficient drainage has occurred to lower the IOP, leading to reversal of any previous optic disc cupping and the condition to *spontaneously arrest*. In light of this, always examine the unaffected 'normal' eye every time to confirm the absence of glaucoma. In aphakia, the angle may be closed with broad, smooth peripheral anterior synechiae. It is therefore important to always systematically identify angle landmarks (specifically the scleral spur) in all cases, as a smoothly closed angle may be difficult to differentiate from the minimally pigmented angle seen in young children.

The purpose of gonioscopy is to differentiate primary from secondary glaucoma. Making the correct diagnosis will guide the clinician to the most appropriate management and prognosis. For example, subtle changes in the angle noted on gonioscopy may indicate that the child has Axenfeld Rieger anomaly rather than PCG and may respond less well to angle surgery. These changes of peripheral iris adhesions to a posterior embryotoxon may not always be visible on slit lamp evaluation (*see* Section 7). PCG is a surgical condition whereas some secondary glaucomas may respond to medical treatment. In cases of uveitic glaucoma, extensive peripheral anterior synechiae identified on gonioscopy preclude angle surgery. For all these reasons, gonioscopy should be performed at least once when possible.

Both direct and indirect gonioscopy can be performed. Direct gonioscopy is performed using a Koeppe lens (appropriate size is determined by the corneal diameter) and a Barkan light with a hand-held binocular microscope or a hand-held portable slit lamp. The hand-held slit lamp comes with the necessary illumination so that no additional external light source is required. Both techniques allow stereoscopic viewing of the angle. Direct gonioscopy can sometimes be performed in the office in a sleeping or swaddled infant. Indirect gonioscopy using a 4-mirror Zeiss goniolens or a Goldmann is a good alternative during EUA or when examining a child on a slit lamp. The angle appearance can be documented photographically by using, for example, the RETCAM® wide-angle lens angled obliquely into a large amount of gonioscopic coupling agent.

Ultrasound biomicroscopy (UBM) can be useful in examining the anterior segment, especially when the cornea is cloudy or opaque.[21]

Hand-held anterior segment optical coherence tomography (OCT) is in early development, but should prove beneficial in understanding both normal and pathologic angle anatomy in infants and young children.

Corneal diameter

The normal horizontal neonatal diameter is around 10 mm, increasing by about 1 mm during the first year of life. A corneal diameter greater than 11 mm in a newborn and 12 mm in an infant less than one year is very suggestive of raised

IOP and with Haab striae it is diagnostic. A measurement of greater than 13 mm in a child of any age is abnormal, as is marked asymmetry in corneal diameters.

During EUA, the corneal diameter is measured with calipers from limbus to limbus and checked with a graduated ruler with estimation to the nearest 0.25 mm. Some clinicians measure only horizontal corneal diameter, whereas others measure both horizontal and vertical. A superior pannus or scarring following surgery may make the vertical measurements indistinct, but in general more measurements provide more information on which to base clinical decisions. Comparison of the two corneal diameters for asymmetric findings is useful. Close-up digital photographs with a millimeter ruler held against the face can be obtained in the office or even by parents, and used to serially track eye size in a patient in whom EUAs are being avoided for medical reasons.

Corneal enlargement secondary to elevated IOP usually occurs before the age of three years, so corneal diameter is an important marker to aid in establishing the diagnosis and in the monitoring of glaucoma progression mainly during infancy. For example, an increasing horizontal corneal diameter over time suggests inadequate IOP control requiring further treatment. In older children, measuring the corneal diameter may be relevant in making the correct diagnosis. For example, an older child presenting with increased corneal diameters, normal IOP and optic discs may indicate previously elevated IOP as an infant and a diagnosis of spontaneously arrested PCG.

An important differential of corneal enlargement is primary megalocornea, a bilateral developmental anomaly where the anterior segment of the eye is larger than normal in the absence of raised IOP.[22] It is a rare, congenital, bilateral, usually X-linked recessive condition.[23] Characteristics include marked corneal enlargement (13-18 mm), thin corneas, normal endothelial cell density and the absence of Haab striae. Typically, the anterior chamber is very deep and the vitreous length short.[22,24] The IOP and optic discs are normal. In older patients, it may be associated with distinctive secondary changes of mosaic corneal degeneration (shagreen) and corneal arcus juvenilis. Furthermore, evidence of pigment dispersion in later childhood can occur with posterior bowing of the iris and peripheral radial iris transillumination defects.[22,23] The diagnosis can now be confirmed by genetic testing or based on repeated examination and should not be made unless all signs of glaucoma are negative – in other words, it is a diagnosis of exclusion. As opposed to glaucoma, the corneal signs are symmetrical and nonprogressive. While these patients do not require treatment, they must be followed lifelong for glaucoma and refractive amblyopia, which may manifest in the future.

Other causes of megalocornea include connective tissue disorders (*e.g.*, Marfan syndrome, osteogenesis imperfecta, brittle cornea syndrome) and recessive *LTBP2* mutations associated with a secondary form of childhood glaucoma. Corneal enlargement may also be present in congenital high myopia but the posterior pole findings such as tilted optic nerve insertion, peripapillary scleral crescent and choroidal mottling characteristic of axial myopia all help distinguish this condition from glaucoma.

Central corneal thickness

Central Corneal Thickness (CCT) has been found to influence the accuracy of most tonometry techniques, especially GAT. Thinner CCT was found to be an important risk factor for the development of glaucoma in ocular hypertensive adults in the Ocular Hypertension Treatment Study.[25] In general, thinner corneas tend to cause tonometers to under-estimate IOP, whereas thicker corneas tend to cause over-estimation of IOP compared to the 'true' value. CCT can be increased from stromal oedema, corneal thickening (congenital or acquired, *e.g.*, postoperative) or scarring.

A recent cross-sectional survey of CCT in normal infants showed that median CCT increases with age from 1 to 11 years. The 50th percentile among White and Hispanic normal infants of one year old was 553 microns, and 5th and 95th percentiles of 493 and 614 microns respectively.[26] African American children had thinner corneas on average than both White and Hispanic children by approximately 20 microns, similar to what has been found among adults.[26,27]

Children with PCG and juvenile open-angle glaucoma (JOAG) have thinner central corneas than normal subjects.[28] In contrast, corneal thickness is known to be thicker in children who have congenital aniridia[29] and who have undergone congenital cataract surgery.[30,31] However, children with aphakia can develop glaucoma and visual field defects despite the theoretical overestimation of IOP that occurs in eyes with thick corneas.[32] It appears this acquired increase in CCT does not necessarily cause an overestimation of IOP in children and it may relate to the corneal properties of a pediatric eye. A recent, small study of 40 eyes with PCG (mean age 13.6 ± 4.8 years) and 40 normal eyes (mean age 14.2 ± 3.6 years) suggested altered corneal biomechanical responses in PCG.[33] There was a significant reduction in corneal hysteresis and corneal response factor in eyes with PCG as measured with the Reichert Ocular Response Analyzer®, supporting the findings of an earlier similar study.[34] Hence in aphakic patients, elevated IOP should be considered primarily within the context of optic disc appearance, corneal diameters, axial lengths, refraction and significant changes to the above, not CCT. Do not discount an elevated IOP (especially when taken under the same circumstances and previously normal), increasing corneal diameters and axial lengths, especially if asymmetric and associated with a myopic shift in refraction. Often, disc examination in these children is difficult due to miosis, lens/capsule remnants or nystagmus and so changes to the optic disc may not be obvious.

There may be cases of 'ocular hypertension' in children with no other ocular pathology or without a history of surgery or glaucoma in the family, whose IOP measures in the 20s but whose CCT is consistently in the 600s. In this setting, pachymetry and continued follow up may help avoid unnecessary treatment.

The definitive role for pachymetry in the evaluation of childhood glaucoma is uncertain. While CCT should be measured in all children with glaucoma or suspected glaucoma, it should not be used to 'adjust' an IOP measurement but rather taken into consideration in the overall context of the examination. Regardless of the CCT, the appearance of the optic disc remains the most important feature of the assessment.

Posterior segment examination

The appearance of the optic disc is by far the most important and sensitive parameter for both diagnosis and progression of glaucoma, as it is influenced neither by anesthesia nor typically by the effect of growth. Richardson noted a cup:disc ratio of > 0.3 in only 3% of 468 normal Caucasian newborn eyes,[35, 36] in contrast to Shaffer who found a cup:disc ratio of > 0.3 in 61% of 85 eyes in infants less than one year with 'congenital glaucoma'.[37] A cup:disc ratio of > 0.3 in a Caucasian infant less than one year or > 0.5 in an older child greatly raises the suspicion of glaucoma.

Dilated fundoscopy is performed once the IOP has been measured and anterior segment examination has been completed, as dilation can spuriously elevate the IOP and alter the angle appearance. It is performed using an indirect ophthalmoscope with a 28D or 20D lens, a direct ophthalmoscope, an operating microscope with a Fuchs lens or using a condensing lens at the slit lamp when the patient is old enough to cooperate. A binocular view is preferable. If angle surgery is contemplated, consider prior dilation in the office or outpatient setting to allow its effects to wear off and so minimize the risk of lens trauma; alternatively, a quick-acting miotic can be instilled into the anterior chamber after ophthalmoscopy and prior to entering the anterior chamber during angle surgery. It may not be possible to visualize the optic disc in infants with significant corneal edema or opacification until once they have cleared. In infants who dilate poorly, the small pupil facility of the indirect ophthalmoscope is useful during an EUA. In these cases, ultrasound may be able to identify advanced cases with deep excavation. In infants with an inadequate view of the optic disc, the monitoring of biometric parameters take on added importance. In fact, biometric parameters can sometimes change before optic nerve changes become obvious.

The optic disc appearance, including its size, cup:disc ratio, focal areas of rim loss and nerve fibre layer defects should be carefully recorded through a dilated pupil with a drawing or preferably a photograph. Comparison of the two optic nerves for asymmetric findings is useful when the optics discs are of equal size. Racial differences in optic disc appearance should also be taken into consideration. Large discs (common in people of African descent) may have physiological cupping, sometimes misdiagnosed as pathological if optic disc size is ignored. With glaucoma suspects it is often informative to examine the optic nerves of the parents or other siblings, as one or more may have a similar nerve appearance to the patient.

Be mindful of other optic disc abnormalities apart from glaucoma, especially when the IOP is normal and there is no other ocular pathology or when the disc appearance does not match the visual field abnormality. These children should be followed up regularly, looking for evidence of change (disc or field appearance) over time. They should be further investigated or referred to exclude a neurological cause when appropriate, especially if there are other findings such as disc pallor and reduced color vision. Common non-glaucomatous congenital causes of optic nerve cupping such as coloboma, morning glory abnormality, and optic nerve pit are usually recognizable by their distinct features. Periventricular leukomalacia, the result of intrauterine hypoxic-ischemic injury to the white matter of the developing brain, can be associated with a unique form of 'optic nerve hypoplasia' in which the disc size remains normal but cupping is increased.[38] It can be mistaken as glaucoma when a premature child is screened for retinopathy of prematurity. This diagnosis should be suspected in any child with optic nerve cupping and a history of perinatal brain hypoxia. Papillorenal syndrome is associated with variable central optic nerve head excavation ('vacant discs') which can be confused with glaucomatous cupping although it does have distinctive features.[39]

In order to be able to assess optic disc change, it is important to have a representative image for baseline comparison. It is best to obtain optic disc photographs whenever possible – clinicians are more likely to detect changes in optic nerve appearance using direct photo-to-photo comparison than when comparing their clinical examination to a drawing or recorded cup:disc ratio. At the time of EUA, this can be achieved with the RETCAM®. A documented increase in disc cupping is definitive evidence of inadequate IOP control and should lead to further intervention regardless of the IOP measurement obtained. Serial photographs can also document reversal of cupping in many successfully treated cases which is thought to represent a 'pre-laminar' phenomenon whereby the neural tissue is stretched but not lost, accompanied by reversible laminar bowing (Fig. 4). Once normal IOP is established, the compression of the pre-laminar tissue is likely relieved and the lamina moves anteriorly, 'filling in' the cupping. A recent digital photographic analysis of eyes with childhood glaucoma identified that a reduction in the size of the scleral canal accompanies the reversal of cupping.[40] Similar phenomenona have been demonstrated *in vivo* by optical coherence tomography (OCT) in adult eyes undergoing trabeculectomy.[41]

In addition to making a detailed assessment of the optic disc appearance, another purpose of fundoscopy is to identify any relevant retinal features of other associated ophthalmic or systemic conditions, such as choroidal hemangioma in Sturge Weber syndrome or pigmentary retinopathy in congenital rubella syndrome.

Refraction

Cycloplegic refraction can be undertaken in the clinic or office. If this is not possible, retinoscopy can be performed during the EUA. A significant reduction of hypermetropia or the presence of myopia in an infant or neonate is additional evidence of glaucoma. Astigmatism at oblique axes and/or irregular astigmatism may occur, especially in the setting of Haab striae. Furthermore, the observation of significant progressive myopia or a myopic shift in aphakic patients indicates inadequate IOP control, especially if seen in the setting of progressive axial length increase.

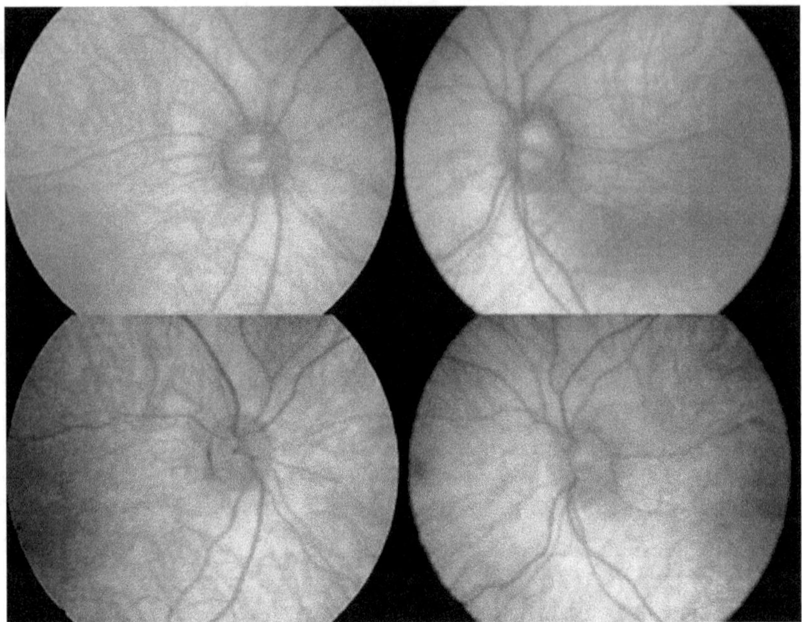

Fig. 4. Reversal of optic disc cupping after successful surgical treatment of primary congenital glaucoma. (Courtesy of Dr. James D. Brandt. Permission has been granted for the reproduction of these figures which were published in Ophthalmology, Yanoff Duker, Congenital Glaucoma, Copyright Elsevier 2013/4.)
Upper row – Preoperative significant optic disc cupping in infant at initial EUA.
Lower row – Postoperative appearance of the same optic nerves with reversal of cupping 6 months after circumferential trabeculotomy and successful lowering of IOP.

Following IOP control, it is important to address ametropia by prescribing glasses or contact lenses and treating amblyopia. Poor visual outcomes despite successful control of IOP are usually due to amblyopia.

General examination

When a diagnosis of an ocular anomaly known to have systemic associations is made, *e.g.*, Axenfeld Rieger anomaly, it is advisable to refer to a pediatrician for medical assessment.

Investigations

Ultrasound

Based on the normal ocular axial growth curve, the steepest growth rate occurs during the first year, followed by a gradual increase in globe elongation during the next four to five years and a plateau by 6-7 years of age.[42] The use of axial length

(AL) measurements in childhood glaucoma is based on the distensibility of the globe in response to raised IOP during early childhood. Measurement of AL can be useful in the baseline assessment for making a diagnosis of glaucoma when the finding is beyond the outer limits of normal range (although there can be cases with AL within the normal range despite raised IOP) and serial measurements can be used to confirm stability, detect progression and/or response to treatment. In children older than about seven years of age, AL measurement monitoring is unlikely to be of significant use as a clinical guide to IOP; nonetheless, in older children who are glaucoma suspects, getting a baseline AL measurement may be useful as it can suggest pathology that occurred during the child's younger years that subsequently arrested.

Axial length can be measured in the clinic or during an EUA. In glaucoma, AL measurements tend to be asymmetrical as compared both to normal eyes and to eyes with megalocornea not related to IOP elevation.[43] Serial AL measurements are best performed regularly at 3-4 month intervals. As AL is influenced also by growth (especially in infancy), axial length measurements, like IOP, AL measurements need to be taken into account with all other clinical parameters (IOP, optic disc appearance, corneal diameter, refraction). Features that suggest poor IOP control include AL beyond normal limits, incremental increase of AL on serial reviews and asymmetrical increase in AL in one eye as compared to the fellow eye. Features that suggest a positive response to glaucoma therapy with good control of IOP include reduction of AL measurement (compared to preoperative values) and stabilization of serial AL measurements (*i.e.*, the AL growth curve begins to parallel the normal axial growth curve).[44-47] Despite reduction of AL after achieving good IOP control, AL is likely to remain above the normal range.

A number of investigators have provided normative data for axial lengths in the pediatric population (Figs. 5 and 6). Both Kiskis and Sampaolesi studied the normal relationship between age and AL in the pediatric population. Kiskis and co-workers recorded the AL in 60 normal eyes of 33 children (age ranged from 0.2 to 9.6 years).[48] Sampaolesi and co-workers recorded 33 normal eyes of infants and children whose ages ranged between 2 and 72 months.[42] Both Kiskis and Sampaolesi generated linear regressions from their data. The disparity in axial length at one month between the two studies is thought to be due to the use of contact A-scan in Kiskis' study, which may artifactually shorten AL measurements. Sampaolesi estimated that at one month of age the 5th percentile and 95th percentile of normal axial length are 17.25 mm and 20.25 mm, respectively. Confounding AL increase from normal growth reduces its sensitivity but these studies provide guidance to the clinician trying to decide if axial lengths are age-appropriate or represent pathologic change.

High-resolution B-scan is useful to detect marked disc cupping in the presence of opaque ocular media or to help exclude posterior segment pathology such as choroidal hemangioma.

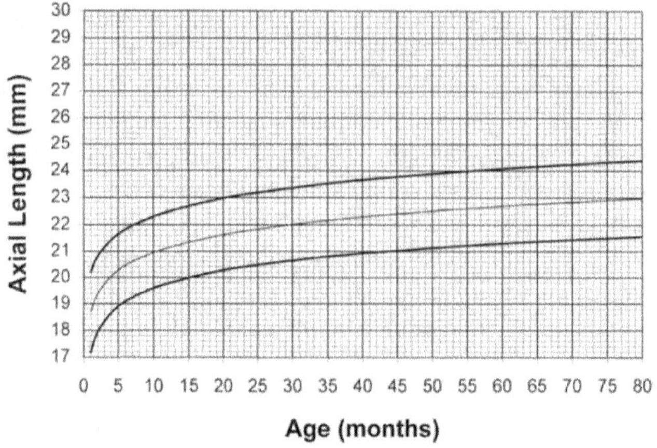

Fig. 5. Axial length in millimeters (y-axis) plotted against linear x axis of age in months. The area within the upper and lower curves represents the standard deviation of axial length with the middle curve representing the mean axial length of normal eyes.
(Adapted from Sampaolesi R, Caruso R. Ocular echometry in the diagnosis of congenital glaucoma. Arch Ophthalmol 1982; 100: 574-577. Courtesy of Drs Simon K. Law and Joseph Caprioli)

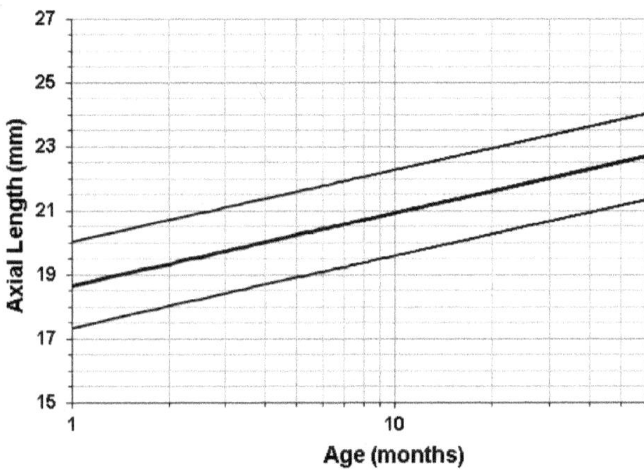

Fig. 6. Axial length in millimeters (y-axis) plotted against log x axis of age in months. The area within the upper and lower lines represents the standard deviation of axial length with the middle line representing the mean axial length of normal eyes.
(Adapted from Sampaolesi R, Caruso R. Ocular echometry in the diagnosis of congenital glaucoma. Arch Ophthalmol 1982; 100: 574-577. Courtesy of Drs Simon K. Law and Joseph Caprioli)

Anterior segment optical coherence tomography (OCT) and ultrasound biomicroscopy (UBM)

Anterior segment OCT and UBM may be particularly useful in cases where corneal edema, dense corneal opacification such as in Peters anomaly, or dense cataract prevents a view of intraocular structures. Both devices are particularly useful for assessing the following: anterior segment in the presence of a significant corneal scar; iridocorneal angle; iris configuration and insertion, and iris tumours/ cysts. UBM uses ultrasound at a higher frequency (50-100 Hz) thereby allowing penetration of ocular tissues with less scatter.[21] As such, UBM can be useful for suspected retro-iridial pathology, *e.g.*, ciliary body masses. One practical limitation of UBM is that it requires the patient to be supine and commonly employs a water bath (or sheathed fluid-containing probe) placed in direct contact with the eye. UBM is therefore only suitable for assessment during an EUA except in much older children. Attempts with a UBM to identify Schlemm canal routinely have failed.

Perimetry

The ability to do a visual field (VF) test depends on child's developmental milestones, maturity, visual acuity, dexterity and coordination. Patterns of visual field loss and progression in children approximates that of adults with glaucoma.[49] Various types of perimetry include:

1. Kinetic perimetry
   a. Manual kinetic perimetry (Goldmann perimetry) is very dependent on a highly-skilled operator. This is possible usually after the age of ten.
   b. Automated kinetic perimetry (available on some models of Octopus perimeters) is less dependent upon the operator and may be feasible in younger children.
2. Automated white-on-white static perimetry
   a. Humphrey SITA 24-2
      i. SITA Standard reduces average testing time by 30-50% as compared with conventional Full-Threshold procedures. SITA Fast adds up to a further 50% reduction in test time. Both SITA Fast and Standard compare very favorably with Full-Threshold procedures.[50] This is feasible in some children beginning around seven years of age, although is possible in younger children.
   b. Octopus tendency oriented perimetry (TOPS)
      i. The TOPS strategy is associated with fast evaluation time, taking about three minutes per eye, and may be suitable for children. This is feasible in some children beginning around seven years of age.
3. Frequency doubling technology (FDT) perimetry
   a. This form of high resolution perimetry does not rely on a white on white target and may be more sensitive to early VF loss. It is fast to perform and

may be more acceptable to children. This is often possible from about age ten.

Static automated perimetry can often be undertaken successfully by the age of seven to eight and is worth introducing at that age even if the initial results are unreliable. As with adults, there is a learning curve, with performance improving with repeated testing. Children can be commenced on HVF SITA Fast and then moved to HVF SITA Standard (24-2). Current normative databases for commercial automated perimeters, from which the mean defect, pattern standard deviation, pattern and total deviation plots are derived, do not include data acquired from child subjects. However, in practical terms, static automated perimetry can be useful for monitoring VF progression in children, assuming the tests undertaken are reliable. Once a visual field deficit is demonstrated, the visual field test should be repeated to confirm its presence. As in adults, in order to attribute a reproducible visual field defect to glaucoma, it should correspond to the disc appearance with there being no other observable cause for the defect. When such correlation is not present, then other causes of visual loss should be considered. These may be neurological in children with relevant systemic disease such as neurofibromatosis with optic nerve gliomas. Testing color vision and checking for an afferent pupillary defect can be done in the office; sometimes neuro-imaging may be indicated.

Quantitative optic disc imaging

As with adult glaucoma, the exact role for semi-automated optic nerve head and retinal nerve fiber layer (RNFL) imaging devices in childhood glaucoma has yet to be fully elucidated. In theory, once a child can be examined comfortably at the slit lamp, then they should be able to undergo optic disc imaging. Optic disc imaging requires cooperation, stable fixation and fairly good visual acuity but generally does not require pupil dilation. Attention and movement remain a problem as with perimetry. Imaging is not possible in the presence of nystagmus or significant media opacity.

One limitation preventing the wider adoption of imaging devices for childhood glaucoma diagnosis is the fact that normative databases for the native classification algorithms do not include measurements obtained from children. This limitation does not apply to the comparison of serial measurements, so these devices can be used for the monitoring of structural change over time as in adults. A prospective, observational study in children with glaucoma confirmed that RNFL thickness and macular thickness measurements decline with increasing severity of glaucomatous disc damage as gauged by stereophotograph examination.[51]

A recent study attempted to establish the normal peripapillary RNFL thickness and macular thickness in 83 healthy children aged 5-15 years using the Spectralis® OCT device.[52] The mean RNFL thickness (107.6 ± 1.2 μm) was thicker than has been reported in adults. It is hoped that such studies will provide the necessary normative data to allow the newer generation of spectral domain OCT (SD-OCT) devices to become useful in assisting in the detection of glaucoma in children. A particular advantage of spectral domain OCT is its rapid image acquisition time, suggesting that it may be useful in younger children where attention and eye movements are problematic. SD-OCT devices have improved axial depth penetration and resolution enabling structures deep to the surface of the cup to be visualized with greater clarity. It seems likely that OCT imaging protocols will find a future place in the assessment of glaucoma in children.

Hand-held SD-OCT devices are now becoming available for use in the operating room which may further expand our ability to assess the optic disc in infants during EUA.

Examination under anesthesia (EUA)

General anesthesia in infants and young children is not benign. Although perioperative cardiac arrest and death is rare in the absence of cardiac disease,[53] even in the hands of expert pediatric anesthesiologists hypoxic events and CNS damage can occur. There is a growing body of evidence that multiple exposures to general anesthetics adversely affect the developing brain and may cause long-term neurocognitive changes.[54-56] To provide more definitive evidence regarding the clinical relevance of anesthetic neurotoxicity in children, the Pediatric Anesthesia Neuro-Development Assessment (PANDA) project is currently underway in the United States. This large multi-center study aims to assess the neurodevelopment and cognitive functions of a group of children exposed to anesthesia compared to another with no exposure.[57] The theoretical concerns of anesthetic neurotoxicity should only be considered within the context of the very real risk of blindness from glaucoma in children not adequately assessed or surgically managed.

For the reasons above, the decision to subject a child to an examination under anesthesia or sedation is not a trivial one. An EUA should be pursued only when the data to be acquired during the EUA will provide a timely diagnosis and opportunity to intervene surgically, or provide important follow-up data that may influence ongoing, consequential clinical decision-making. Preferably the ophthalmologist undertaking the initial EUA should be capable of performing the definitive surgery under the same anesthetic, to avoid unnecessary anesthesia and a delay in treatment. The IOP can be reduced in the meantime with medical treatment by the referring ophthalmologist.

Obtaining as much information as possible before committing an infant to a EUA is important. Doing so allows you to carefully counsel the parents with regard to the level of suspicion or certainty that their child has glaucoma, which will be confirmed at the time of the EUA, and also affords the opportunity to discuss intended surgical options, risks and benefits. Even if uncertainty exists preoperatively, appropriate consent for any anticipated procedures should be obtained. If the diagnosis is tentative and substantiation is being sought by an EUA, it is sometimes worth ceasing antiglaucoma medication a few days day prior to the EUA.

Even if the diagnosis remains uncertain, an EUA offers the opportunity to acquire good baseline data (*e.g.*, untreated IOPs, axial length, disc photographs, etc.) for comparison with future data. Furthermore, it is useful to establish an 'EUA routine' to avoid missing essential details (Table 1).

Table 1. Examination under anesthesia – essential data and instrumentation.

Essential EUA data	Essential EUA instrumentation	Optional
Date	Tonometer, *e.g.*, Perkins, iCare®	Ultrasound pachymeter
Visual acuity	Pediatric Lang speculum	Autorefractor
Anesthetic agent	Calipers and a ruler	UBM
Tonometer	Squint hook and forceps (to manipulate eye)	B scan
IOP measurements		OCT
Corneal diameter	Koeppe or 4-mirror goniolens	
Axial length	Direct or indirect ophthalmoscope and condensing lenses	
Examination findings		
Anterior segment (including gonioscopy when indicated)	Retinoscope and lenses	
Posterior segment (optic disc, retina)	Hand held slit lamp *e.g.*, Kowa portable SL	
Refraction (if not possible/inaccurate in office/clinic)		
Optic disc digital photos (preferable), *e.g.*, Retcam II®		

Anesthetic choices

As a general rule, all anesthetics and sedating agents lower the IOP with the exceptions of ketamine, chloral hydrate and the benzodiazapenes.[58] The degree of IOP lowering is unpredictable and relates to factors such as the agent chosen, route of administration, depth of anesthesia and the starting IOP. Inhaled anesthetics may significantly lower the IOP (by up to 30 mmHg over the course of an anesthetic), which can have a profound impact on the diagnosis and management of these patients.[59,60] Sevoflurane causes progressive reduction in IOP with time from induction[61] hence it is important to document the time IOP is measured after induction with inhalational anesthetics. It follows that tonometry under anesthesia generally provides us only with an approximation of the true IOP. The finding of a normal IOP with the use of anesthetic agents known to reduce IOP does not exclude glaucoma. For example, when the IOP is normal but buphthalmos, corneal enlargement with Haab striae and pathological optic cupping are present, it may be a case of falsely low IOP related to anesthesia.

With ketamine hydrochloride the IOP measurements are thought to be similar to those taken in awake infants.[61] The drug can cause a transient rise in IOP for a few minutes[62] so the IOP should be measured several times in both eyes. Ketamine hydrochloride can be administered intravenously (following the use of local anesthetic patches) in conjunction with an agent that reduces bronchial secretions (atropine or glycopyrolate) and midazolam, which acts as a sedative and as an amnesic agent. This IOP rise can be minimized by pre-medication with anxiolytics and titrating the dose rather than using an intramuscular bolus. If a surgical procedure needs to be undertaken at the end of the EUA, the anesthetist can switch to the standard preferred regime of inhaled and intravenous anesthesia. Sedation with chloral hydrate may be best suitable for younger children in settings where suitable infrastructure is in place, such as appropriate nursing expertise and inpatient monitoring. Pre-medication alone with an oral or intra-nasal benzodiazapene such as midazolam often results in a drowsy child willing to cooperate with tonometry as long as the lights are dimmed and noises kept to a minimum; as midazolam does not appear to affect IOP when used at sedating doses,[63] IOPs acquired in this manner are probably among the most accurate in young children.

A recent international survey, querying ophthalmologists of the Childhood Glaucoma Research Network (CGRN), UK Paediatric Glaucoma Society and International and UK Pediatric Ophthalmology web groups regarding their anesthetic preferences, showed that sevoflurane is the most widely used inhaled agent due to its convenience and safety profile. Ketamine is the second most commonly used agent because it is believed to give the best representation of a non-anesthetized IOP. It was particularly favored by those measuring IOPs most frequently under EUA. A minority of CGRN members use chloral hydrate. The choice of agents will be dictated by a number of factors including hospital policies and regional preferences.

It is crucial that the ophthalmologist have a good working relationship with the team administering the anesthetic, so that they understand the importance of controlling variables which can falsely raise (raised mean arterial pressure, raised pCO_2 and endotracheal intubation) and lower IOP. IOPs measured even minutes after a child is intubated during a sevofluorane anesthetic can be artificially lowered into the single digits. No anesthetic medication should be administered without the ophthalmologist present and ready to acquire IOP measurements the moment the child stops moving. Although maintenance of an airway is paramount, the anesthesia team should know that the major point of the trip to the operating room that day is to acquire an IOP measurement during those crucial few moments. Arriving in the operating room only to find your patient intubated and asleep represents a misunderstanding of the goals for the EUA.

The choice of an appropriate anesthetic and how it is administered is vital in the assessment of children with glaucoma, especially in subtle cases where early diagnosis can have a profound impact on the visual prognosis. Regardless of the anesthetic used, it is important to have a consistent approach. Using the same agent for serial examinations and measuring the IOP at the same time with inhaled general anesthesia, preferably as soon as possible after initiation of anesthesia (prior to intubation), helps reduce at least some of the variability between EUAs. Refer to Figure 7 for an approach to the evaluation of a child with glaucoma or suspected glaucoma.

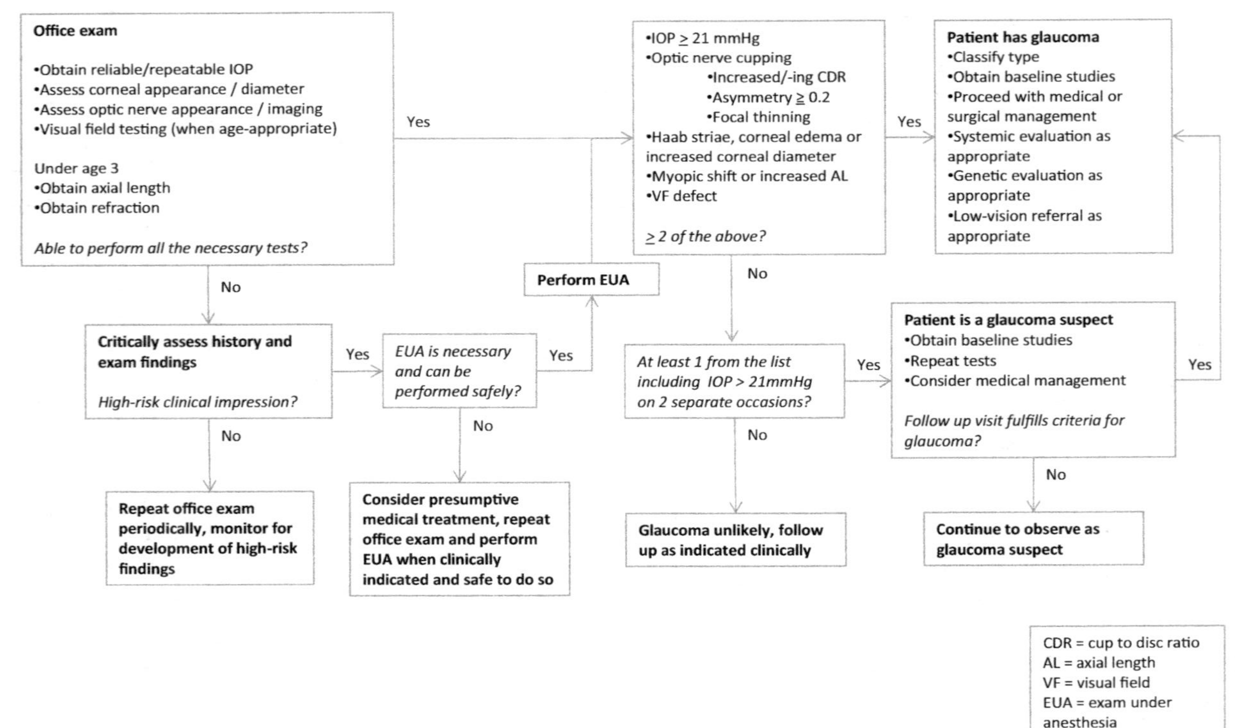

Fig. 7. A suggested approach to the evaluation of a child with glaucoma or suspected glaucoma. (It will be influenced by clinician preference/experience and local facilities/equipment availability.)

References

1. Radtke ND, Cohan BE. Intraocular pressure measurement in the newborn. Am J Ophthalmol 1974; 78: 501-504.
2. Sihota R, Tuli D, Dada T, et al. Distribution and determinants of intraocular pressure in a normal pediatric population. J Pediatr Ophthalmol Strabismus 2006; 43: 14-18; quiz 36-37.
3. Levy J, Lifshitz T, Rosen S, et al. Is the tono-pen accurate for measuring intraocular pressure in young children with congenital glaucoma? J AAPOS 2005; 9: 321-325.
4. Garcia-Resua C, Gonzalez-Meijome JM, Gilino J, Yebra-Pimentel E. Accuracy of the new ICare rebound tonometer vs. other portable tonometers in healthy eyes. Optom Vis Sci 2006; 83: 102-107.
5. Bradfield YS, Kaminski BM, Repka MX, et al. Comparison of Tono-Pen and Goldmann applanation tonometers for measurement of intraocular pressure in healthy children. J AAPOS 2012; 16: 242-248.
6. Eisenberg DL, Sherman BG, McKeown CA, Schuman JS. Tonometry in adults and children. A manometric evaluation of pneumatonometry, applanation, and TonoPen in vitro and in vivo. Ophthalmology 1998; 105: 1173-1181.
7. Kageyama M, Hirooka K, Baba T, Shiraga F. Comparison of ICare rebound tonometer with noncontact tonometer in healthy children. J Glaucoma 2011; 20: 63-66.
8. Lundvall A, Svedberg H, Chen E. Application of the ICare rebound tonometer in healthy infants. J Glaucoma 2011; 20: 7-9.
9. Flemmons MS, Hsiao YC, Dzau J, et al. Icare rebound tonometry in children with known and suspected glaucoma. J AAPOS 2011; 15: 153-157.
10. Dahlmann-Noor AH, Puertas R, Tabasa-Lim S, et al. Comparison of handheld rebound tonometry with Goldmann applanation tonometry in children with glaucoma: a cohort study. BMJ Open 2013; 3(4).
11. Poostchi A, Mitchell R, Nicholas S, et al. The iCare rebound tonometer: comparisons with Goldmann tonometry, and influence of central corneal thickness. Clin Experiment Ophthalmol 2009; 37: 687-691.
12. Martinez-de-la-Casa JM, Garcia-Feijoo J, Saenz-Frances F, et al. Comparison of rebound tonometer and Goldmann handheld applanation tonometer in congenital glaucoma. J Glaucoma 2009; 18: 49-52.
13. Lambert SR, Melia M, Buffenn AN, et al. Rebound tonometry in children: a report by the American Academy of Ophthalmology. Ophthalmology 2013; 120: e21-27.
14. Honig MA, Barraquer J, Perry HD, et al. Forceps and vacuum injuries to the cornea: histopathologic features of twelve cases and review of the literature. Cornea 1996; 15: 463-472.
15. Cibis GW, Tripathi RC. The differential diagnosis of Descemet's tears (Haab's striae) and posterior polymorpous dystrophy bands. A clinicopathologic study. Ophthalmology 1982; 89: 614-620.
16. Khan AO, Al-Shehah A, Ghadhfan FE. High measured intraocular pressure in children with recessive congenital hereditary endothelial dystrophy. J Pediatr Ophthalmol Strabismus 2010; 47: 29-33.
17. Ramamurthy B, Sachdeva V, Mandal AK, et al. Coexistent congenital hereditary endothelial dystrophy and congenital glaucoma. Cornea 2007; 26: 647-649.
18. Khan AO. Conditions that can be mistaken as early childhood glaucoma. Ophthalmic Genet 2011; 32: 129-137.
19. Anderson DR. The development of the trabecular meshwork and its abnormality in primary infantile glaucoma. Trans Am Ophthalmol Soc 1981; 79: 458-485.
20. Anderson DR. Pathology of the glaucomas. Br J Ophthalmol 1972; 56: 146-157.
21. Gupta V, Jha R, Srinivasan G, et al. Ultrasound biomicroscopic characteristics of the anterior segment in primary congenital glaucoma. J AAPOS 2007; 11: 546-550.

22. Ho CL, Walton DS. Primary megalocornea: clinical features for differentiation from infantile glaucoma. J Pediatr Ophthalmol Strabismus 2004; 41: 11-17; quiz 46-47.
23. Webb TR, Matarin M, Gardner JC, et al. X-linked megalocornea caused by mutations in CHRDL1 identifies an essential role for ventroptin in anterior segment development. Am J Hum Genet 2012; 90: 247-259.
24. Meire FM, Delleman JW. Biometry in X linked megalocornea: pathognomonic findings. Br J Ophthalmol 1994; 78: 781-785.
25. Gordon MO, Beiser JA, Brandt JD, et al. The Ocular Hypertension Treatment Study: Baseline Factors That Predict the Onset of Primary Open-Angle Glaucoma. Arch Ophthalmol 2002; 120: 714-720.
26. Pediatric Eye Disease Investigator Group, Bradfield YS, Melia BM, et al. Central corneal thickness in children. Arch Ophthalmol 2011; 129: 1132-1138.
27. Brandt JD, Beiser JA, Kass MA, Gordon MO. Central Corneal Thickness in the Ocular Hypertension Treatment Study (OHTS). Ophthalmology 2001; 108: 1779-1788.
28. Wygnanski-Jaffe T, Barequet IS. Central corneal thickness in congenital glaucoma. Cornea 2006; 25: 923-925.
29. Brandt JD, Casuso LA, Budenz DL. Markedly increased central corneal thickness: an unrecognized finding in congenital aniridia. Am J Ophthalmol 2004; 137: 348-350.
30. Muir KW, Duncan L, Enyedi LB, et al. Central corneal thickness: congenital cataracts and aphakia. Am J Ophthalmol 2007; 144: 502-506.
31. Lupinacci AP, da Silva Jordao ML, Massa G, et al. Central corneal thickness in children with congenital cataract and children with surgical aphakia: a case-control study. Br J Ophthalmol 2009; 93: 337-341.
32. Chen TC, Walton DS, Bhatia LS. Aphakic glaucoma after congenital cataract surgery. Arch Ophthalmol 2004; 122: 1819-1825.
33. Gatzioufas Z, Labiris G, Stachs O, et al. Biomechanical profile of the cornea in primary congenital glaucoma. Acta Ophthalmol 2012.
34. Kirwan C, O'Keefe M, Lanigan B. Corneal hysteresis and intraocular pressure measurement in children using the Reichert Ocular Response Analyzer. Am J Ophthalmol 2006; 142: 990-992.
35. Richardson KT. Optic cup symmetry in normal newborn infants. Invest Ophthalmol 1968; 7: 137-140.
36. Richardson KT, Shaffer RN. Optic-nerve cupping in congenital glaucoma. Am J Ophthalmol 1966; 62: 507-509.
37. Shaffer RN. New concepts in infantile glaucoma. Can J Ophthalmol 1967; 2: 243-248.
38. Jacobson L, Hellstrom A, Flodmark O. Large cups in normal-sized optic discs: a variant of optic nerve hypoplasia in children with periventricular leukomalacia. Arch Ophthalmol 1997; 115: 1263-1269.
39. Khan AO, Nowilaty SR. Early diagnosis of the papillorenal syndrome by optic disc morphology. J Neuroophthalmol 2005; 25: 209-211.
40. Mochizuki H, Lesley AG, Brandt JD. Shrinkage of the scleral canal during cupping reversal in children. Ophthalmology 2011; 118: 2008-2013.
41. Lee EJ, Kim TW, Weinreb RN. Reversal of lamina cribrosa displacement and thickness after trabeculectomy in glaucoma. Ophthalmology 2012; 119: 1359-1366.
42. Sampaolesi R, Caruso R. Ocular echometry in the diagnosis of congenital glaucoma. Arch Ophthalmol 1982; 100: 574-577.
43. Sampaolesi R. Corneal diameter and axial length in congenital glaucoma. Can J Ophthalmol 1988; 23: 42-44.
44. Law SK, Bui D, Caprioli J. Serial axial length measurements in congenital glaucoma. Am J Ophthalmol 2001; 132: 926-928.
45. Kiefer G, Schwenn O, Grehn F. Correlation of postoperative axial length growth and intraocular pressure in congenital glaucoma--a retrospective study in trabeculotomy and goniotomy. Graefes Arch Clin Exp Ophthalmol 2001; 239: 893-899.

46. Panarello SM, Priolo E, Vittone P. Pediatric ultrasound: a personal experience during the period 1991-1994. Ophthalmologica 1998; 212 Suppl 1: 115-117.
47. Carvalho CA, Betinjane AJ. Ultrasonographic echometry in the control of congenital glaucoma. In: Krieglstein GK, Leidheker W (Eds.), Glaucoma Update II. Berlin: Springer-Verlag 1983.
48. Kiskis AA, Markowitz SN, Morin JD. Corneal diameter and axial length in congenital glaucoma. Can J Ophthalmol 1985; 20: 93-97.
49. Robin AL, Quigley HA, Pollack IP, et al. An analysis of visual acuity, visual fields, and disk cupping in childhood glaucoma. Am J Ophthalmol 1979; 88: 847-58.
50. Johnson CA. Recent developments in automated perimetry in glaucoma diagnosis and management. Curr Opin Ophthalmol 2002; 13: 77-84.
51. El-Dairi MA, Holgado S, Asrani SG, et al. Correlation between optical coherence tomography and glaucomatous optic nerve head damage in children. Br J Ophthalmol 2009; 93: 1325-1330.
52. Yanni SE, Wang J, Cheng CS, et al. Normative reference ranges for the retinal nerve fiber layer, macula, and retinal layer thicknesses in children. Am J Ophthalmol 2013; 155: 354-360 e1.
53. Flick RP, Sprung J, Harrison TE, et al. Perioperative cardiac arrests in children between 1988 and 2005 at a tertiary referral center: a study of 92,881 patients. Anesthesiology 2007; 106: 226-237; quiz 413-414.
54. DiMaggio C, Sun LS, Li G. Early childhood exposure to anesthesia and risk of developmental and behavioral disorders in a sibling birth cohort. Anesth Analg 2011; 113: 1143-1151.
55. Sun L. Early childhood general anaesthesia exposure and neurocognitive development. Br J Anaesth 2010; 105 Suppl 1: i61-68.
56. McCann ME, Soriano SG. Is anesthesia bad for the newborn brain? Anesthesiol Clin 2009; 27: 269-284.
57. Sun LS, Li G, DiMaggio CJ, et al. Feasibility and pilot study of the Pediatric Anesthesia NeuroDevelopment Assessment (PANDA) project. J Neurosurg Anesthesiol 2012; 24: 382-388.
58. Self WG, Ellis PP. The effect of general anesthetic agents on intraocular pressure. Surv Ophthalmol 1977; 21: 494-500.
59. Quigley HA. Childhood glaucoma: results with trabeculotomy and study of reversible cupping. Ophthalmology 1982; 89: 219-226.
60. Ausinsch B, Munson ES, Levy NS. Intraocular pressures in children with glaucoma during halothane anesthesia. Ann Ophthalmol 1977; 9: 1391-1394.
61. Blumberg D, Congdon N, Jampel H, et al. The effects of sevoflurane and ketamine on intraocular pressure in children during examination under anesthesia. Am J Ophthalmol 2007; 143: 494-499.
62. Yoshikawa K, Murai Y. The effect of ketamine on intraocular pressure in children. Anesth Analg 1971; 50: 199-202.
63. Oberacher-Velten I, Prasser C, Rochon J, et al. The effects of midazolam on intraocular pressure in children during examination under sedation. Br J Ophthalmol 2011; 95: 1102-1105.

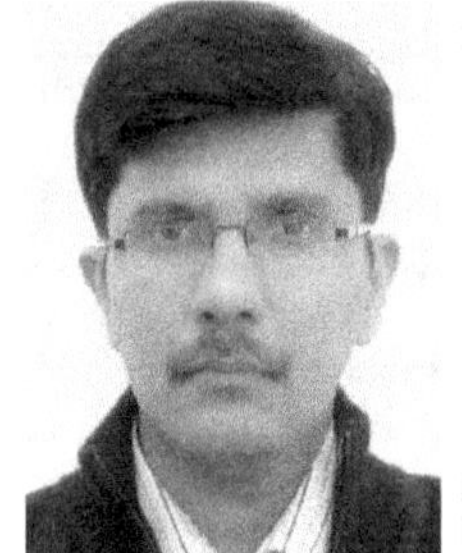

Viney Gupta

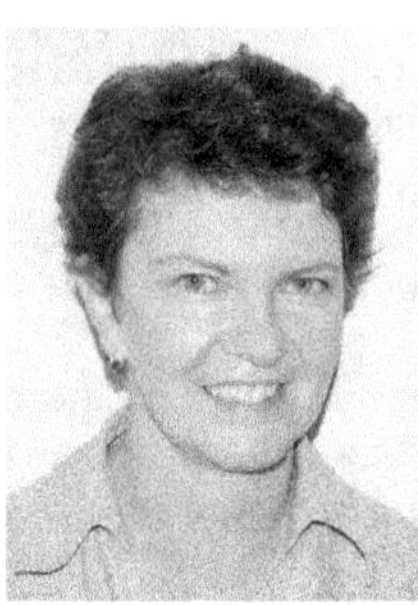

Robyn Jamieson

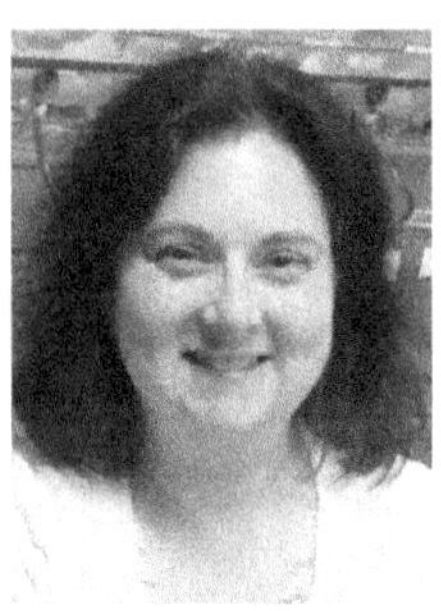

Lisa Schimmenti

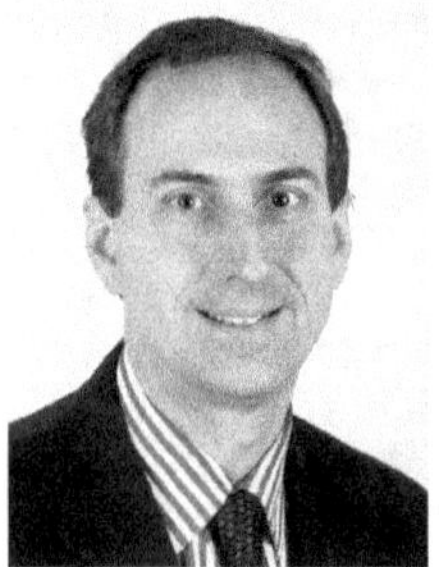

John Grigg

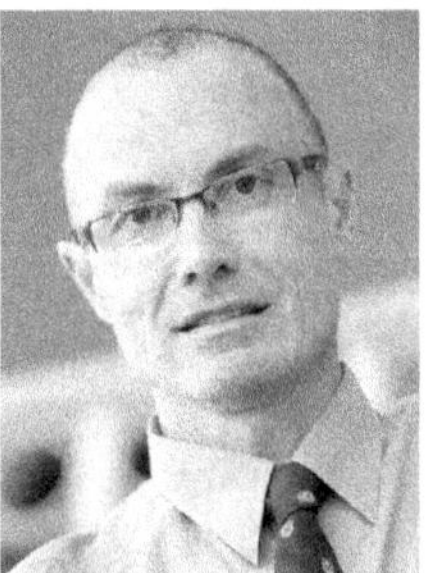

David Mackey

3. GENETICS

Viney Gupta, Robyn Jamieson, Lisa Schimmenti, John Grigg, David Mackey

Section Leaders: John Grigg, Viney Gupta
Contributors: Arif Khan, Tanuj Dada, Mansoor Sarfarazi

Consensus statements

1. Genetic evaluation of childhood glaucoma is especially important in those types of glaucoma when genotype phenotype correlations are known to exist.
   Comment: The results of these tests may be important in counseling, prognosis and management.
2. There is a known correlation between primary congenital glaucoma (PCG) and mutations in the *CYP1B1* gene.
   Comment: Performing carrier testing for at risk relatives is possible if both disease causing alleles of an affected family member have been identified.
3. Families affected by autosomal dominant juvenile open angle glaucoma (JOAG) have been found to have mutations in the *MYOC* gene.
   Comment: Genetic screening and genetic counseling could be considered in these patients to help diagnose pre-symptomatic cases among first and second-degree relatives of these patients.
4. Axenfeld-Rieger anomaly and syndrome have been associated with *PITX2* and *FOXC1* mutations.
   Comment: *PITX2* mutations are more likely to be associated with systemic findings, while the risk of glaucoma is increased with *FOXC1* duplications and *PITX2* mutations.
   Comment: Prospective parents may consider genetic counseling for risk calculation.
5. Aniridia is usually inherited in an autosomal-dominant fashion with high penetrance and variable expressivity, and it is almost exclusively caused by *PAX6* mutations.
   Comment: A child with sporadic aniridia should have ultrasound surveillance for Wilms tumor unless genetic testing rules out a microdeletion involving the Wilms tumor gene.

Childhood Glaucoma, pp. 43-60
Edited by Robert N. Weinreb, Alana L. Grajewski, Maria Papadopoulos, John Grigg,
and Sharon Freedman
2013 © Kugler Publications, Amsterdam, The Netherlands

6. The *LTBP2* mutations seem to be involved in complex ocular phenotypes including ectopia lentis, megalocornea (unrelated to elevated intraocular pressure), microspherophakia and associated secondary glaucoma.
7. To optimize genetic counseling for families, accurate clinical ophthalmic diagnosis is critical.
   Comment: Marked variation in penetrance and expression in primary and secondary childhood glaucomas exist, so parents and siblings of an affected child should be examined to provide maximally accurate phenotypic diagnoses for the clinical geneticist.
8. General pediatric assessment forms an important part of the management for children with glaucoma and can greatly assist in identifying systemic associations and initiating early management.
9. Genetics review plays a number of important roles including confirming or identifying syndromic diagnoses, recurrence risk assessment, genetic diagnosis, interpretation of molecular data, and reproductive counseling where this may be requested by the family after appropriate genetic counseling.

Introduction

The genetics of glaucoma is an evolving area of research with most of the genetic risk for the glaucomas yet to be discovered. Thus any recommendations may change significantly as new information comes to light. Genetic evaluation of childhood glaucoma is especially important in those types of glaucoma where genotype phenotype correlations are known to exist. (Table 1) Currently, for identified genes no definitive correlation exists between a mutation in the affected gene and the severity of the condition. The cost-benefit ratio of genetic testing in all primary childhood glaucomas and syndromic forms of childhood glaucoma is not well established. This is because in most populations the majority of cases do not have an identified genetic mutation and, where the mutation is known, the genes account for often only a small proportion of cases.

In evaluating patients with childhood glaucoma it is important to assess other family members to assist in establishing inheritance patterns. Sporadic cases are those where there is no identifiable family history. These cases may be the first presentation in a family and so have a genetic basis with implications for future generations.

Table 1. Genes associated with childhood glaucoma

Primary congenital glaucoma	*CYP1B1*
Juvenile open-angle glaucoma	*MYOC*
Aniridia	*PAX6*
Axenfeld-Rieger	*PITX2, FOXC1*
Peters anomaly	*PAX6, CYP1B1, PITX2, FOXC1*

In addition to improving understanding of the natural history and response to treatment, genetic testing can predict children at increased risk of developing glaucoma in childhood (and ensure clinical follow up) and raises the possibility of prenatal and pre-implantation interventions and may further allow us to devise specific treatments.

Genetics of primary childhood glaucoma

Primary congenital glaucoma (PCG)

CYP1B1 gene

The *CYP1B1* gene has been most commonly associated with the pathogenesis of primary congenital glaucoma (PCG). It contains three exons and is mapped to chromosome 2p22-p21.[1,2] It was speculated that *CYP1B1* participates in the metabolism of an unknown biologically active molecule that is a participant in eye development. Schwartzman *et al.* implicated a cytochrome-P450-dependent arachidonate metabolite that inhibits Na^+/K^+-ATPase in the cornea in regulating corneal transparency and aqueous humor secretion.[3] This finding is consistent with the clouding of the cornea and increased intraocular pressure (IOP), the two major diagnostic criteria for PCG. Additionally contributory effects of mitochondrial DNA variations in PCG patients are being analyzed to see what effect these may have on growth and differentiation of the anterior segment.[4]

The proportion of patients with PCG whose disease is due to *CYP1B1* mutation varies from 20% to 100% in various populations.[5] They are more commonly seen among familial than among sporadic cases. Variable expressivity and penetrance are known to be associated with a varied phenotype associated with *CYP1B1* mutations.[6,7] While those presenting as neonatal PCG are more likely to have *CYP1B1* mutations, there could be others with less severe PCG or no glaucoma as children who nonetheless have the same mutations.[8] Thus this exhibits incomplete penetrance and variable expressivity (Fig. 1).

Inheritance patterns are autosomal recessive and prevalence is higher in populations with higher rates of consanguinity. The presence of recessive *CYP1B1* mutation does not predict a severe phenotype.[8] Attempts at genotype-phenotype correlations have been inconclusive. Surgical outcomes and a relationship to genotype have also proved inconclusive.[9,10] Hollander *et al.* demonstrated varying severity of goniodysgenesis among PCG patients with different *CYP1B1* mutations.[11] Considering that up to 40% of PCG is heritable in an autosomal recessive fashion,[12] parents with one affected child without genetic screening have a 10% (0.4 x 0.25) chance of having another affected child with their next pregnancy. If the first affected child is screened for *CYP1B1* mutations and none are found, there would be 2% chance of an affected child being born out of the next pregnancy.

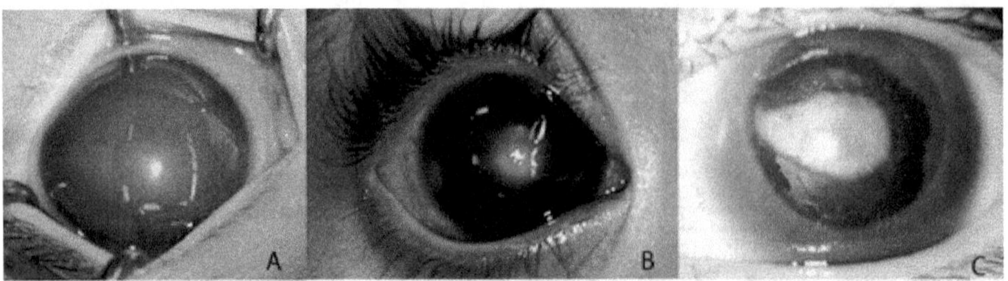

Fig. 1. CYP1B1 mutations and variable phenotypes. A. Primary congenital glaucoma buphthalmos and generalized corneal haze; B. Buphthalmos and persistent corneal haze denser centrally, no lens or iris anomalies; C. Peters anomaly post corneal graft showing anterior lens plaque.

However, if mutations (one inherited from each parent) are found, the risk for the next child is 25%, although there may not be complete penetrance.[12]

Performing a carrier test for at risk relatives and prenatal diagnosis for pregnancies at increased risk is possible if both disease causing alleles in an affected family member have been identified.

Juvenile open-angle glaucoma (JOAG)

Myocilin gene

In 1997, Stone and colleagues identified mutations in the *Myocilin* (*MYOC*) gene (also called the *trabecular meshwork-induced glucocorticoid response* or *TIGR* gene) in families affected by autosomal dominant primary open angle glaucoma.[13] Independently, Kubota *et al.* discovered the myocilin protein and determined that the *MYOC* gene contains three coding exons.[14] They identified an imperfect palindromic glucocorticoid response associated with this gene. It has been implicated in the pathogenesis of glaucoma by a mutation-dependent, gain-of-function association causing mutant forms of the Myocilin protein being misfolded and aggregating in the endoplasmic reticulum of trabecular meshwork cells.[15]

The genetic mutations in the *MYOC* gene have been associated with certain phenotypic characteristics. Although in general, genotype-phenotype correlation is highly variable. An online catalog of *myocilin* variants and their associated phenotypes is available at www.myocilin.com. The phenotype of *MYOC* mutations can range from a mild ocular hypertension to blindness at presentation. Such is the variation that the phenotype can vary significantly in the same individual (one eye being more severely affected than the other).[16,17]

Mutations in the *CYP1B1* gene have also been associated with cases of juvenile and adult onset glaucoma in some families in which other members have PCG, suggesting that shared or overlapping mechanisms may predispose to both forms of glaucoma.[18] Digenic inheritance in JOAG was shown by Vincent *et al.*, due to mutations in both the *MYOC* and the *CYP1B1* genes.[19]

Compared to adult primary open-angle glaucoma, JOAG has a much higher percentage of familial cases as it is known to exhibit an autosomal dominant inheritance.[20-22] Hence genetic screening and genetic counseling could be considered in these patients to help diagnose pre-symptomatic cases among first and second-degree relatives.

Genetics of secondary childhood glaucoma

Axenfeld Rieger (AR) anomaly and syndrome[23]

Recent advances in molecular genetics have identified two major genes, *PITX2* and *FOXC1* (formerly named *FKHL7*). *PITX2* at 4q25 was the first gene identified by Semina *et al.*[24] *PITX2*, mutations can be identified in 10% to 60% of probands affected with AR syndrome.[25,26] Other implicated loci include those at 13q14 and 16q24,[26,27] but mutations in a causative gene have not been identified.[28]

Mutations in *PITX2* or *FOXC1* can cause phenotypic variants such as AR anomaly, AR syndrome, and Congenital iris hypoplasia. *PITX2* mutations are more likely to be associated with systemic findings, while the risk of glaucoma is greatest with *FOXC1* duplication, followed by *PITX2* mutations and then *FOXC1* mutations.[28]

When the diagnosis of AR is suspected, parents and other family members should be examined as the presence of anomalous anterior segment features may facilitate a diagnosis (Fig. 2).[28] Further examinations of the pedigree often disclose the autosomal dominant inheritance pattern (70%), though sporadic cases of AR do occur.

Prenatal testing for pregnancies at increased risk is possible if the disease-causing mutation in the family has been identified. Prospective parents might consider genetic counseling for risk calculation. Clinical management might be facilitated as genotype-phenotype correlations can be made to some extent.[29]

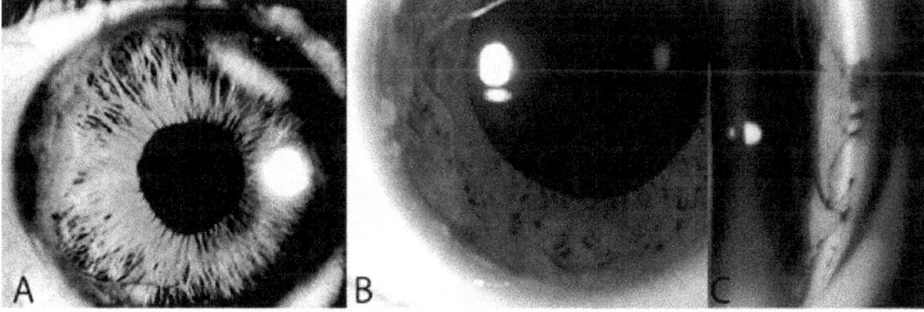

Fig. 2. Family history and examination. A. Child referred with corneal opacity and iris changes initially thought to be related to birth trauma; B and C. Anterior segment examination, including gonioscopy, identified features of AR anomaly in the father.

Peters anomaly

Peters anomaly consists of a central corneal opacity (leukoma) with iridocorneal attachments to the posterior edges of the defect and posterior corneal thinning involving the posterior stroma, Descemet membrane and endothelium.[30] Peters anomaly usually occurs sporadically, but there are reported cases of autosomal recessive inheritance and less commonly autosomal dominant inheritance. Peters anomaly is genetically heterogeneous. It can be caused by genetic mutations in *PAX6*, *PITX2*,[31] *FOXC1*, *CYP1B1*[19,32,33] and *FOXE3*[34,35] genes.

Peters anomaly associated with systemic features is referred to as Peters plus syndrome.[36] The genetic origin of the syndrome was confirmed by the discovery of mutations identified in the beta- 1,3-galactosyltransferase-like glycosyltransferase (*B3GALTL*) gene.[37]

Aniridia

Aniridia is a severe, congenital ocular malformation inherited in an autosomal-dominant fashion with high penetrance and variable expression. The phenotype ranges from complete absence of the iris, partial absence or normal iris[38] (Fig. 3)

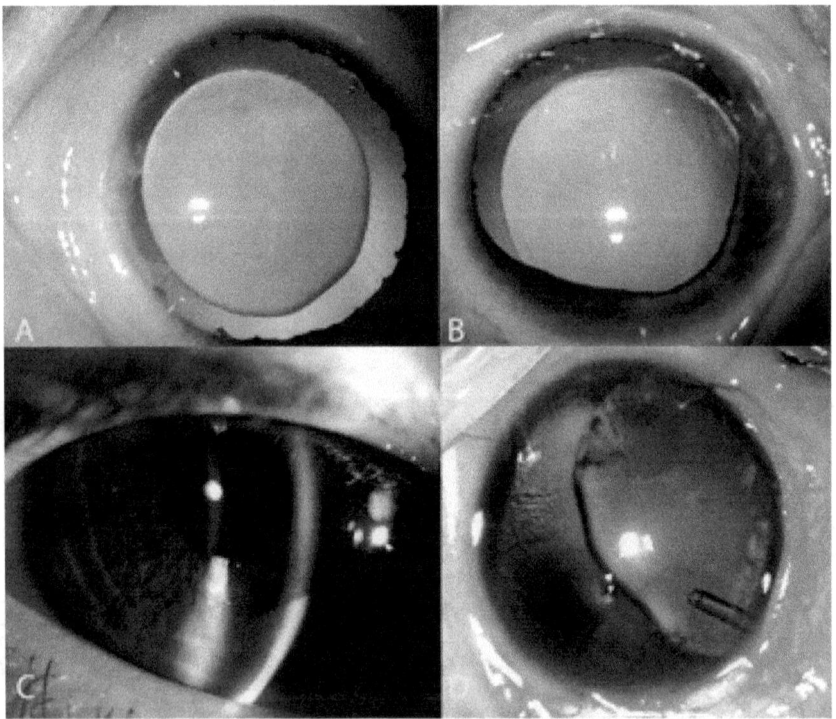

Fig. 3. Spectrum of *PAX6* phenotypes. A. Complete absence of iris; B. Partial absence of iris; C. Mild iris hypoplasia and ectropion uvea; D. Minimal iris tissue and ectopia lentis.

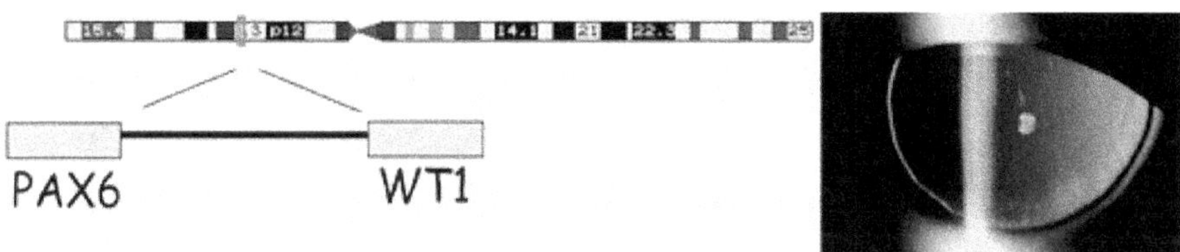

Fig. 4. Chromosome 11 diagram illustrating location of PAX6 gene and proximity of WT1 (Wilms tumour gene) and complete aniridia phenotype in a patient with deletion of both genes.

along with other ocular features including limbal stem cell failure, optic nerve hypoplasia[39] and foveal hypoplasia.[40,41]

Aniridia exists in both sporadic and familial forms. In humans, aniridia is almost exclusively caused by *PAX6* mutations,[42] which include nonsense (37%); frame shift (23%); and splice site, missense, anti-termination mutations, and in-frame deletions or insertions (39%).[43,44] *PAX6* is located on chromosome 11p13, and its mutations lead to a variety of hereditary ocular malformations of the anterior and posterior segment, including aniridia and foveal hypoplasia. The *PAX6* gene is adjacent to the Wilms tumour gene, so it is possible that sporadic cases of aniridia may have a deletion of both genes (Fig. 4). Sporadic cases are at markedly increased risk of Wilms tumor (nephroblastoma). WAGR syndrome is the name given to the constellation of clinical findings including Wilms tumor (80% before the age of 5), aniridia, genitourinary abnormalities and mental retardation.

A study found no difference in the clinical phenotype between aniridia patients with and without detectable mutations in the *PAX6* gene.[45] Though most *PAX6* nonsense mutations lead to aniridia, many missense mutations may result in Peters anomaly.[46]

LTBP2 mutations

LTBP2 (Latent transforming growth factor-beta-binding protein 2) is the largest member of the latent transforming growth factor (TGF)-β binding protein family. These are extracellular matrix proteins with multi-domain structure.[47] High *LTBP2* expression occurs in human eyes, including in the trabecular meshwork and ciliary processes that are thought to be relevant to the etiology of primary congenital glaucoma. The *LTBP2* mutations seem to be involved in non-syndromic glaucoma as well as those with complex ocular phenotypes including ectopia lentis and microspherophakia,[48,49] suggesting a lens pathology as part of the phenotype besides megalocornea (unrelated to elevated IOP) and secondary pupillary block glaucoma.[50]

Important conditions in the differential diagnosis of childhood glaucoma

X-linked megalocornea

X-linked megalocornea is an inherited eye disorder in which the corneal diameter is bilaterally enlarged (> 13 mm) without an increase in intraocular pressure. Features of megalocornea in addition to a deep anterior chamber include astigmatic refractive errors, atrophy of the iris stroma, miosis secondary to decreased function of the dilator muscle, iridodonesis and tremulousness, subluxation, or dislocation of the lens.[51] Webb *et al.*[52] identified *CHRDL1* as a disease causing gene for megalocornea.

Congenital hereditary endothelial dystrophy (CHED)

CHED is characterized by thickening and opacification of the cornea, altered morphology of the endothelium, and secretion of an abnormal collagenous layer at the Descemet membrane (Fig. 5). There are both autosomal dominant (CHED1) and autosomal recessive (CHED2) forms, with the latter being more common and more severe.[53] Mutations have been identified in the recessive form in the gene *SLC4A11*.[53] Genetic testing may be helpful in confirming the diagnosis of CHED; however, the diagnosis remains clinical as a negative result does not rule out the condition.[54]

In the recessive form corneal clouding is observed at birth or within the neonatal period, nystagmus is often present, but no photophobia or epiphora is seen. In the dominant form, corneal opacification is usually seen in the first or second year of life and progresses slowly, photophobia and epiphora may be the first signs of the dystrophy, and nystagmus is infrequently seen.[55] Some authors argue that CHED and glaucoma can co-exist,[56,57] although others dispute this.[54,58] A normal eye size and corneal thickness measurements, respectively, help to differentiate this condition from primary congenital glaucoma.

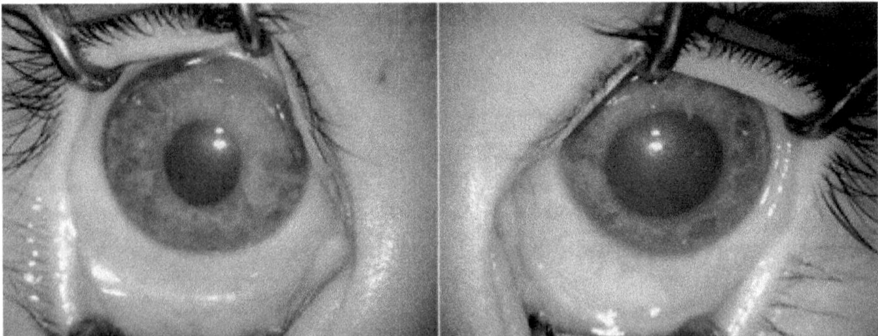

Fig. 5. Congenital hereditary endothelial dystrophy in a child aged eight months illustrating persistent corneal haze, no Haab striae, central corneal thickness 1084 μ and 1113 μ, horizontal corneal diameter 11.5 mm OU, refraction +2.0 diopters OU (pupils partly dilated during examination under anesthesia).

Syndromic forms of glaucoma

Table 2 presents some of the better recognized syndromes which have glaucoma as part of their clinical picture. For some syndromes, glaucoma may be the presenting feature.

Table 2. Syndromic forms of glaucoma

Syndrome	Clinical features	Gene
Nail-patella syndrome (AD)[59]	Dysplasia of the nails, absent or hypoplastic patellae, renal anomalies and prevalence of glaucoma (9.6%). *Lester sign*, consists of a zone of darker pigmentation of roughly cloverleaf shape around the central iris.	*LMX1B*[60]
Oculodentodigital dysplasia (AD)[61]	Typical facial appearance, variable involvement of the dentition, fingers and eyes (microphthalmia, microcornea, glaucoma).	connexin-43 gene (*GJA1*)[62]
Frank-ter Haar syndrome (AR)[63]	Brachycephaly, wide fontanels, prominent forehead, hypertelorism, prominent eyes, macrocornea with or without glaucoma.	*TKS4* gene (*SH3PXD2B*)[64]
Rubinstein-Taybi syndrome (AR)[65]	Mental retardation, postnatal growth deficiency, microcephaly, broad thumbs, dysmorphic facial features, refractive error, strabismus, glaucoma and cataract.	*CREBBP*[66,67]
Ehlers-Danlos type VI[68]	Severe muscle hypotonia at birth, generalized joint laxity, scoliosis at birth, scleral fragility ± rupture of the ocular globe or glaucoma.[69]	*PLOD1*[70,71]
Neurofibromatosis, type 1 (AD)[72]	Tumor development of the nerve sheaths, Lisch nodules, plexiform neurofibroma of lid, sphenoid wing dysplasia, optic nerve glioma, glaucoma.	neurofibromin gene (*NF1*)[73]
Peters plus syndrome (AR)c[74]	Mental delay, short of stature, brachymorphism, abnormal ears and Peters anomaly.	*B3GALTL*[37]
Zellweger (Peroxisome biogenesis disorder 1a)(AR)[75]	Severe neurologic dysfunction, craniofacial abnormalities, liver dysfunction, and the absence of peroxisomes diagnosed biochemically. Corneal clouding, cataracts, pigmentary retinopathy, glaucoma and nystagmus.	*PEX1*[76]
Marfan syndrome (AD)[77]	Increased height, disproportionately long limbs and digits, anterior chest deformity, ectopia lentis and dilatation of the aortic root.	fibrillin-1 gene (*FBN1*)[78]
Klippel-Trenaunay-Weber Syndrome[79]	Large cutaneous hemangiomata with hypertrophy of related bones and soft tissues. Resembles Sturge-Weber syndrome clinically.	gene disputed

Table 2. Cont.

Syndrome	Clinical features	Gene
Charcot-Marie-Tooth disease type 4B2 (CMT4B2) (AR)[80]	Demyelinating hereditary motor and sensory neuropathy characterized by abnormal folding of myelin sheaths.	*SBF2*[81]
Walker Warburg Syndrome (Muscular Dystrophy-Dystroglycanopathy (Congenital With Brain And Eye Anomalies), Type A, 1; Mddga1) (AR)[82]	Congenital muscular dystrophy-dystroglycanopathy with brain and eye anomalies.	*POMT1*[83] *ISPD*[84]
MIDAS (microphthalmia, dermal aplasia, and sclerocornea) syndrome (XL-Dominant)[85]	Unilateral or bilateral microphthalmia and linear skin defects which are limited to the face and neck.	*HCCS*[86]
Renal Tubular Acidosis, Proximal, with Ocular Abnormalities and Mental Retardation (AR)[87]	Proximal renal tubular acidosis, growth retardation, mental retardation, nystagmus, cataract, corneal opacities and glaucoma.	*SLC4A4*[88]

Clinical genetics

For accurate genetic information for families, accurate clinical ophthalmic diagnosis is critical. The ophthalmologist needs to provide clear information to the clinical geneticist regarding the nature of the ophthalmic abnormality. For example, rather than saying the child has congenital glaucoma, it is important that as far as possible, the ophthalmologist provides information about whether the child has primary congenital glaucoma, or whether there may be other changes such as iris hypoplasia or iris strands that may indicate AR anomaly, since these indicate different genetic counseling and testing scenarios.

As noted in the preceding sections, there can be marked variation in penetrance and expression in primary and secondary childhood glaucomas, hence to provide accurate genetic counseling, parents and siblings of an affected child should be examined by the ophthalmologist to determine if anyone else in the family may have subtle features of the condition in the proband. This can make a significant difference to the genetic counseling information. For example, for a couple with one affected child with AR anomaly – if one of the parents is found to have previously unrecognized features of the condition – then there is an up to 50% recurrence risk for a future child to be affected (Fig. 6). However, if neither parent is affected, then the recurrence risk is more likely in the vicinity of < 5-10%, since this may be a new autosomal dominant condition in the child with an expected very low recurrence risk. In another scenario, there may be gonosomal mosaicism in a parent, meaning that one parent has a mutation in a subset of their cells, including those of their reproductive organs, or one of the parents may have a mutation in the contributing disease gene but be non-penetrant for the condition.

The ophthalmologist needs to consider if referral to a pediatrician in addition to referral for genetic information may be beneficial. If there is any concern about developmental milestones, growth parameters or dysmorphic features then involvement of a pediatrician can be helpful for the patient's overall management. In any infant or young child with features indicating sporadic aniridia, an urgent renal ultrasound is required to check for the presence of Wilms tumor and a plan needs to be in place for three monthly renal ultrasounds, until testing can be arranged to determine if the child has a deletion involving PAX6 and WT1 or not. This testing can be undertaken using CGH microarray or FISH probes in the PAX6/WT1 region depending on the available genetic testing services.

On referral to a clinical geneticist, there should be examination of the child for any associated syndromic features as outlined in the Table 2 delineating syndromic conditions where glaucoma may be a feature. If a syndromic diagnosis is made, then recurrence risk information can be based on the inheritance pattern associated with that disorder. If the underlying disease gene is known for the particular syndrome and testing is available, genetic testing can be undertaken if clinically indicated in the family. For those with an isolated ocular condition, recurrence risk information should be provided to families on the basis of the most likely mode of inheritance associated with the condition, in concert with any relevant ocular findings in other family members.

Genetic testing is particularly indicated when this may impact upon future reproductive decisions. An example where this may be helpful is where there may be a child affected with Peters anomaly. If the parents and siblings are examined and there is no evidence of ocular disease, this may be a new autosomal dominant condition or it could be an autosomal recessive condition in the child (Fig. 6). Hence the recurrence risk given to the parents will be from < 1% to 25%. To clarify this risk, genetic testing can be undertaken. For example, if in one family a *de novo* heterozygous mutation is identified in *PAX6* in the proband, while in another family the proband is found to have compound heterozygous mutations in *CYP1B1*: members of the first family have a definite recurrence risk information of < 1% with the small residual risk due to the possibility of gonosomal mosaicism in an unaffected parent. And members of the second family have definite recurrence risk information of 25% for future offspring (Fig. 7). Identification of the mutations allows the possibility of prenatal or pre-implantation genetic diagnosis where this may be requested by the family after appropriate genetic counseling.

It is important to keep in mind that recurrence risk information varies depending upon a person's position in the pedigree. Many ophthalmologists treating children with childhood glaucoma will manage these individuals through to late teenage/early adult years. In the scenarios described above, the parents in the first family were given a low recurrence risk of having another child affected with Peters anomaly, since their child's Peters anomaly was due to a de novo heterozygous mutation in PAX6. It needs to be remembered that the affected child has a new

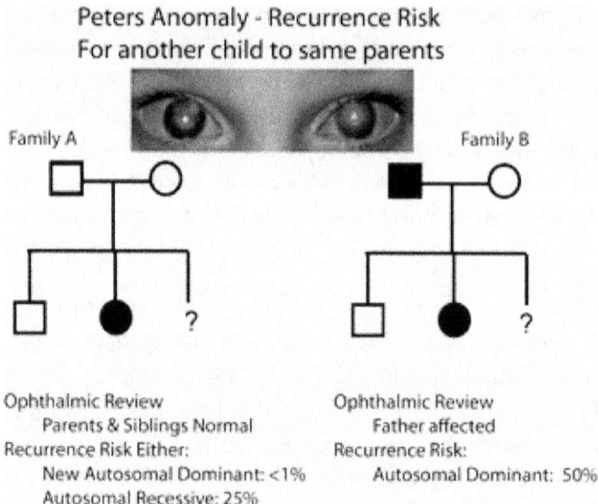

Fig. 6. Recurrence risk for parents with affected child – importance of ophthalmic review of family members.

Fig. 7. Recurrence risk for an affected individual – genetic diagnosis guides recurrence risk.

autosomal dominant condition, so the risk for them of having an affected child in the future is 50%, and referral for genetic counseling for such a patient is recommended at an appropriate time in late teenage/early adult years. By contrast, the child with Peters anomaly with compound heterozygous mutations in CYP1B1 has a low recurrence risk for an affected child if they have children with someone unaffected with eye disease and to whom they are unrelated, since the carrier frequency for CYP1B1 mutations in the general population may be expected to be relatively low (Fig. 7). Again, referral for genetic counseling would be recommended at an appropriate time for discussion of the genetic issues (Fig. 8).

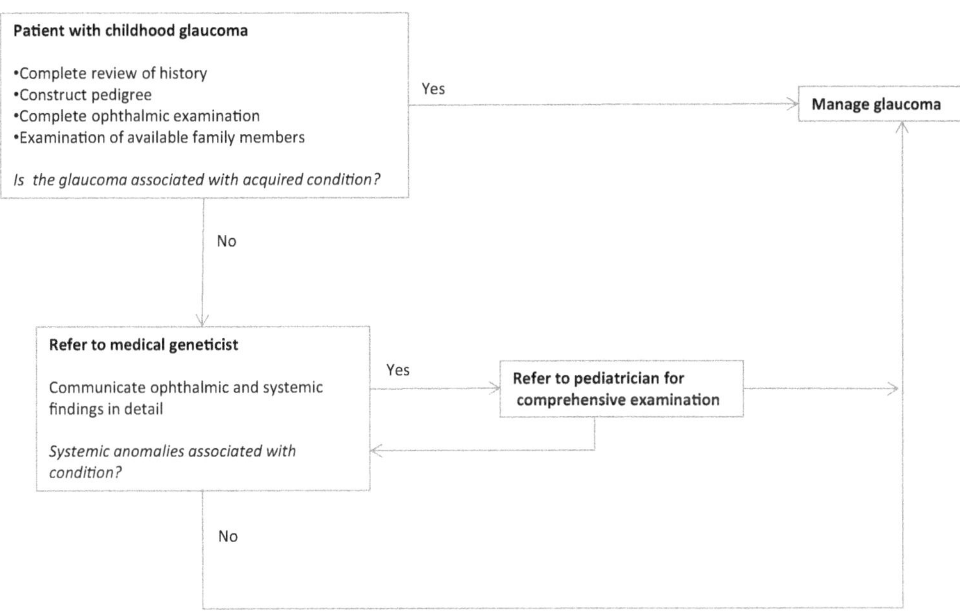

Fig. 8. An approach to managing a child with glaucoma.

Next-generation sequencing

There are three billion base pairs in the haploid human genome, with approximately 45 million base pairs found in the coding regions of the approximate 23,000 genes. Up until recently, sequencing of genes has only been possible on a gene by gene basis, after coding exons were amplified by PCR and base pairs sequenced sequentially in a process called Sanger sequencing. This is labor-intensive and costly, particularly for genetically heterogeneous conditions where a number of different genes may cause a similar phenotype.

Through next-generation sequencing (NGS) platforms, massively parallel sequencing is undertaken where parts or all of the genome are sequenced simultaneously. This can be undertaken in a targeted manner, so that certain groups of genes that may cause a particular disorder can be sequenced together, called targeted NGS, or all exons in the genome can be selected and sequenced together, called whole exome sequencing (WES). In whole genome sequencing, the entire genome is fragmented and all exons and non-coding regions are sequenced simultaneously. These approaches reduce sequencing costs where there are large scale sequencing requirements, but there is a need for extensive computing and bio-informatic resources for the storage, analysis and interpretation of sequencing data.

NGS is starting to be introduced for clinical testing in genetic eye disease. There are a number of targeted NGS panels available for disorders causing genetically heterogeneous retinal diseases including retinitis pigmentosa. Such panels will be particularly valuable in glaucomatous conditions such as Peters anomaly where a number of disease genes may underlie the condition. Exome and whole genome sequencing are currently mostly in use in research settings where novel disease genes are being sought. As costs of exome and whole genome sequencing fall and bioinformatics resources improve, it is likely that these approaches will be increasingly undertaken in the clinical setting to be followed by filtering of the data to look particularly at the known disease genes, especially in genetically heterogeneous conditions. These approaches raise concerns about the possibility of incidental medically relevant genetic findings unrelated to the disease under investigation, for example a mutation in one of the breast cancer genes, and how these should be handled. Patients will need to be informed of this possibility as part of their consent to these investigations, and recent guidelines have been proposed to manage these possible findings (American College of Medical Genetics and Genomics Recommendations for Reporting of Incidental Findings in Clinical Exome and Genome Sequencing, March 2013).

Direct to consumer (DTC) DNA testing

At present, most of the DTC testing does not include the rare mutations associated with childhood glaucoma. Thus clinicians and patients should not rely on this to identify genes associated with childhood glaucomas. The Academy of Ophthalmology (AAO) has recently published guidelines on testing.[89] This also includes recommendations for the testing of asymptomatic children.

References

1. Sutter T, Tang Y, Hayes C, et al. Complete cDNA sequence of a human dioxin-inducible mRNA identifies a new gene subfamily of cytochrome P450 that maps to chromosome 2. J Biol Chem 1994; 269: 13092-13099.
2. Tang Y, Wo Y, Stewart J, et al. Isolation and characterization of the human cytochrome P450 CYP1B1 gene. J Biol Chem 1996; 271: 28324-28330.
3. Schwartzman M, Abraham N, Masferrer J, et al. Cytochrome P450-dependent arachidonate metabolism in corneal epithelium: formation of biologically active compounds. Adv Prostaglandin Thromboxane Leukot Res 1987; 17A: 78-83.
4. Kumar M, Tanwar M, Faiq M, et al. Mitochondrial DNA nucleotide changes in primary congenital glaucoma patients. Mol Vis 2013; 19: 220-230.
5. Sarfarazi M, Stoilov I, Schenkman J. Genetics and biochemistry of primary congenital glaucoma. Ophthalmol Clin North Am 2003; 16: 543-554.
6. Suri F, Yazdani S, Narooie-Nejhad M, et al. Variable expressivity and high penetrance of CYP1B1 mutations associated with primary congenital glaucoma. Ophthalmology 2009; 116: 2101-2109.
7. Bejjani B, Stockton D, Lewis R, et al. Multiple CYP1B1 mutations and incomplete penetrance in an inbred population segregating primary congenital glaucoma suggest frequent de novo events and a dominant modifier locus. Hum Molec Genet 2000; 9: 367-374.

8.   Khan A. Genetics of primary glaucoma. Curr Opin Ophthalmol 2011; 22: 347-355.

9.   Abu-Amero K, Osman E, Mousa A, et al. Screening of CYP1B1 and LTBP2 genes in Saudi families with primary congenital glaucoma: genotype-phenotype correlation. Mol Vis 2011; 17: 2911-2919.

10   Tanwar M, Dada T, Sihota R, et al. Mutation spectrum of CYP1B1 in North Indian congenital glaucoma patients. Mol Vis 2009; 15: 1200-1209.

11   Hollander D, Sarfarazi M, Stoilov I, et al. Genotype and phenotype correlations in congenital glaucoma: CYP1B1 mutations, goniodysgenesis, and clinical characteristics. Am J Ophthalmol 2006; 142: 993-1004.

12   Sarfarazi M, Stoilov I. Molecular genetics of primary congenital glaucoma. Eye 2004; 14: 422-428.

13   Stone E, Fingert J, Alward W, et al. Identification of a gene that causes primary open angle glaucoma. Science 1997; 275(5300): 668-670.

14   Kubota R, Noda S, Wang Y, et al. A novel myosin like protein (myocilin) expressed in the connecting cilium of the photoreceptor: molecular cloning, tissue expression and chromosomal mapping. Genomics 1997; 41: 360-369.

15   Shepard A, Jacobson N, Millar JC, et al. Glaucoma-causing myocilin mutants require the Peroxisomal targeting signal-1 receptor (PTS1R) to elevate intraocular pressure. Hum Mol Genet 2007; 16: 609-617.

16   Walton DS, Katsavounidou G. Newborn primary congenital glaucoma: 2005 update. J Pediatr Ophthalmol Strabismus 2005; 42: 333-341.

17   Gupta V, Gupta S, Dhawan M, et al. Inter ocular asymmetry in juvenile onset primary open angle glaucoma. Clin Exp Ophthalmol 2011; 39: 633-638.

18   Melki R, Colomb E, Lefort N, et al. CYP1B1 mutations in French patients with early-onset primary open-angle glaucoma. J Med Genet 2004; 41: 647-651.

19   Vincent AL, Billingsley G, Buys Y, et al. Digenic inheritance of early-onset glaucoma: CYP1B1, a potential modifier gene. Am J Hum Genet 2002; 70: 448-460.

20   Richards JE, Lichter P, Boehnke M, et al. Mapping of a gene for autosomal dominant juvenile-onset open-angle glaucoma to chromosome 1q. Am J Hum Genet 1994; 54: 62-70.

21   Johnson AT, Drack A, Kwitek A, et al. Clinical features and linkage analysis of a family with autosomal dominant juvenile glaucoma. Ophthalmology 1993; 100: 524-529.

22   Wiggs JL, Del Bono E, Schuman J, et al. Genetic linkage of autosomal dominant juvenile glaucoma to 1q21-q31 in three affected pedigrees. Genomics 1994; 21: 299-303.

23   Reis LM, Semina EV. Genetics of anterior segment dysgenesis disorders. Current Opinion in Ophthalmology 2011; 22: 314-324.

24   Semina EV, Reiter R, Leysens NJ, et al. Cloning and characterization of a novel bicoid-related homeobox transcription factor gene, RIEG, involved in Rieger syndrome. Nature Genetics 1996; 14: 392-399.

25   Borges A, Susanna RJ, Carani J, et al. Genetic analysis of PITX2 and FOXC1 in Rieger Syndrome patients from Brazil. J Glaucoma 2002; 11: 51-56.

26   Lines M, Kozlowski K, Kulak S, et al. Characterization and prevalence of PITX2 microdeletions and mutations in Axenfeld-Rieger malformations. Invest Ophthalmol Vis Sci 2004; 45: 828-833.

27   Phillips J, del Bono E, Haines J, et al. A second locus for Rieger syndrome maps to chromosome 13q14. Am J Hum Genet 1996; 59: 613-619.

28   Chang T, Summers C, Schimmenti L, Grajewski AL. Axenfeld-Rieger syndrome: new perspectives. Br J Ophthalmol 2012; 96: 318-322.

29   Weisschuh N, De Baere E, Wissinger B, Tümer Z. Clinical utility gene card for: Axenfeld-Rieger syndrome. Eur J Hum Genet 2011; 19(3).

30   Stone D, Kenyon K, Green W, Ryan S. Congenital central corneal leukoma (Peters anomaly). Am J Ophthalmol 1976; 81: 173-193.

31   Doward W, Perveen R, Lloyd IC, et al. A mutation in the RIEG1 gene associated with Peters anomaly. J Med Genet 1999; 36: 152-155.

32 Vincent A, Billingsley G, Priston M, et al. Phenotypic heterogeneity of CYP1B1: mutations in a patient with Peters anomaly. J Med Genet 2001; 38: 324-326.

33 Vincent A, Billingsley G, Priston M, et al. Further support of the role of CYP1B1 in patients with Peters anomaly. Molecular Vision 2006; 12: 506-510.

34 Doucette L, Green J, Fernandez B, et al. A novel, non-stop mutation in FOXE3 causes an autosomal dominant form of variable anterior segment dysgenesis including Peters anomaly. Eur J Hum Genet 2011; 19: 293-299.

35 Ormestad M, Blixt A, Churchill A, et al. Foxe3 haploinsufficiency in mice: a model for Peters anomaly. Invest Ophthalmol Vis Sci 2002; 43: 1350-1357.

36 Aliferis K, Marsal C, Pelletier V, et al. A novel nonsense B3GALTL mutation confirms Peters plus syndrome in a patient with multiple malformations and Peters anomaly. Ophthalmic Genet 2010; 31: 205-208.

37 Lesnik Oberstein S, Kriek M, White S, et al. Peters Plus syndrome is caused by mutations in B3GALTL, a putative glycosyltransferase. Am J Hum Genet 2006; 79: 562-566.

38 Willcock C, Grigg J, Wilson M, et al. Congenital iris ectropion as an indicator of variant aniridia. Brit J Ophthalmol 2006; 90: 658-569.

39 McCulley TJ, Mayer K, Dahr SS, et al. Aniridia and optic nerve hypoplasia. Eye 2005; 19: 762-764.

40 Dharmaraj N, Reddy A, Kiran V, et al. PAX6 gene mutations and genotype-phenotype correlations in sporadic cases of aniridia from India. Ophthalmic Genet 2003; 24: 161-165.

41 Tzoulaki I, White IM, Hanson IM. PAX6 mutations: genotype-phenotype correlations. BMC Genet 2005; 6: 27.

42 Jordan T, Hanson I, Zaletayev D, et al. The human PAX6 gene is mutated in two patients with aniridia. Nature Genetics 1992; 1: 328-332.

43 Hanson I, Seawrigh A, Hardman K, et al. PAX6 mutations in aniridia. Hum Molec Gen 1993; 2: 915-920.

44 Hanson I. Review PAX6 and congenital eye malformations. Pediatr Res 2003; 54: 791.

45 Lim H, Seo E, Kim G, et al. Comparison between aniridia with and without PAX6 mutations: clinical and molecular analysis in 14 Korean patients with aniridia. Ophthalmology 2012; 119: 1258-1264.

46 Azuma N, Yamada M. Missense mutation at the C terminus of the PAX6 gene in ocular anterior segment anomalies. Invest Ophthalmol Vis Sci 1998; 39: 828-830.

47 Narooie-Nejad M, Paylakhi SH, Shojaee S, et al. Loss of function mutations in the gene encoding latent transforming growth factor beta binding protein 2, LTBP2, cause primary congenital glaucoma. Hum Molec Genet 2009; 18: 3969-3977.

48 Kumar A, Duvvari MR, Prabhakaran VC, et al. A homozygous mutation in LTBP2 causes isolated microspherophakia. Hum Genet 2010; 128: 365-371.

49 Haji-Seyed-Javadi R, Jelodari-Mamaghani S, Paylakhi SH, et al. LTBP2 mutations cause Weill-Marchesani and Weill-Marchesani-like syndrome and affect disruptions in the extracellular matrix. Hum Mutat 2012; 33: 1182-1187.

50 Azmanov DN, Dimitrova S, Florez L, et al. LTBP2 and CYP1B1 mutations and associated ocular phenotypes in the Roma/Gypsy founder population. Europ J Hum Genet 2011; 19: 326-333.

51 Skuta GL, Sugar J, Ericson ES. Corneal endothelial cell measurements in megalocornea. Arch Ophthalmol 1983; 101: 51-53.

52 Webb TR, Matarin M, Gardner JC, et al. X-linked megalocornea caused by mutations in CHRDL1 identifies an essential role for ventroptin in anterior segment development. Am J Hum Genet 2012; 90: 247-259.

53 Vithana EN, Morgan P, Sundaresan P, et al. Mutations in sodium-borate cotransporter SLC4A11 cause recessive congenital hereditary endothelial dystrophy (CHED2). Nature Genet 2006; 38: 755-757.

54 Khan AO, Al-Shehah A, Ghadhfan, FE. High measured intraocular pressure in children with recessive congenital hereditary endothelial dystrophy. J Pediatr Ophthalmol Strabismus 2010; 47: 29-33.

55 Judisch GF, Maumenee IH. Clinical differentiation of recessive congenital hereditary endothelial dystrophy and dominant hereditary endothelial dystrophy. Am J Ophthalmol 1978; 85: 606-612.

56 Ramamurthy B, Sachdeva V, Mandal AK, et al. Coexistent congenital hereditary endothelial dystrophy and congenital glaucoma. Cornea 2007; 26: 647-649.

57 Mullaney PB, Risco JM, Teichmann K, Millar L. Congenital hereditary endothelial dystrophy associated with glaucoma. Ophthalmology 1995; 102: 186-192.

58 Khan A. Conditions that can be mistaken as early childhood glaucoma. Ophthalmic Genet 2011; 32: 129-137.

59 Sweeney E, Fryer A, Mountford R, Green A, McIntosh I. Nail patella syndrome: a review of the phenotype aided by developmental biology. J Med Genet 2003; 40: 153-162.

60 Vollrath D, Jaramillo-Babb VL, Clough MV, et al. Loss-of-function mutations in the LIM-homeodomain gene, LMX1B, in nail-patella syndrome. Hum Molec Genet 1998; 7: 1091-1098.

61. Gabriel LAR, Sachdeva R, Marcotty A, et al. Oculodentodigital dysplasia: new ocular findings and a novel connexin 43 mutation. Arch Ophthal 2011; 129: 781-784.

62 Paznekas WA, Boyadjiev SA, Shapiro RE, et al. Connexin 43 (GJA1) mutations cause the pleiotropic phenotype of oculodentodigital dysplasia. Am J Hum Genet 2003; 72: 408-418.

63 Maas SM, Kayserili II, Lam J, et al. Further delineation of Frank-ter-Haar syndrome. Am J Med Genet 2004; 131A: 127-133.

64 Iqbal Z, Cejudo-Martin P, de Brouwer A, et al. Disruption of the podosome adaptor protein TKS4 (SH3PXD2B) causes the skeletal dysplasia, eye, and cardiac abnormalities of Frank-ter Haar syndrome. Am J Hum Genet 2010; 86: 254-261.

65 Stevens CA, Pouncey J, Knowles D. Adults with Rubinstein-Taybi syndrome. Am J Med Genet 2011; 155A: 1680-1684.

66 Petrij F, Giles RH, Dauwerse HG, et al. Rubinstein-Taybi syndrome caused by mutations in the transcriptional co-activator CBP. Nature 1995; 376: 348-351.

67 Schorry EK, Keddache M, Lanphear N, et al. Genotype-phenotype correlations in Rubinstein-Taybi syndrome. Am J Med Genet 2008; 146A: 2512-2519.

68 Beighton P, De Paepe A, Steinmann B, et al. Ehlers-Danlos syndromes: revised nosology, Villefranche, 1997. Am J Med Genet 1998; 77: 31-37.

69 Wenstrup RJ, Murad, S, Pinnell, SR. Ehlers-Danlos syndrome type VI: clinical manifestations of collagen lysyl hydroxylase deficiency. J Pediat 1989; 115: 405-409.

70 Pinnell SR, Krane SM, Kenzora JE, Glimcher MJ. Heritable disorder with hydroxylysine-deficient collagen: hydroxylysine-deficient collagen disease New Eng J Med 1972; 286: 1013-1020.

71 Pousi B, Hautala T, Heikkinen J, et al. Alu-alu recombination results in a duplication of seven exons in the lysyl hydroxylase gene in a patient with the type VI variant of Ehlers-Danlos syndrome. Am J Hum Genet 1994; 55: 899-906.

72 Kissil JL, Blakeley JO, Ferner RE, et al. What's new in neurofibromatosis? Proceedings from the 2009 NF Conference: new frontiers. Am J Med Genet A 2010; 152A: 269-283.

73 Wallace MR, Andersen LB, Saulino AM, et al. A de novo Alu insertion results in neurofibromatosis type 1. Nature 1991; 353: 864-866.

74 Maillette de Buy Wenniger-Prick LJ, Hennekam RC. The Peters plus syndrome: a review. Ann Genet 2002; 45: 97-103.

75 Wanders RJA. Metabolic and molecular basis of peroxisomal disorders: a review. Am J Med Genet 2004; 126A: 355-375.

76 Ebberink MS, Mooijer PAW, Gootjes J, et al. Genetic classification and mutational spectrum of more than 600 patients with a Zellweger syndrome spectrum disorder. Hum Mut 2010; 32: 59-69.

77 Gray JR, Davies SJ. Marfan syndrome. J Med Genet 1996; 33: 403-408.

78 Maslen CL, Corson GM, Maddox BK, et al. Partial sequence of a candidate gene for the Marfan syndrome. Nature 1991; 352: 334-337.

79 Oduber C, van der Horst CM, Hennekam R. Klippel-Trenaunay syndrome: diagnostic criteria and hypothesis on etiology. Annals of Plastic Surgery 2008; 60: 217-223.

80 Kiwaki T, Umehara F, Takashima H, et al. Hereditary motor and sensory neuropathy with myelin folding and juvenile onset glaucoma. Neurology 2000; 55: 392-397.

81 Azzedine H, Bolino A, Taieb T, et al. Mutations in MTMR13, a new pseudophosphatase homologue of MTMR2 and Sbf1, in two families with an autosomal recessive demyelinating form of Charcot-Marie-Tooth disease associated with early-onset glaucoma. Am J Hum Genet 2003; 72: 1141-1153.

82 Dobyns WB, Pagon RA, Armstrong D, et al. Diagnostic criteria for Walker-Warburg syndrome. Am J Med Genet 1989; 32: 195-210.

83 Currier SC, Lee CK, Chang BS, et al. Mutations in POMT1 are found in a minority of patients with Walker-Warburg syndrome. Am J Med Genet 2005; 133A: 53-57.

84 Roscioli T, Kamsteeg EJ, Buysse K, et al. Mutations in ISPD cause Walker-Warburg syndrome and defective glycosylation of alpha-dystroglycan. Nat Genet 2012 Apr 22.

85 Morleo M, Pramparo T, Perone L, et al. Microphthalmia with linear skin defects (MLS) syndrome: clinical, cytogenetic, and molecular characterization of 11 cases. Am J Med Genet 2005; 137A: 190-198.

86 Wimplinger I, Morleo M, Rosenberger G, et al. Mutations of the mitochondrial holocytochrome c-type synthase in X-linked dominant microphthalmia with linear skin defects syndrome. Am J Hum Genet 2006; 79: 878-889.

87 Igarashi T, Ishii T, Watanabe K, et al. Persistent isolated proximal renal tubular acidosis – a systemic disease with a distinct clinical entity. Pediat Nephrol 1994; 8: 70-71.

88 Igarashi T, Inatomi J, Sekine T, et al. Mutations in SLC4A4 cause permanent isolated proximal renal tubular acidosis with ocular abnormalities. Nature Genet 1999; 23: 264-265.

89 Stone E, Aldave AJ, Drack AV, et al. Recommendations for genetic testing of inherited eye diseases. Report of the American Academy of Ophthalmology task force on genetic testing. Ophthalmology 2012; 119: 2408-2401.

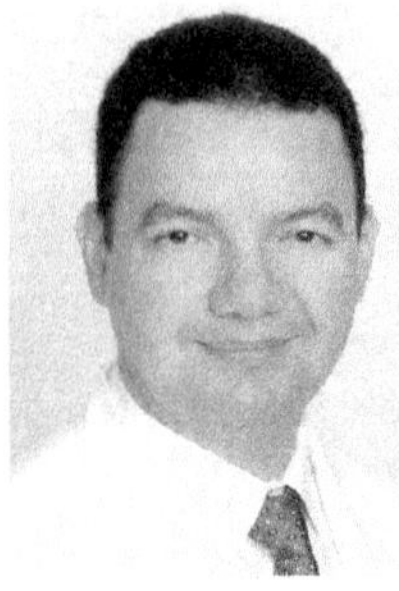

Oscar Albis-Donado

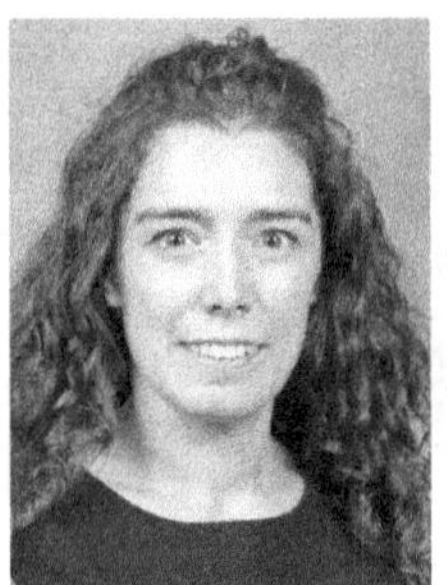

Elena Bitrian

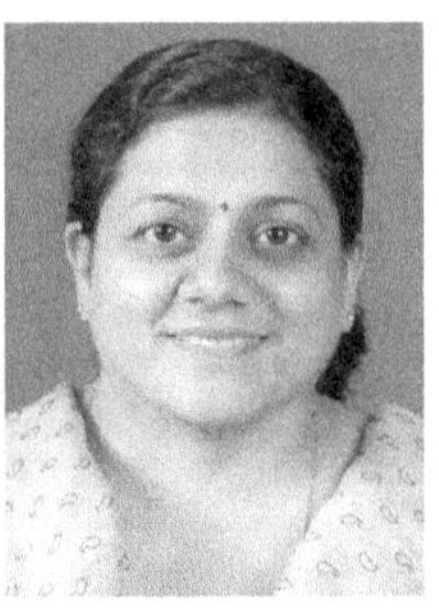

Manju Anilkumar

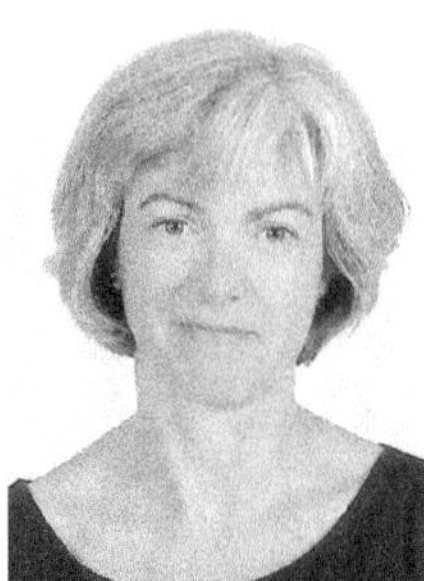

Maria Cristina Brito

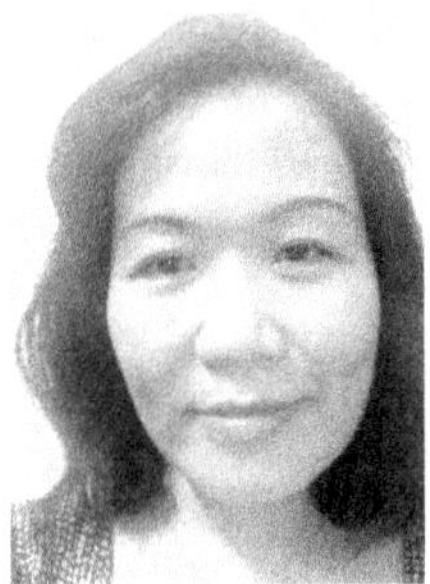

Tam Dang

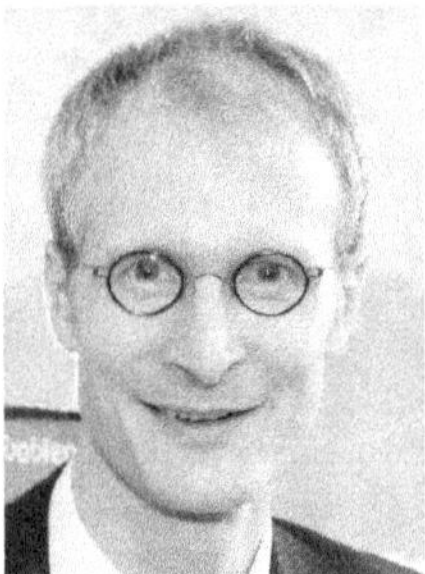

Thomas Klink

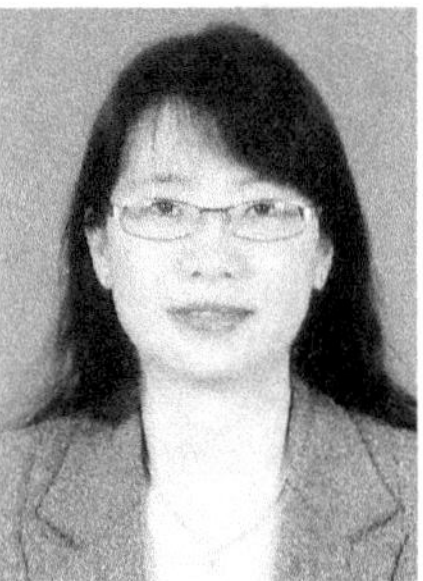

Ming-Yueh Lee

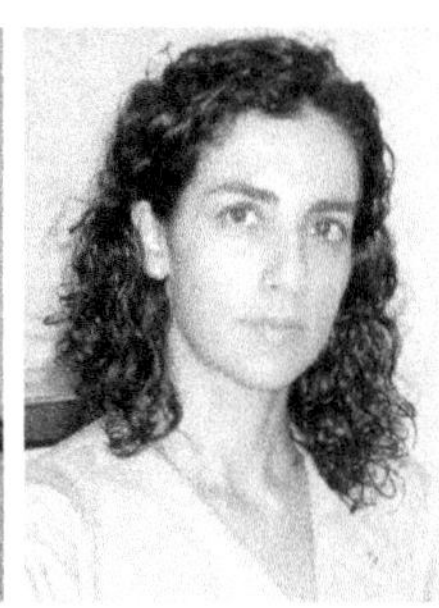

Carmen Mendez Hernandez

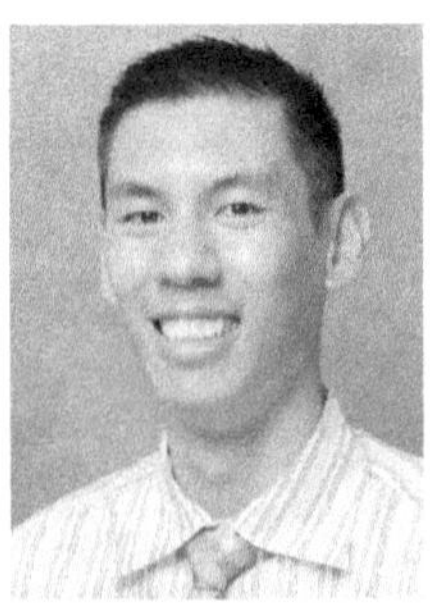

Ta Chen Peter Chang

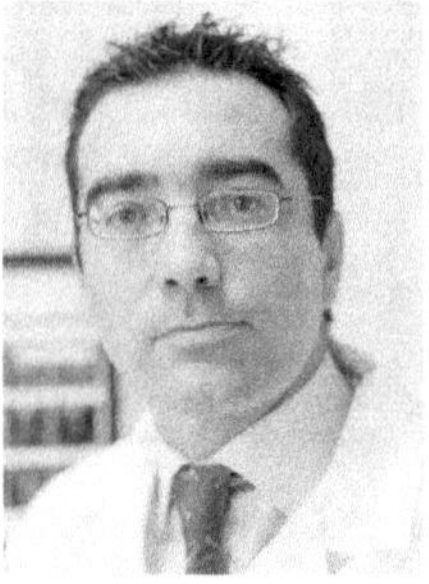

Julian Garcia Feijoo

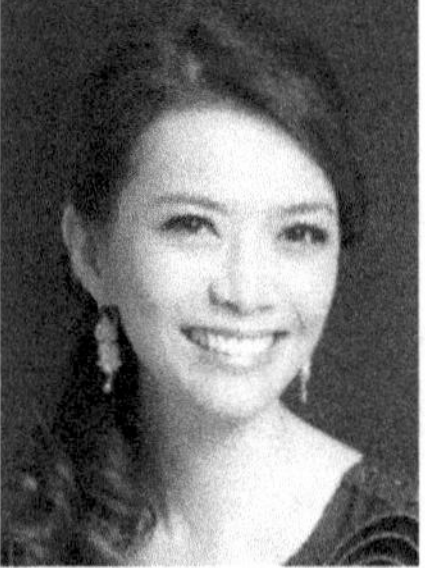

Ching Lin Ho

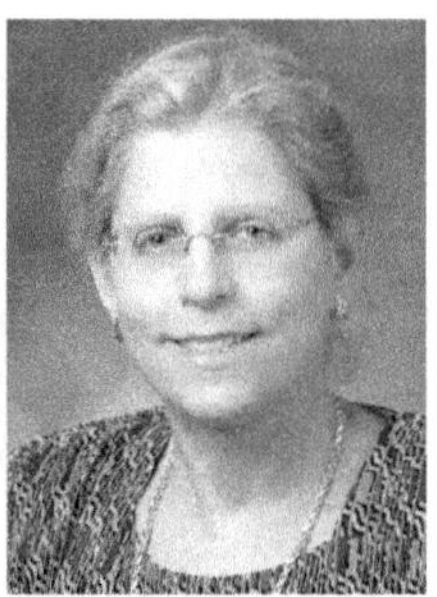

Sharon Freedman

4. MEDICATIONS

Oscar Albis-Donado, Elena Bitrian, Manju Anilkumar, Maria Cristina Brito, Tam Dang, Thomas Klink, Ming-Yueh Lee, Carmen Mendez Hernandez, Ta Chen Peter Chang, Julian Garcia Feijoo, Ching Lin Ho, Sharon Freedman

Section Leaders: Sharon Freedman, Julian Garcia Feijoo, Ching Lin Ho
Contributors: David Plager, Tomomi Higashide, Gwen Hofman

Consensus statements

1. Medications alone rarely show sustained efficacy as primary treatment for glaucoma in infants and young children, especially in primary congenital glaucoma (PCG).
   Comment: Medical therapy is frequently needed as temporizing intraocular pressure (IOP) lowering treatment before surgery or as adjuvant therapy after partially successful surgical procedures in childhood glaucoma.
   Comment: IOP-reducing medication may help reduce corneal edema prior to surgery for childhood glaucoma.
   Comment: Medical therapy should be considered first-line for some cases of childhood glaucoma (*e.g.*, uveitis-related, glaucoma after cataract removal).
2. Childhood glaucomas are heterogeneous in their causation as well as in their responses to different glaucoma medications.
3. Systemic pharmocokinetics for glaucoma medications are different in children than in adults.
   Comment: Systemic absorption can be significant and may be reduced by advising parents to close the lids (if possible), remove excess periocular liquid and perform naso-lacrimal occlusion.
   Comment: Use minimum frequency and concentration to achieve target IOP.
4. Potentially serious or fatal systemic adverse reactions which are rarely seen in adults may occur in young children after exposure to glaucoma medications.
   Comment: Adverse side effects may manifest atypically in children (*e.g.*, nocturnal cough with beta blockers rather than wheeze with reactive airways).
   Comment: Brimonidine should be avoided in young children.
   Comment: Children are more vulnerable to adverse effects of medications as they may be unable to verbalize symptoms and parents may not readily recognize them.
   Comment: Parents must be informed of the potential side effects.

Childhood Glaucoma, pp. 63-90
Edited by Robert N. Weinreb, Alana L. Grajewski, Maria Papadopoulos, John Grigg,
and Sharon Freedman
2013 © Kugler Publications, Amsterdam, The Netherlands

5. Compliance and adherence issues are greater and more complex in children due to their dependence on caregivers or parents, possible lack of cooperation in the administration of treatment, as well as concurrent medical conditions that may complicate medical therapy.
6. Target pressure must be chosen and reassessed with all available information concerning whether glaucoma is adequately controlled.
   Comment: Limitations on ability to perform structural and functional testing of optic nerve make verification of glaucoma control more difficult in children.
7. Consider surgery when medical treatment fails to control glaucoma.
   Comment: Glaucoma therapy in children has to be individualized, especially in situations where the risk of surgery outweighs the benefits of continuing medical therapy.

Introduction and challenges of medical therapy in childhood glaucoma

While surgery is the mainstay of glaucoma treatment in infants and young children, medical therapy has an important role to play in the management of childhood glaucoma. The role of medical treatment in the armamentarium of childhood glaucoma treatment varies with the type of glaucoma, as well as specific features of the affected child and eye(s). For example, medications alone rarely show sustained efficacy as primary treatment for glaucoma in infants and young children, especially in cases of PCG. In this scenario, glaucoma medications can help reduce the IOP and sufficiently clear corneal edema to enable angle surgery (goniotomy). In general, medical therapy is frequently useful as a temporizing IOP-lowering treatment prior to surgery, or as adjuvant therapy after partially-successful surgical procedures in refractory childhood glaucoma.

Medical therapy in children differs in several important respects from treatment of adult patients. Childhood glaucomas are heterogeneous in their causation as well as in their responses to different glaucoma medications. In addition, systemic pharmacokinetics for glaucoma medications are different in children compared with in adults. Only a few drugs have been evaluated for pharmacokinetics in children. The child's plasma volume is generally much reduced compared with that of an adult, while the ocular volumes of a child and an adult are much more similar in magnitude, often resulting in higher systemic exposure of the child to topically-applied glaucoma medications. Several simple maneuvers can help reduce systemic absorption of topical medications: (1) having care providers close the lids, remove excess liquid and perform nasolacrimal occlusion after drop instillation, when possible; and (2) using the minimum frequency and lowest concentration of a given glaucoma drug that is needed to achieve the target intraocular pressure.

There is a lack of safety and comparative efficacy testing in children for almost all drugs, although safety and efficacy data are emerging from their widespread clinical use as well as from small numbers of prospective trials. Potentially serious or fatal systemic adverse reactions, which are rarely seen in adults, may occur in young children after exposure to glaucoma medications. Adverse side effects may manifest atypically in children (*e.g.*, nocturnal cough rather than frank wheezing in children with reactive airways exposed to beta blockers). Children are more vulnerable to adverse effects of medications as they may be unable to verbalize symptoms and parents may not readily recognize them; parents must be well-informed about potential side effects of prescribed glaucoma medications, and providers must regularly inquire about possible contraindications and side effects of treated pediatric patients.

Compliance and adherence issues are greater and more complex in children due to their dependence on caregivers or parents, possible lack of cooperation in the administration of treatment, as well as concurrent medical conditions that may complicate medical therapy. Setting a target pressure and determining when glaucoma control has been achieved can additionally be challenging in children, for a variety of reasons. Among these include limited ability to perform structural and functional testing of the optic nerve. As a result, all available information must be considered when assessing glaucoma stability.

The availability and cost of medications, especially in developing countries, may be additional barriers to successful long-term medical therapy. There may be selected, especially refractory cases, where the risks of additional surgery are high enough that partial control of the glaucoma by medical therapy may be preferable to risking devastating surgical complications (especially in monocular cases where the fellow eye was lost as complication of glaucoma surgery).

Medications in the treatment strategy (Table 1)

Disease/type of glaucoma – role of medications

Childhood glaucomas are heterogeneous in their causation as well as in their responses to different glaucoma medications. The role of medications in childhood glaucoma is summarized here.

1. Primary childhood glaucoma
   - Primary congenital glaucoma (PCG)
     (i) to temporize before surgery;
     (ii) as an adjunct after surgery if IOP reduction is insufficient.
   - Juvenile open-angle glaucoma (JOAG)
     (i) first-line;
     (ii) adjunctive after surgery.

Table 1. Medication use in childhood glaucoma*

Medication type	Indications	Contra-indications/Side effects
β-Blockers Non-selective (timolol, levobunolol, carteolol) β_1 Selective (betaxolol)	1st-line therapy for many, 2nd-line for some older children. Non-selective drugs more effective than selective drugs, but the latter relatively safer in children with asthma.	Systemic effects: bronchospasm, bradycardia. Avoid in premature or tiny infants, and in children with history of reactive airways. Start with 0.1% or 0.25% in smaller children.
Carbonic anhydrase inhibitors Topical (dorzolamide, brinzolamide), 2x- or 3x-daily dosing Oral (acetazolamide, 10-20 mg/kg/d, given 2-4 times daily; methazolamide)	1st- or 2nd-line in young children, add well to other classes. Topical therapy better tolerated but not as effective; may use both if needed.	Topical systemically safe. May wish to avoid, or use as later option, in children with compromised corneas, especially with corneal transplant. Dorzolamide stings. Metabolic acidosis may occur with oral therapy, rarely in newborns with topical.
Miotics Echothiophate iodide Pilocarpine	Echothiophate rarely used, sometimes in aphakia; pilocarpine after angle surgery and sometimes with JOAG; less effective IOP reduction in congenital glaucoma.	Systemic effects (echothiophate): sometimes diarrhea, warn about use of succinyl choline with echothiophate; (both) headache; both may induce myopic shift; possible pro-inflammatory effect (echothiophate).
Adrenergic agonists Epinephrine compounds	Rarely used, limited effectiveness.	Systemic effects: hypertension, tachycardia in small children.
α_2-Agonists Apraclonidine, 0.5%	Helps during/after angle surgery; useful in the short term in infants and after corneal transplantation.	Systemically safe; effect may wear off; rarely local allergy or red eye.
Brimonidine (use lowest concentration, *e.g.*, 0.10%, in smaller children)	Use only in older children: 2nd- or 3rd-line therapy with JOAG, aphakia, older children with other glaucoma types.	**Do not use in infants/small children** weighing < 40 lbs. (approx.), as may cause bradycardia, hypotension, hypothermia, hypotonia, apnea – especially if used with β-blocker.
Prostaglandins and similar Latanoprost, travoprost, bimatoprost, tafluprost	1st-, 2nd-, or 3rd-line with JOAG; usually 2nd- or 3rd-line (after β-blockers and topical CAIs) in others.	Systemically safe in children; long eyelashes will result (beware unilateral use); redness common (especially with bimatoprost); trial use with uveitic glaucoma as last resort.

* approx. = approximately; CAI = carbonic anhydrase inhibitor; JOAG = juvenile open-angle glaucoma.

2. Secondary childhood glaucoma
    (i) first-line as long as the glaucoma is open-angle (secondary glaucomas
        with angle closure (*e.g.*, pupillary block in uveitis) usually do not respond
        to medical therapy alone);
    (ii) adjunctive if surgery is needed but insufficient.

Details regarding medical therapy related to specific diagnosis

Primary congenital glaucoma (PCG)

PCG is a surgical condition, however, medications can be helpful before planned
angle surgery, to attenuate symptoms (photophobia and pain) and to help clear the
cornea for a better view of the angle especially when goniosurgery is planned.
Preoperative use of pilocarpine 1-2% in angle surgery can improve angle acces-
sibility and many surgeons use the drug for two to three weeks post angle surgery
(tid or bid) to induce miosis in the hope of decreasing anterior synechiae across
the cleft. Side effects such as diarrhea can occur in neonates with higher concentrations and frequency. With regards to beta-blockers, the lowest doses (timolol 0.1%
or 0.25%) and frequency along with gel formulations are preferred whenever available. Carbonic anhydrase inhibitors (CAIs) oral formulations can have significant
IOP-lowering effect, but possible metabolic acidosis and other systemic side effects
call for caution. Topical CAIs are safer but less potent. Brinzolamide is better
tolerated than dorzolamide in some cases, due to stinging of the latter drug. Prostaglandin analogues do not have a large role in the early medical treatment of these
infants and children, but can be useful adjunctive medication.

   In neonates, beta-blocker and carbonic anhydrase inhibitors (oral or topical) can
be used preoperatively but with special attention to side effects. Caregivers should
be instructed about systemic effects and how to minimize drop absorption. Pediatricians must be informed of their use. Neonates on oral carbonic anhydrase inhibitors are especially vulnerable to metabolic acidosis with compensative
respiratory alkalosis, which sometimes complicates feeding and anesthesia. In this
group, topical therapy is preferable unless prolonged delays are needed before
surgical IOP-reducing surgery. Brimonidine must be avoided in neonates, infants
and young children (Fig. 1).

Juvenile open-angle glaucoma (JOAG)

JOAG is more responsive to topical hypotensive treatment than PCG. The first
drug to prescribe is usually either a prostaglandin analogue or a beta-blocker. Both
work well for this type of glaucoma, with prostaglandin analogues particularly
effective in these eyes. In a stepwise fashion other drugs can be added until the
target IOP has been reached. For example, if a prostaglandin analogue was first-
line, then a beta blocker would be second-line, followed by a topical carbonic
anhydrase inhibitor as third-line (often in combination with the beta blocker in
one bottle), and finally by an adrenergic agonist fourth-line. Pilocarpine can

reduce IOP, but has many ocular side effects that usually prevent its use for JOAG patients (Fig. 1).

Glaucoma following cataract surgery

Pharmacologic treatment of glaucoma following cataract surgery can be similar to that of JOAG, provided the angle is open (Fig. 1). Additional considerations include the possibility of macular edema with prostaglandin use, but this is rare in practice. Pilocarpine may be useful in selected cases, as can phospholine iodide.

Adjuvant role for surgery- pre and postoperative considerations

There is little consensus about the role of medications specifically related to surgery, but some general agreement was found on these considerations:

- Many use aqueous suppression to help reduce IOP and cause reduced corneal edema prior to surgery for PCG (*see* above).
- Alpha-adrenergic agents (apraclonidine 0.5%) may have a role in reducing angle bleeding if used before and in the early postoperative period with angle surgery.
- Brimonidine should be avoided in infants and small children.
- Pilocarpine is frequently used before and after angle surgery in the hope that miosis will facilitate angle surgery and reduce cleft closure by synechiae.

In many cases, one operation is not enough to control glaucoma. Glaucoma medications play an important adjunctive role in the early postoperative period, 'between' surgeries, especially with angle surgery, and when the IOP after surgery is improved but thought to be inadequate for long-term safety. There is no good consensus about the use of long-term medications in PCG, where some surgeons strive for complete medication-free control, while others stop after angle surgery and control with medications if possible, reserving further surgery for refractory cases. Some specific examples include:

- Post-angle surgery with high IOP – miotics and aqueous suppressants. These are often discontinued purposefully prior to the next EUA, especially if the decision for further angle surgery will depend upon the IOP measured at the EUA without the influence of hypotensive medications.
- Post-trabeculectomy with IOP elevation – medical therapy including glaucoma medications and steroids can be used before bleb manipulation or revisions.
- Post-tube shunt hypertensive phase – aqueous suppressants are preferred.

Age of patients

Infants and very young children tend to be less responsive to topical glaucoma medications compared to older children and adolescents. This may be due to age as well as severity of disease as the more severe the anomaly leading to glaucoma, the more likely it will manifest at a younger age. Furthermore, side effects of medication may be more prominent in small children. They may be related to the combination of smaller plasma volume in young children and metabolic immaturity leading to increased drug blood levels, as well as lack of the child's ability to report side effects.

Scenario 1 – 3 month old baby, full-term and otherwise well, with bilaterally large and cloudy corneas, suspected of having primary congenital glaucoma. Pressures are in the 30s both eyes, and angle surgery is planned in the next few days.

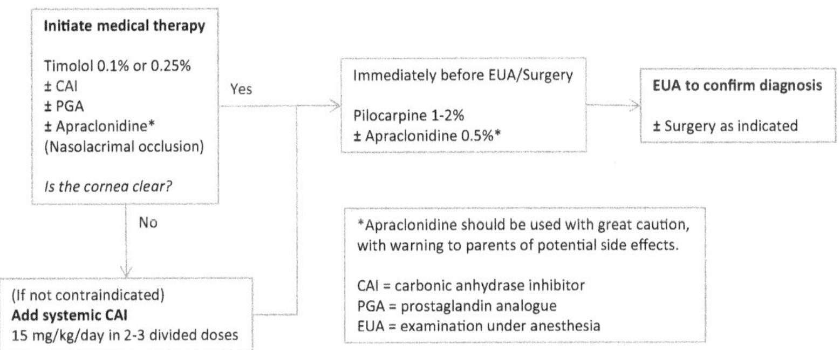

Scenario 2 – 6 month old baby with bilateral aphakia, just noted to have elevated IOP to the 30s and mild corneal haze and slight enlargement of one eye. Optic nerve looks normal without cupping. The other eye is unremarkable with IOP of 15mmHg. Anterior chamber is deep and iris plane is flat in both eyes.
a)   Baby is healthy otherwise and full-term.
b)   Baby has had respiratory syncytial virus (RSV) infection and requires use of a nebulizer periodically

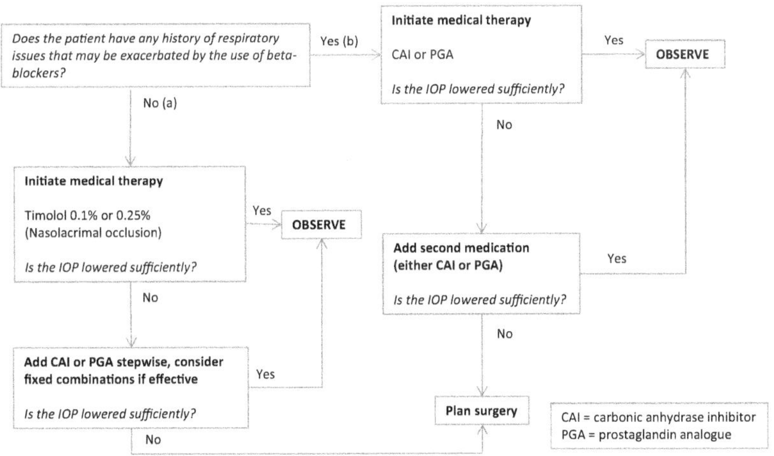

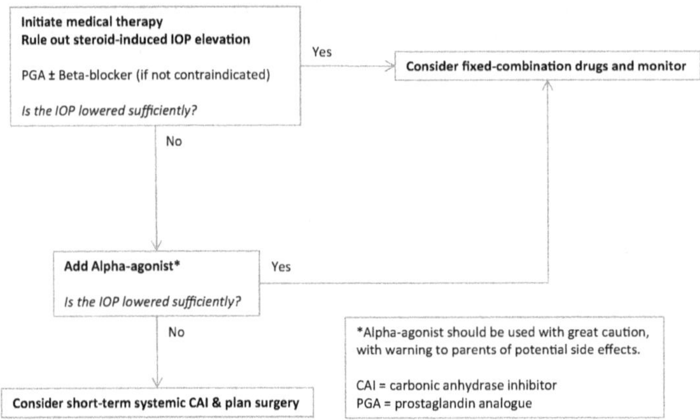

Fig. 1. Suggested approaches to different clinical scenarios. (They will be influenced by doctor preference/experience and local availability/ affordability of medication.)

Drug safety in children

Most drugs have been used in children without specifically designed studies and so prescription is based on adult safety and effectiveness. Most anti-glaucoma drugs were approved without requiring pediatric data. Studies show that bio-availability of drugs varies in children related to the child's maturity, weight and organ development. So, as a result, the child may receive ineffective drugs, doses that are too high or too low, or may experience deleterious side effects.

Implementation of pediatric legislation in the USA and the EU has encouraged pediatric-specific product development and testing. There has been a recent trend towards collaboration between the FDA and the EMEA. The USA Congress passed the Best Pharmaceuticals for Children Act (BPCA) of 2002 and the Pediatric Research Equity Act (PREA) of 2003 to encourage drug manufacturers to develop and label drugs for pediatric use. BPCA offers manufacturers incentives to conduct pediatric-specific research. PREA requires certain pediatric use information in products' labeling. By making BPCA and PREA permanent (in 2012) under the FDA authority, the law ensures that children will have a permanent place on the agenda for drug research and development. In 2007, the European Union's Pediatric Regulation gave the European Medicines Agency (EMA) new responsibilities to stimulate research into the uses of medicines in children and to lead to their authorization in all ages. Product development programs should include pediatric studies when pediatric use is anticipated. Development of product information in pediatric patients should be timely and, often requires the development of pediatric formulations. It was largely as a result of this that latanoprost was the first drug to be tested in a multi-center trial (in the EU) for use in children. Recently, articles on drug safety and efficacy in pediatric patients have been published.[1-5] Current trials on drug safety and efficacy in children include:

- Treatment of Pediatric Glaucoma
  Sponsor: Azienda Ospedaliera Spedali Civili di Brescia.

The study will assess the ocular hypotensive effect of latanoprost and dorzolamide in a selected sample of patients affected by primary pediatric glaucoma (PG), refractory to surgical procedures. Safety will also be assessed.

- Pharmacokinetic and Safety Study of Travoprost 0.004% in Pediatric Glaucoma Patients
  Sponsor: Alcon Research.

The purpose of this study is to assess the safety and describe the steady state plasma pharmacokinetic profiles of Travoprost ophthalmic solution, 0.004% (new formulation) following a once-daily administration for seven days in pediatric glaucoma or ocular hypertension patients.

- Study of Travoprost Ophthalmic Solution, 0.004% Compared to Timolol (0.5% or 0.25%) in Pediatric Glaucoma Patients
  Sponsor: Alcon Research.

The primary objective of this study is to demonstrate that the IOP-lowering efficacy of Travoprost ophthalmic solution, 0.004% (new formulation) is non-inferior to Timolol ophthalmic solution (0.5% or 0.25%) in pediatric glaucoma patients.

- Long-Term Non-Interventional Latanoprost Study (LYNX)
  Sponsor: Pfizer.

This is a non-interventional, prospective, longitudinal cohort study. A total of 200 pediatric subjects with glaucoma or elevated IOP, including 150 latanoprost-treated subjects and 50 non-topical prostaglandin analogue treated subjects, will be enrolled from ophthalmic hospital clinics and academic ophthalmic centers. As a non-interventional study, the study subjects' continued use of latanoprost and assessments of ocular events will be obtained through the routine medical follow-up with treating ophthalmologists or other designated members of the medical care team.

- A Study of the Safety and Efficacy of Bimatoprost Ophthalmic Solution in Pediatric Patients With Glaucoma
  Sponsor: Allergan.

The purpose of this study is to assess the safety and efficacy of a new formulation of bimatoprost ophthalmic solution compared to timolol ophthalmic solution in the treatment of pediatric patients with glaucoma.

Lactation and pregnancy

Glaucoma during pregnancy is a relatively uncommon situation and little is known regarding the fetal effects of glaucoma medications. Appropriate management of the pregnant/lactating glaucoma patient requires balancing the risk to the fetus of treatment against the risk to the mother if treatment is reduced or suspended.[6] The mother should make decisions regarding appropriate glaucoma management, once she has been informed of the potential risks to the fetus and to herself from the various options.

Like all systemically absorbed medications that are used during pregnancy and lactation, the maternal use of topical anti-glaucoma medications carries risks of teratogenicity, of interference with establishment or maintenance of pregnancy, or of side effects in the neonate. According to the FDA classification of drug risk categories in pregnancy, most drugs in use for glaucoma fall in category C (*animal reproduction studies have shown an adverse effect on the fetus and there are no adequate and well-controlled studies in humans, but potential benefits may warrant use of the drug in pregnant women despite potential risks*) with the only exception for brimonidine and dipivefrin, that fall in category B (*animal reproduction studies have failed to demonstrate a risk to the fetus and there are no adequate and well-controlled studies in pregnant women*) and are safer drugs to use, except during parturition as brimonidine can cross the placenta and cause apnea in the neonate.[7]

While there is a lack of prospective human data, publications on clinical experiences provide a guide to this decision-making process.[8,9] It is important to inform women of childbearing years about the possibility of pregnancy before prescribing and to try to address glaucoma management options before conception. During the first trimester, all medications should be avoided as much as is possible, with special attempt to avoid prostaglandin analogues due to their theoretical ability to increase risk of miscarriage. In the second and third trimester beta-blockers, alpha agonists, topical CAIs, parasympathomimetics (miotics) have been used. Alpha agonists should preferably be stopped before labor and it should be considered to stop beta-blockers during labor. Topical CAIs are generally well-tolerated during pregnancy, but oral CAIs should not be used. The treating obstetrician should be fully involved in all discussions of medication use in pregnant women taking glaucoma medications. Laser trabeculoplasty can be a reasonable initial or adjunctive intervention in pregnant and nursing women. Filtering surgery, preferably without antiscarring agents, can be considered in certain cases. During lactation, alpha agonists and oral CAIs should be avoided. Topical CAIs, prostaglandin analogues and miotics may be a valid alternative. Topical beta-blockers are considered acceptable during lactation by some but not all.[10] Punctal occlusion and even punctal plugs may reduce systemic absorption (and therefore presumably also fetal exposure or breast milk exposure) of glaucoma medications.

Side effects that have been attributed to anti-glaucoma drugs in the mother and baby include:[7]

- Beta-blockers – bradycardia and cardiac arrhythmia in fetus or breastfed child.[11] The American Academy of Pediatrics has approved the use of timolol during lactation with punctal occlusion.[12]
- Alpha-agonists – CNS depression, apnea and hypotension in the neonate or and infants.[13,14]
- Carbonic anhydrase inhibitors – possible teratogenicity, metabolic acidosis in the breastfed child. It is not known if they are excreted in the milk. Dorzolamide is approved for use with punctal occlusion during lactation by the American Academy of Pediatrics.[12]
- Prostaglandin analogues – uterine contractions and premature labor.
- Parasympathomimetics – cholinergic effects in the newborn.

The medication menu and specific considerations in children (Table 1)

1. Beta-adrenergic antagonists (beta-blockers)
2. Carbonic anhydrase inhibitors (CAIs)
3. Adrenergic agonists
4. Prostaglandin analogues (PGAs)
5. Miotics (Pilocarpine, Phospholine iodide)
6. Combination drugs and non-preserved drugs
7. Preservative-free drugs

Beta adrenergic antagonists (beta-blockers)

These often serve as first-line agents in appropriate pediatric glaucoma cases, but systemic side effects must be respected and minimized.

Mechanism of action

The beta-adrenergic antagonists act primarily to decrease aqueous production. Since the mechanism of these drugs has been well studied in adults, we will limit our discussion to specific use of this class of medications in children. Beta-adrenergic antagonists probably mainly exert their effect directly on the ciliary epithelium. They also may bind to beta-2-adrenoceptors in the anterior ciliary artery wall, causing vasoconstriction and thus indirectly decreasing aqueous humor secretion.

The choices (non-selective, selective, concentrations, combinations)

Timolol
Non-selective beta-1 and beta-2 blocker, available in 0.1% (in some countries, but not the USA, for example), 0.25% and 0.5% concentrations. These drugs are intended to be bid-medications. It has been suggested that the 0.25% concentration is the top of the dose-response curve for most individuals with lightly pigmented

irises, whereas the 0.5% concentration is more effective for patients with dark irises. The 0.5% and 0.25% preparations are also available as a viscous formulation, gel-forming solution, which makes them possible to dose as once daily drugs. These viscous preparations are not recommended for use with contact lenses.

Betaxolol
Relatively selective beta-1-blocker, available in 0.25% and 0.5% concentrations, and may have a favorable effect on ocular perfusion (which may or may not have clinical relevance). It has less effect on airways than non-selective beta-blockers.

Other beta-blockers
Levobunolol is a nonselective beta-1- and beta-2-blocker, and is available in 0.25% and 0.5% concentrations. Other beta blockers, *e.g., carteolol, metipranolol, propranolol* have a side-effect profile similar to timolol, but efficacy and safety data in children is not available.

Effectiveness (20-25% IOP reduction)

Often the response to the first few doses is a reduction in IOP of 40% or more.[15] However, this effect may diminish over several days to a few weeks. This decline in efficacy has been termed the 'short-term escape' and may relate to an increase in the number of beta-adrenergic receptors in the ciliary processes under the condition of prolonged beta-adrenergic blockade. In children the response rate and IOP reduction has been reported to be less than in adults.[16] In adults, 10-20% of patients demonstrate some loss of drug effect over subsequent months. This process has been termed the 'long-term drift' and may be explained by a time-dependent decrease in cellular sensitivity to adrenergic antagonists. So after the initial response, an increase in IOP over time may occur in childhood glaucoma.

Additive to many drug classes

Beta-blockers combine well with most other classes of drug in terms of their IOP-reducing effect (*e.g.*, CAIs, alpha agonists, PGA). There is, however, a point of 'diminishing returns', especially when drugs of similar mechanism are combined (*e.g.*, aqueous suppressants, such as beta-blockers and CAIs or alpha-adrenergic agonists).

Side effects (ocular and systemic)

Numerous side effects have been reported with use of ocular and systemic beta-blockers, but most are well known. Beta-blockers should not be used or used only with extreme caution in premature infants and newborns, in whom apnea and bradycardia are most likely to occur as a result of high systemic drug levels.[11]

The ocular volume of the neonate is approximately half that of the adult, while the blood volume of the neonate (as a function of body weight) is only a small fraction of that of the adult. Because of the relatively large ocular volume in a child, it may seem reasonable to administer the usual adult ocular dosage to reach local therapeutic levels. However, when it is systemically absorbed (mostly through the nasal mucosa), the beta-blocker (and other topical drugs) dosage is diluted by a much smaller volume of blood, leading to higher systemic concentrations in children than in their adult counterparts.[17]

Contra-indications for the use of beta-blockers include bradycardia, second- or third-degree atrioventricular block, and active bronchoconstrictive disease (at least for non-selective beta-antagonists). Serious adverse events such as apnea have been reported in younger children. Asthma can occur in pediatric patients with topical timolol treatment. Exacerbation of respiratory symptoms may occur in infants and even older children who have known or undiagnosed 'reactive airways' or in whom a viral respiratory illness renders airways more susceptible to beta blockage. Sometimes children manifest bronchospasm as a persistent cough, rather than frank wheezing.

The beta-2 selective beta-blocker, betaxolol, may cause less bronchospasm than the non-selective beta-blockers, but is slightly less effective at IOP reduction, and can also trigger or worsen reactive airways in children.

Practical considerations

- Begin with lowest dose timolol (0.1%, 0.25%) or betaxolol (0.25%).

The introduction of timolol 0.1% has been useful in neonates and infants due to its superior risk profile. This formulation is not universally commercially available, however. In children, the gel-forming solutions are preferred to drops by some providers because gel is theoretically less absorbed into the systemic circulation. The 0.1% (or 0.25% where the 0.1% is unavailable) timolol or timolol gel-forming solution is often sufficient and is the preferred agent in infants with childhood glaucoma, because of the lower concentration, decreased systemic absorption, and once-daily dosing.[1] Hoskins *et al.*[15] recommended starting with 0.25% and stepping up to 0.5% only if desired response was not obtained with lower dosage, and observed that most of the patients were controlled with 0.25% and most of the complications were seen in 0.5% dosage in children. Plasma timolol levels in children after 0.25% drops greatly exceed those in adults after 0.5% drops, especially in infants, whose blood levels of timolol reached above the level of systemic beta blockade targeted in adults on systemic beta-blockers.[17]

- Minimize systemic absorption and observe after first dose.

Blotting off of excess drops and nasolacrimal occlusion or forced eyelid closure may greatly reduce systemic absorption (up to 40%) and should be taught to parents. Using the lowest possible concentration of the drug and the fewest administrations necessary to control IOP can reduce systemic drug levels. Instructing patients to limit instillation to one drop of medication per eye and to use eyelid closure after administration can also lower drug concentrations in plasma. Neonates and small infants must be monitored carefully for the development of apnea. Clinicians should inform pediatricians when topical beta-blockers are used in young glaucoma patients as many pediatricians may not be aware of the potential systemic effects of topical medications.

Carbonic anhydrase inhibitors (CAIs)

Available both as oral and topical formulations, are good adjunctive agents, and are often first-line drugs in selected children with contraindications to beta blockers and prostaglandin analogues.

Mechanism of action

CAIs inhibit aqueous production by preventing rapid interconversion of bicarbonate and carbon dioxide.

The choices

Oral CAIs: Acetazolamide (Diamox) and Methazolamide (Neptazane)
- Acetazolamide (Diamox) tablets: 125 mg, 250 mg, 500 mg and sustained release capsule 250 mg, 500 mg.
- Methazolamide (Neptazane) 25 mg, 50 mg tablets.

Dose

- Acetazolamide: 10-15 mg/kg/day (maximum dose 20 mg/kg/day) with meals, divided bid to qd. The recommended childhood glaucoma dose for acetazolamide appears to be empiric and varies from 5 to 10 mg/kg every 6 to 12 hours. To prepare the medication, the pharmacist must crush the tablets and suspend the powder in flavored syrup, with a convenient final concentration of 50 mg/ml. Many children can also take the tablets crushed up with applesauce or a similar food and with liquids.
- Methazolamide: < 2 mg/kg/day, divided bid.

Effectiveness ($\geq$ 25% IOP reduction)

The maximum oral acetazolamide-induced IOP decrease is approximately 40%, and clinical trials show an efficacy ranging from 25 to 30%.

Additive to other drug classes

Often considered as a temporizing measure prior to surgery, but reasonable longer term drug for refractory cases.

Side effects ($\geq$ 40%)

Lethargy, loss of appetite, gastrointestinal disturbance, diarrhea, metabolic acidosis, failure to thrive, bed wetting, cross reactivity with sulfa allergy.

Systemic CAIs would be expected to have similar side effects compared with those seen in adults. It is said that only about one third of patients can tolerate oral acetazolamide for over a month due to various systemic adverse events. These include but are not limited to headache, dizziness, paresthesia, asthenia, sinusitis, rhinitis, nausea, lethargy, hypersensitivity reactions (including urticaria, angio-edema, and bronchospasm), bitter taste, epistaxis, urolithiasis, and growth suppression. Other possible side effects (reported in adults) include neutropenia (with possible but very rarely occurring aplastic anemia, thought to be idiosyncratic but more likely with very long-term use of oral CAIs), gastrointestinal distress, Stevens-Johnson syndrome, photosensitivity, purpura, erythema multiforme, Lyell syndrome, globus hystericus (feeling of lump in throat), malaise syndrome, metabolic acidosis, anorexia, weight loss, depression, somnolence, confusion, nephrolithiasis, polyuria, hematuria, glycosuria, and seizures. Topical acetazolamide has inadequate effect for lowering IOP, although systemic side effects would be expected to be less, a change to modern formulations would be needed to increase penetration and effectiveness.[18]

Systemic CAIs, more commonly acetazolamide, should be avoided in children with sickle cell disease and used with great caution in those with sickle cell trait, since the metabolic acidosis might induce sickling, especially if treating hyphema-induced ocular hypertension.[19]

Side effects due to systemic CAIs in infants and young children are not commonly reported, although pediatric patients often cannot verbalize or recognize these side effects unless specifically asked. Small infants will sometimes manifest respiratory alkalosis as a compensatory mechanism for metabolic acidosis. Failure to thrive, enuresis, and lethargy are common in children.

Methazolamide more readily penetrates the blood aqueous and blood brain barriers. It is a potent CAI effective in lower dosage than acetazolamide, with recommended dose 5 mg/kg/day. It is more selectively concentrated in erythrocytes and is metabolized primarily in liver. In addition, methazolamide is only 55% bound to plasma protein, whereas acetazolamide is 95% bound. In practical terms, this means that a far smaller quantity of oral methazolamide is needed to produce therapeutic levels in target tissue (presumably the ciliary processes), compared with acetazolamide. Because of this difference in dose, the renal effects of carbonic anhydrase inhibition can be minimized with administration of methazolamide at doses of less than 2 mg/kg/day. Another advantage is serum half-life of 15 hours, compared with the four-hour half-life of acetazolamide. It is therefore unnecessary to give methazolamide more often than every 12 hours, in contrast to the common dosing of oral acetazolamide three or four times daily by many providers. Side effects in children are not well documented, but are expected to be similar to those encountered with oral acetazolamide, although perhaps less severe in some children.

The choices

Topical CAIs (Dorzolamide 2% [Trusopt], Brinzolamide 1% [Azopt])
- Dorzolamide 2% (Trusopt)
- Brinzolamide 1% (Azopt)

Effectiveness

Less than oral CAIs. Dorzolamide 2% had a significant IOP-lowering effect of 27% in patients with childhood glaucoma who previously showed a substantial IOP reduction of 36% while taking oral acetazolamide, even when these patients were already receiving topical beta-blocker therapy.[20] Long-term, dorzolamide seems to maintain its effectiveness without tachyphylaxis and is reasonably well tolerated.[21]

Additive to other drug classes

Dorzolamide has been used successfully both alone and in a fixed combination with timolol. It lowers IOP an additional 13-16% when added to twice-daily timolol maleate therapy. The combination certainly is more convenient than using either alone and may improve adherence compared to using both agents separately. Also, topical CAIs suppresses IOP spikes at night, while timolol does not. Dorzolamide tends to sting upon application, and some children object to it on this basis.

Brinzolamide is often better tolerated by children who object to the sting of dorzolamide, but otherwise seems similar in its IOP-reducing properties to dorzolamide.[2] The latter drug is now generic in many locales. The topical CAIs are additive to drugs acting on the outflow system such as pilocarpine and prostaglandin analogues.

Oral CAI has demonstrated an additive IOP lowering effect when used with topical CAI in children with childhood glaucoma, a result not consistently found in adult population (in whom the additive effect is minimal).[22]

Side effects

- Systemic effects are possible but uncommon.
- Use with caution in decompensated/vulnerable corneas.

When an infant is receiving topical CAIs, it should be determined whether the child is feeding well and gaining weight. If either of these does not occur, the topical CAI should be stopped, pending investigations, because these may be the presenting symptoms of acidosis in an infant.

Even topically applied, CAIs accumulate in the red blood cells and inhibit approximately 21% of the carbonic anhydrase II content of the cells. This inhibition does not cause any clinically detectable side effects in adults, but in newborns or premature newborns that have fetal hemoglobin, topical CAIs may lead to acidosis.[23] Thus, administration of topical CAIs in newborns requires some caution.

The corneal endothelium is rich in carbonic anhydrase; this fact caused concern that carbonic anhydrase inhibition by topical agents might interfere with endothelial function, theoretically causing corneal thickening and even decompensation in diseased corneas. Using ultrasonic pachymetry, Wilkerson and co-workers showed that topical dorzolamide administered over four weeks increases the corneal thickness very slightly compared with placebo;[24] however, it is unlikely that this small change is clinically significant in normal corneas, but one should use caution when applying topical CAIs to compromised corneas, although there have been no published case series finding a significant irreversible negative effect of topical carbonic anhydrase inhibitors on the cornea except for one.[25] The topical CAIs are therefore often avoided when possible in children with corneal edema and corneal transplants.

Practical considerations

- Good first-line drug if beta-blocker not safe.

They are useful as second-line drugs or when beta-blockers are contraindicated. Brinzolamide could be a better choice for children than dorzolamide because its topical use causes less burning, stinging, and itching. In a short randomized, controlled, double-masked, multicenter trial, dorzolamide was found to be well tolerated and effective for up to 3 months in children younger than six years.[21]

- Bid vs. tid administration of topical CAIs.

Because of the 8- to 10-hour duration of dorzolamide (brinzolamide), it does seem that there is a small but definite increase in efficacy with three-times-daily monotherapy compared to twice daily. Many ophthalmologists use dorzolamide twice daily as both monotherapy and adjunctive therapy, but there is an occasional patient who benefits from three times daily administration of topical CAIs.

Adrenergic agonists

Mechanism of action

Adrenergic agonists increase uveoscleral outflow and decrease aqueous humor production.

The choices

There are non-selective agonists (epinephrine and dipivefrin) and alpha-2 selective agonists (apraclonidine and brimonidine).

Non-selective agonists (epinephrine, dipivefrin [Propine])
Both epinephrine and dipivefrin are infrequently used today for glaucoma treatment in children due to their limited effectiveness and common ocular side effects (including burning, stinging, follicular conjunctivitis, mydriasis, blurry vision, and allergic reaction, and adrenochrome deposits) as well as systemic side effects (including tachycardia, arrhythmias, and elevated systolic blood pressure). Dipivefrin is a prodrug of epinephrine, and therefore has fewer ocular and systemic side effects, but is similarly rarely used in childhood glaucoma treatment.

Apraclonidine (Iopidine 0.5%)
Apraclonidine is usually used as a short-term adjunctive therapy before surgery or laser and produces an allergic reaction in 40% of adult patients. Apraclonidine is less alpha-2 selective than brimonidine but it is more hydrophilic,[26] greatly reduc-

ing penetration through the blood-brain barrier. While this drug is considered safer in children than brimonidine,[27] it must still be used with caution in infants, and especially in infants and young children who are on concurrent beta blocker therapy. In these cases, systemic side effects similar to those seen with brimonidine can result (*see* below). Apraclonidine is very effective in short- and intermediate-term IOP reduction in selected pediatric cases, but tachyphylaxis and topical allergy often limit its effectiveness. Some surgeons use topical apraclonidine prior to angle surgery to help prevent bleeding.[27] Care must be taken to counter the pupil-dilating effects of this drug with pilocarpine, however, in phakic eyes before angle surgery. Rebound redness often occurs between doses, and this drug is often used bid, although tid dosing is permitted.

Brimonidine (generic brimonidine 0.2 %, Alphagan P 0.15, 0.10%)

Brimonidine is effective in lowering IOP in children, but side effects are frequent and more common than with other glaucoma medications in children. Because brimonidine is an alpha-2 specific agonist, it does not affect pulmonary function and heart rate. Since it is highly lipophilic, brimonidine is absorbed through the cornea and also passes through the blood-brain barrier in neonates and infants, producing central nervous system toxicity. Neurological symptoms reported are somnolence, respiratory depression, apnea and even coma. Those effects usually happen 30-60 minutes after administration, and recover without sequelae.[13] Naloxone has been reported to reverse those symptoms after been administered in cases of severe central nervous system involvement.[28]

Use in children

Since children have smaller plasma volumes, excessive systemic absorption, immature metabolism and excretion, immature blood-brain barrier and increased receptor sensitivity, they are at a higher risk of having central nervous system effects. For this reason, alternative therapies should be considered for children younger than six years and weighting less than about 20 kg, or in those with cognitive impairment in whom central nervous system suppression might go unrecognized.[29] Brimonidine is unquestionably contra-indicated for children younger than two years old.[30] The central nervous system side effects can be exacerbated in children taking topical beta blockers and brimonidine together.[14,31]

The weight of the child is the more accurate factor in predicting central nervous system side effects, especially excessive sleepiness and lethargy. All children and their parents should be warned of the potential for fatigue and lethargy when brimonidine is prescribed.[32] Other strategies for reducing risk of systemic adverse effects are administer the lowest effective dose, dose reduction or dilution by the pharmacist, removal of excess drops from the eyelids and application of digital pressure to the lacrimal puncti for several minutes after instillation.[33]

Summary

Apraclonidine and brimonidine are usually administered as second- or third-line in anti-glaucoma therapy and are useful as short term adjunct therapy pre and post-surgery. While most topical anti-glaucoma medications are safe to use in children despite not being licensed for such use,[34] the central suppressive effects of brimonidine can have severe effects.[35-38]

Prostaglandin analogues (PGAs)

Mechanism of action

The most accepted mechanism of action for all the prostaglandin analogues/prostamides is the increase of the uveoscleral outflow. For prostamides a complementary mechanism of action has been proposed: increase of the trabecular outflow.

The choices

Latanoprost 0,005%, travoprost 0,004%, bimatoprost 0,03%-0,01% (prostamide), tafluprost (preservative-free), rescula (unoprostone).
Preservative-free latanoprost,[39] travoprost and bimatoprost are available, but little experience exists in using preservative free PGAs in children. Generic latanoprost is also now available.

Use in children

For Latanoprost Phase I and Phase III studies have been performed and its use in children has been approved in Europe, although not in the United States. There are ongoing phase I and Phase III for Travoprost in Europe. Some reports of travoprost in children suggest it to be effective and with similar side effect profile to latanoprost. Anecdotally, bimatoprost is less well tolerated, due to increased ocular side effects (*see* below), possibly with increased IOP reduction in selected cases. There is little data on the use of tafluprost in children at present.

Effectiveness

In adults on PGA monotherapy, reported IOP reduction ranges from 25-35%. In children, PGAs have a significant ocular hypotensive effect, although some patients do not respond well. In PCG latanoprost is marginally more effective than timolol (response rate and IOP reduction), but was reported to be higher in other childhood glaucomas.[5] Responders are more likely to be older than non-responders and are more likely to have JOAG.[3]

Prostaglandin analogues can be considered appropriate first-line therapy in selected cases such as JOAG. Some use this drug as monotherapy in PCG also, although there is controversy in the latter situation. These drugs are relatively, but not absolutely, contra-indicated in uveitis, but may be used with caution in well controlled cases when other medical therapy has proven inadequate.

Recent studies (phase I and phase III prospective clinical trials) have demonstrated the safety profile and the efficacy of latanoprost in childhood glaucoma.[4] Latanoprost efficacy and tolerability have been evaluated in studies of a variety of glaucoma diagnoses, including PCG, JOAG, glaucoma after cataract removal, and glaucoma associated with port-wine stain. Latanoprost may be less efficacious in children in combination with other medications as compared with its use as monotherapy (as with many other topical medications).

Interactions with other drops

A counterproductive interaction between PGAs and pilocarpine is theoretically possible as pilocarpine contracts the ciliary muscle decreasing the uveoscleral outflow. In practice, it is unclear that this affects the IOP lowering effect of the PGAs. In adults there is evidence of an additive effect of PGAs when used in combination with pilocarpine. The angular/ciliary body characteristics in childhood glaucoma (PCG and non-PCG) differ from the adults (POAG) so this interaction/antagonism could affect the IOP lowering effect of the PGAs in a different way. However the use of miotics in children has declined and there are other more convenient combinations. Miotics are used only for a short period in some centers after angle surgery. In this early postoperative period, PGAs are not usually used to avoid theoretical pro-inflammatory effects or bleeding.

Side effects

The systemic safety profile of PGAs in children dosed qhs, has been recently studied in prospective pediatric trials, and has been excellent. Frequent ocular side effects include lash growth and hyperemia, with less common local side effects including reported iris pigmentation change, hyperemia, allergy, uveitis, periocular hyperpigmentation.[41] More side effects (ocular) seem to occur with travoprost and bimatoprost compared with latanoprost (mostly anecdotal), so most providers prefer to begin PGA treatment with latanoprost. Parents should be advised about the possibility of longer, thicker hyperpigmented eyelashes and the potential for permanent iris color change.[42,43] The very long-term side effects of PGA therapy are still unknown. Orbital fat atrophy has been described in adults.[44]

Use in children

Studies have been performed for latanoprost Phase I and Phase III, and its use in children has been approved in Europe, although not in the USA. There are ongoing Phase I and Phase III studies for travoprost in Europe. Some reports of travoprost in children suggest it to be effective and with similar side effect profile to latanoprost.[40] Anecdotally, bimatoprost is less well tolerated, due to increased ocular side effects (*see* below), possibly with increased IOP reduction in selected cases. At present, there is little data on the use of tafluprost in children.

Miotics

These drugs are rarely used as first-line agents, but have a limited role in treating selected cases of childhood glaucoma.
Miotics are infrequently used (especially in treating adults with glaucoma) and several formulations have been discontinued by industry due to decreased popularity. This varies by region but amongst them are: Carbachol, Pilogel, Ocusert and physostigmine.

Mechanism of action

These drugs are irreversible inhibitors of cholinesterase and pseudocholinesterase, with a long duration of action. Thus, unlike pilocarpine (which is a direct parasympathomimetic), echothiophate indirectly prolongs the presence of acetylcholine at the parasympathomimetic synapses. By increasing the tone of the ciliary muscle, the drug increases pull on the scleral spur, thereby increasing aqueous outflow through the trabecular meshwork in selected cases.

The choices

Echothiophate or Phospholine Iodide
Not readily available (in the USA it is available only in 0.125% and is dosed qid).

Side effects

In common with pilocarpine 4-6%, this drug can theoretically cause cataract formation and retinal detachment. Its other side effects, especially in small children or small individuals generally are apnea, decreased heart rate, increased sweating, miosis, and hypersalivation. These result from lowering of serum cholinesterase and pseudocholinesterase. Children tolerate this drug better than adults but are prone to diarrhea and the above side effects. Common to all ages, echothiophate leaves all patients susceptible to anaesthetic complications when succinylcholine is used for neuromuscular blockade.

Use in children

Its most common use is in children with accommodative esotropia and a high accommodative convergence to accommodation ratio, but it is also useful for its efficacy in treating refractory glaucoma associated with aphakia and pseudophakia. Although sometimes effective in children with JOAG, the ciliary spasm, miosis, and induced myopia are usually poorly tolerated.

Pilocarpine
Pilocarpine is available in 0.5- 6% solutions but is commonly used only in 1-2% concentrations.[45] Drops are instilled one to four times per day and often two to three times per day in children.

Mechanism of action

Pilocarpine is a direct-acting parasympathomimetic or stimulant to the parasympathetic system in the eye. Like phospholine iodide, its main action is to stimulate the ciliary muscle thus altering the trabecular meshwork outflow channels. There does not seem to be any effect on aqueous production or the uveoscleral outflow channels. Other effects are to cause ciliary spasm (myopic shift) in younger patients plus miosis. Pilocarpine is hence often used to produce miosis for angle surgery.

Side effects

Pilocarpine at low dose produces few systemic side effects, but can cause brow ache, miosis, and variably increased myopia. The systemic effects are few unless overdosing with increased percentage or number of drops per day occurs.

Use in children

IOP lowering is not expected in a large percentage of pediatric eyes due to the abnormal angle structures including high insertion of the iris root. An exception may occur in selected cases of glaucoma after childhood cataract removal. The main uses are for induced miosis in preoperative preparation for laser iridotomies or angle surgery, and for its use post-angle surgery, hopefully to minimize synechiae formation.

Summary

More modern drugs in the field of the childhood glaucomas have almost replaced miotics. But, in selected cases, they may still play a part. Most literature is at least a decade old and will probably not be increased for this subgroup of medical options in glaucoma. That which exists is not robust often because patients were not adequately categorized into clinical diagnoses for treatment or their numbers were too small. The clinician is therefore left with "trials" on neonates and children to see if the drug works in selected cases. They appear to be most effective in aphakic / pseudophakic eyes but may also be used preoperatively and postoperatively with angle surgery.

Fixed combination drugs

Advantages

Convenient for children and caregivers, presumably better adherence, combination of timolol 0.5%, dorzolamide, brinzolamide, brimonidine, and latanoprost available (fixed combination, off-label use for children). Preservative-free dorzolamide-timolol (*Cosopt PF*) has recently become available. The availability of combination drugs varies greatly by location worldwide.

Disadvantages

All fixed combinations containing timolol use the 0.5% rather than lower dosage, in several health systems fixed combinations are too expensive or not available, and fixed combinations of timolol-brimonidine should be avoided in young children (due to risks of bradycardia, hypotension, apnea and coma).

Summary

There are insufficient data on fixed combinations in childhood glaucoma therapy. Before using fixed combinations in small children, the timolol dosage should be increased stepwise beginning with 0.1% (where available), followed by 0.25% and finally 0.5%. There are no data concerning adherence and compliance in childhood glaucoma with combination versus component drug therapy, but the probability of an increase with fixed combinations seems reasonable, especially in cases where multiple drops must be used to control IOP, where children are uncooperative with drop administration, and where older children are self-administering medications.

Preservative-free drugs

Advantages

All classes of topical anti-glaucoma drugs are available without benzalkonium chloride (BAC). Beta-blockers are available from 0.1-0.5% (in some locales) and some have an approval for childhood glaucoma. Preservative-free drugs might reduce ocular surface changes, and therefore be useful in childhood glaucoma accompanied by ocular surface diseases, *e.g.*, aniridia. Preservative-free drugs also have the theoretically possibility of inducing fewer conjunctival changes over time, perhaps rendering eyes more amenable to future incisional glaucoma surgery.

Disadvantages

There are no data available concerning preservative-free anti-glaucoma drugs in childhood glaucoma. Some BAC-free drugs have other preservatives. All preservative-free agents are more costly than their preserved counterparts and many are not approved by insurance carriers of many patients. Most of the preservative-free medication is not available in every country.

Summary

Beta-blockers, CAIs, alpha-agonists and PGAs are available without BAC. Some have different preservatives, *e.g.*, Purite. Many of the preservative-free drugs are not approved for use in children, not all are available in every locale, and all of the preservative-free agents are more costly than preserved medication. Against the background that in many patients anti-glaucoma medication will be given lifelong, preservative-free agents should be prescribed whenever possible and affordable. If resources are limited, preservative-free agents might be reserved for selected childhood glaucoma cases with accompanying ocular surface diseases: inflammatory surface diseases, blepharitis, chronic or allergic conjunctivitis, limbal stem cell deficiency, after corneal transplant, multiple glaucoma surgeries and aniridia (theoretically to reduce the risk or progression of corneal pannus).

Overall considerations for medical therapy in children

'Target pressure'

Set the 'target pressure' and reassess often: initial target pressure should be set according to the initial IOP at presentation and severity of glaucomatous damage. Rate of progression, medical history, family history and life expectancy should be given due importance in setting target IOP. Initial target pressure ranges from 25% reduction for patients with mild glaucoma to 35% for severe damage seem reasonable, although there is little data available to assist with setting target pressures in children, and providers are often left to draw upon personal experience and data derived from studies of adults with open angle glaucoma.

Target IOP range should ideally be documented in each clinical chart and reassessed if clinical parameters dictate. The adequacy of the chosen target pressure should be checked often, ideally at every visit, by comparing the optic nerve appearance to the initial presentation, along with visual fields or biometric parameters in infants/young children. If progression occurs at the target pressure, undetected IOP fluctuations and adherence to therapy can be re-evaluated before adjusting the target IOP. During the re-evaluation, it is essential to determine whether the IOP target is appropriate or should be changed (lowered or raised). In determining and assessing the adequacy of target IOP, consideration should also be given to the adequacy of the IOP measurement itself, which can be affected by corneal conditions (scarring, irregular surface, edema, microcornea) as well as by nystagmus, photophobia, or other child-specific issues (anxiety, method of tonometry [rebound often reads higher than Goldmann applanation, for example, *see* Section 2]). In addition, glaucoma stability itself is often difficult to assess, especially when accurate visual fields and nerve fiber layer analysis are not possible, or optic nerve cupping is severe at baseline, so all available information must be considered. Further, large diurnal fluctuations in IOP have been reported in children with glaucoma, and must be suspected if progression occurs despite IOP readings lower than the target IOP.[46]

Medication adherence

Medical adherence is a topic with many facets and little documented data. Related topics to medical adherence include: ability and available resources to assess and improve adherence to medical therapy; the impact of caregivers and systemic status.

There have been many suggestions to improve medical adherence but with no proof of their relative value. Each provider must work with his/her specific pediatric patients and families depending upon the situation. Suggestions have included:

- Watching your patients (the parent or the child) administer a drop to ensure they are capable of accurate delivery.
- Assuming poor adherence, especially during rebellious adolescence, when individualization is the key to success. While often the teenager with chronic illness and/or visual disability does not want to be different, he/she is also afraid of becoming blind. There is no 'one size fits all' here.
- Using patient (or parent) education: reinforce regularly, use verbal and written delivery.
- Reviewing drug administration and its difficulties at each visit.
- Explaining to the parents that drugs applied when patient is crying/ squeezing eyes may not be as effective.
- Advising against instilling two or more drops at a time; considering controlled drug delivering droppers (as available with some drugs).

Monocular trial

Although no data have been documented supporting the strategy of a monocular trial in children, it seems reasonable in many situations, especially in cases where side effects may be expected and efficacy unknown. Monocular trial presumes that IOP response in untreated eye will mirror that of treated eye and one eye serves as a control for other eye. Uses are limited due to contralateral cross over IOP reduction, non-symmetrical response of IOP in both eyes and non-compliance. It has the advantage of potentially reducing the serious drug-related systemic side effects by halving the amount of drug reaching systemic circulation.

Simplify regimen

Simplify and tailor regimen to individual patient using lowest concentration, lowest frequency and nasolacrimal occlusion where possible to reduce the side effects. Also, rather than adding medications, try substituting medications for the less than ideally effective medication, *e.g.*, using timolol 0.50% instead of 0.25%. Discontinue drugs that demonstrate no IOP-lowering effect.

Side effects

It is important to enquire about and examine for possible contraindications and side effects. Most caretakers do not attribute systemic effects to the ocular medication; hence, providing specific side effect details to care providers and the child's pediatrician (written, where possible) and asking about these periodically at scheduled visits, may help.

Sub-optimal medical control

Sub-optimal control is not a substitute for surgery in most cases, although there are selected situations where it may seem preferable to partially control glaucoma rather than risking sudden blindness with surgery in eyes that have end stage disease, or in cases where devastating surgical complications have caused blindness/loss of the fellow eye.[47] Each of these cases must be taken individually, and preferably with involvement of the family and even the child if he/she is old enough to participate in the decision-making at some level.

References

General textbook references

Stamper RL, Lieberman MF, Drake MV. Becker-Shaffer's Diagnosis and Therapy of the Glaucoma's. 8th Edition. Maryland Heights, MO: Mosby 2009.

Netland PA, Allen RC. Glaucoma Medical Therapy: Principles and Management. Second edition. New York, NY: Oxford University Press 2008.

Schacknow PN, Samples JR. The Glaucoma Book: A Practical, Evidence-Based Approach to Patient Care. New York, NY: Springer 2010.

Zimmerman TJ, Kooner KS, Sharir M, Fechtner RD (Eds.), Textbook of Ocular Pharmacology. 3rd edition. Hagerstown, MD: Lippincott-Raven 1997.

Shaarawy TM, Sherwood MB, Hitchings RA, Crowston JG. Glaucoma medical diagnosis and therapy, volume one. Philadelpjia, PA: Saunders Elsevier 2009.

Specific literature references

1. Plager DA, Whitson JT, Netland PA, et al. Betaxolol hydrochloride ophthalmic suspension 0.25% and timolol gel-forming solution 0.25% and 0.5% in paediatric glaucoma: a randomized clinical trial. J AAPOS 2009; 13: 384-390.

2. Whitson JT, Roarty JD, Vijaya L, et al. Brinzolamide Pediatric Study Group. Efficacy of brinzolamide and levobetaxolol in pediatric glaucomas: a randomized clinical trial. J AAPOS 2008; 12: 239-246.

3. Black AC, Jones S, Yanovitch TL, et al. Latanoprost in pediatric glaucoma--pediatric exposure over a decade. J AAPOS 2009; 13: 558-562.

4. Raber S, Courtney R, Maeda-Chubachi T, et al. A6111139 Study Group. Latanoprost systemic exposure in pediatric and adult patients with glaucoma: a phase 1, open-label study. Ophthalmology 2011; 118: 2022-2027.

5. Maeda-Chubachi T, Chi-Burris K, Simons BD, et al.; A6111137 Study Group. Comparison of latanoprost and timolol in pediatric glaucoma: a phase 3, 12-week, randomized, double-masked multicenter study. Ophthalmology 2011; 118: 2014-2021.

6. Maris PJ Jr, Mandal AK, Netland PA. Medical therapy of pediatric glaucoma and glaucoma in pregnancy. Ophthalmol Clin North Am 2005; 18: 461-468, vii.

7. Razeghinejad MR, Tania Tai TY, Fudemberg SJ, Katz LJ. Pregnancy and glaucoma. Surv Ophthalmol 2011; 56: 324-335.

8. Brauner SC, Chen TC, Hutchinson BT, et al. The course of glaucoma during pregnancy: a retrospective case series. Arch Ophthalmol 2006; 124: 1089-1094.

9. Mendez-Hernandez C, Garcia-Feijoo J, Saenz-Frances F, et al. Topical intraocular pressure therapy effects on pregnancy. Clin Ophthalmol 2012; 6: 1629-1632.

10. [http://www.clevelandclinicmeded.com/medicalpubs/diseasemanagement/cardiology/pregnancy-and-heart-disease/]. Last accessed April 2013.
11. Olson RJ, Bromberg BB, Zimmerman TJ. Apneic spells associated with timolol therapy in a neonate. Am J Ophthalmol 1979; 88: 120-122.
12. American Academy of Pediatrics Committee on Drugs: The transfer of drugs and other chemicals into human milk. Pediatrics 1994; 193: 1137-1150.
13. Carlsen JO, Zabriskie NA, Kwon YH, et al. Apparent central nervous system depression in infants after the use of topical brimonidine. Am J Ophthalmol 1999; 128: 255-256.
14. Mungan NK, Wilson TW, Nischal KK, et al. Hypotension and bradycardia in infants after the use of topical brimonidine and beta-blockers. J AAPOS 2003; 7: 69-70.
15. Hoskins HD Jr, Hetherington J Jr, Magee SD, et al. Clinical experience with timolol in childhood glaucoma. Arch Ophthalmol 1985; 103: 1163-1165.
16. Zimmerman TJ, Kooner KS, Morgan KS. Safety and efficacy of timolol in pediatric glaucoma. Surv Ophthalmol 1983; 28 Suppl: 262-264.
17. Passo MS, Palmer EA, Van Buskirk EM. Plasma timolol in glaucoma patients. Ophthalmology 1984; 91: 1361-1363.
18. Kaur IP, Smitha R, Aggarwal D, et al. Acetazolamide: future perspective in topical glaucoma therapeutics. Int J Pharm 2002; 248: 1-14.
19. Deutsch TA, Weinreb RN, Goldberg MF: Indications for surgical management of hyphema in patients with sickle cell trait. Arch Ophthalmol 1984; 102: 566-569.
20. Portellos M, Buckley EG, Freedman SF. Topical versus oral carbonic anhydrase inhibitor therapy for pediatric glaucoma. J AAPOS 1998; 2: 43-47.
21. Ott EZ, Mills MD, Arango S, at al. A randomized trial assessing dorzolamide in patients with glaucoma who are younger than 6 years. Arch Ophthalmol 2005; 123: 1177-1186.
22. Sabri K, Levin AV. The additive effect of topical dorzolamide and systemic acetazolamide in pediatric glaucoma. J AAPOS 2006; 10: 464-468.
23. Morris S, Geh V, Nischal KK, et al.Topical dorzolamide and metabolic acidosis in a neonate. Br J Ophthalmol 2003; 87: 1052-1053.
24. Wilkerson M, Cyrlin M, Lippa EA, et al. Four-week safety and efficacy study of dorzolamide, a novel, active topical carbonic anhydrase inhibitor. Arch Ophthalmol 1993; 111: 1343-1350.
25. Konowal A, Morrison JC, Brown SV, et al. Irreversible corneal decompensation in patients treated with topical dorzolamide. Am J Ophthalmol. 1999; 127: 403-406.
26. Chien D-S, Homsy JJ, Gluchowski C, Tang-Liu DD. Corneal and conjunctival/scleral penetration of p-aminoclonidine, AGN 190342, and clonidine in rabbit eyes. Curr Eye Research 1990; 9: 1051-1059.
27. Wright TM, Freedman SF. Exposure to topical apraclonidine in children with glaucoma. J Glaucoma 2009; 18: 395-398.
28. Lai Becker M, Huntington N, Woolf AD. Brimonidine tartrate poisoning in children: frequency, trends, and use of naloxone as an antidote. Pediatrics 2009; 123: e305-311.
29. Al-Shahwan S, Al-Torbak AA, Turkmani S, et al. Side-effect profile of brimonidine tartrate in children. Ophthalmology 2005; 112: 2143.
30. Coppens G, Stalmans I, Zeyen T, Casteels I. The safety and efficacy of glaucoma medication in the pediatric population. J Pediatr Ophthalmol Strabismus 2009; 46: 12-18.
31. Moore W, Nischal KK. Pharmacologic management of glaucoma in childhood. Pediatr Drugs 2007; 9: 71-79.
32. Bowman RJ, Cope J, Nischal KK. Ocular and systemic side effects of brimonidine 0.2% eye drops (Alphagan) in children. Eye (Lond) 2004; 18: 24-26.
33. Myers TM, Wallace, DK, Johnson SM. Ophthalmic medications in paediatric patients. Compr Ophthalmol Update 2005; 6: 85-101.
34. Fortinguerra F, Clavenna A, Bonati M. Ocular medicines in children: the regulatory situation related to clinical research. BMC Pediatr 2012; 20; 12-18.
35. Enyedi LB, Freedman SF. Safety and efficacy of brimonidine in children with glaucoma. J AAPOS 2001; 5: 281-284.

36. Rahman MQ, Ramaesh K, Montgomery DM. Brimonidine for glaucoma. Expert Opin Drug Saf 2010; 9: 483-4891.

37. Vanhaesebrouck S, Cossey V, Cosaert K, et al. Cardiorespiratory depression and hyperglycemia after unintentional ingestion of brimonidine in a neonate. Eur J Ophthalmol 2009; 19: 694-695.

38. Berlin RJ, Lee UT, Samples JR, et al. Ophthalmic drops causing coma in an infant. J Pediatr 2001; 138: 441-443.

39. Rouland JF, Traverso CE, Stalmans I, et al. T2345 Study Group. Efficacy and safety of preservative-free latanoprost eyedrops, compared with BAK-preserved latanoprost in patients with ocular hypertension or glaucoma. Br J Ophthalmol 2013; 97: 196-200.

40. Yanovitch TL, Enyedi LB, Schotthoeffer EO, Freedman SF. Travoprost in children: adverse effects and intraocular pressure response. J AAPOS 2009; 13: 91-93.

41. Enyedi LB, Freedman SF. Latanoprost for the treatment of pediatric glaucoma. Surv Ophthalmol 2002; 47 Suppl 1: S129-132.

42. Brown SM. Increased iris pigment in a child due to latanoprost. Arch Ophthalmol 1998; 116: 1683-1684.

43. Elgin U, Batman A, Berker N, Ilhan B. The comparison of eyelash lengthening effect of latanoprost therapy in adults and children. Eur J Ophthalmol 2006; 16: 247-250.

44. Park J, Cho HK, Moon JI. Changes to upper eyelid orbital fat from use of topical bimatoprost, travoprost, and latanoprost. Jpn J Ophthalmol 2011; 55: 22-27.

45. Mauger TF, Craig EL. Havener's ocular pharmacology. 6th edition. St. Louis: Mosby 1994.

46. Flemmons MS, Hsiao YC, Dzau J, et al. Home tonometry for management of pediatric glaucoma. Am J Ophthalmol 2011; 152: 470-478.

47. Papadopoulos M, Khaw PT. Advances in the management of paediatric glaucoma. Eye (Lond) 2007; 21: 1319-1325.

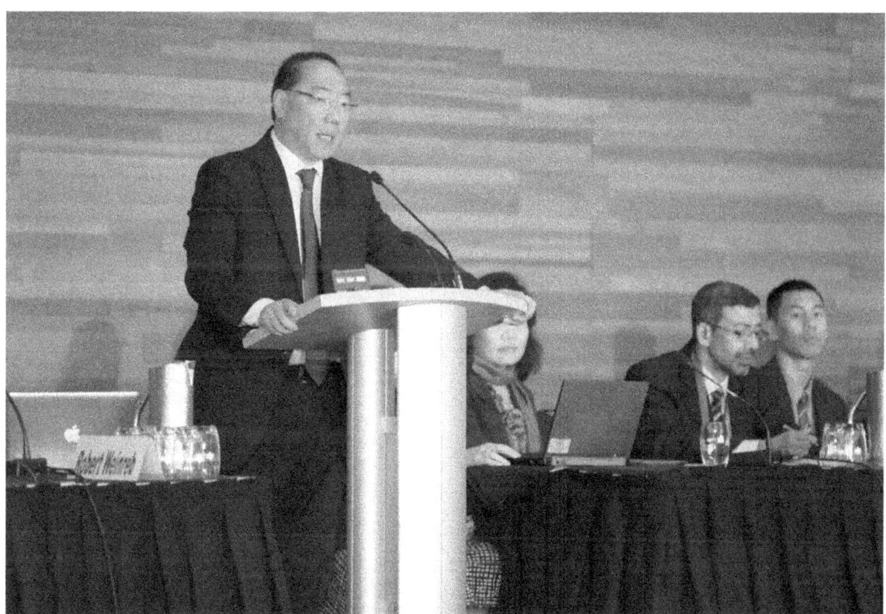

Peng T. Khaw

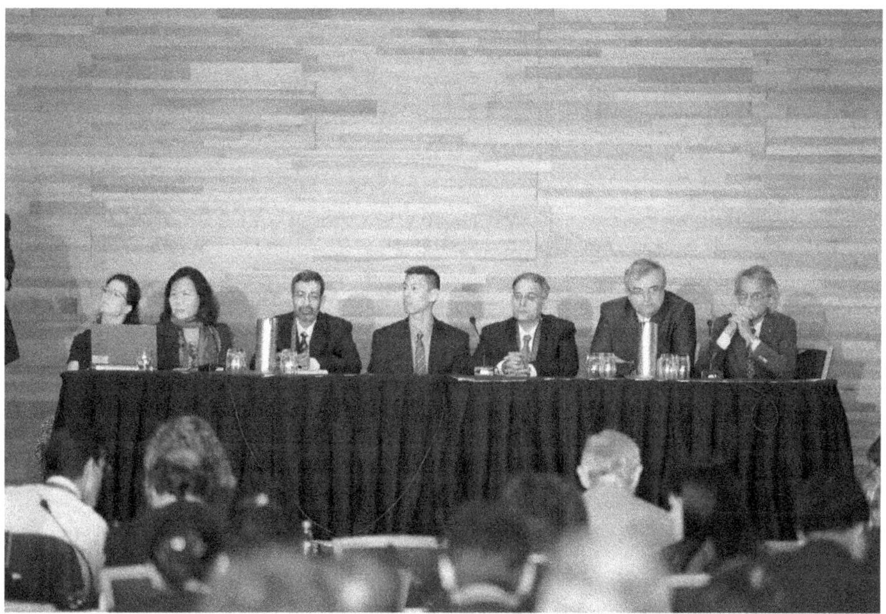

Beth Edmunds, Tam Dang, Anil Mandal, Ta Chen Peter Chang, Tanuj Dada, Stefano Gandolfi, Giorgio Marchini (L-R)

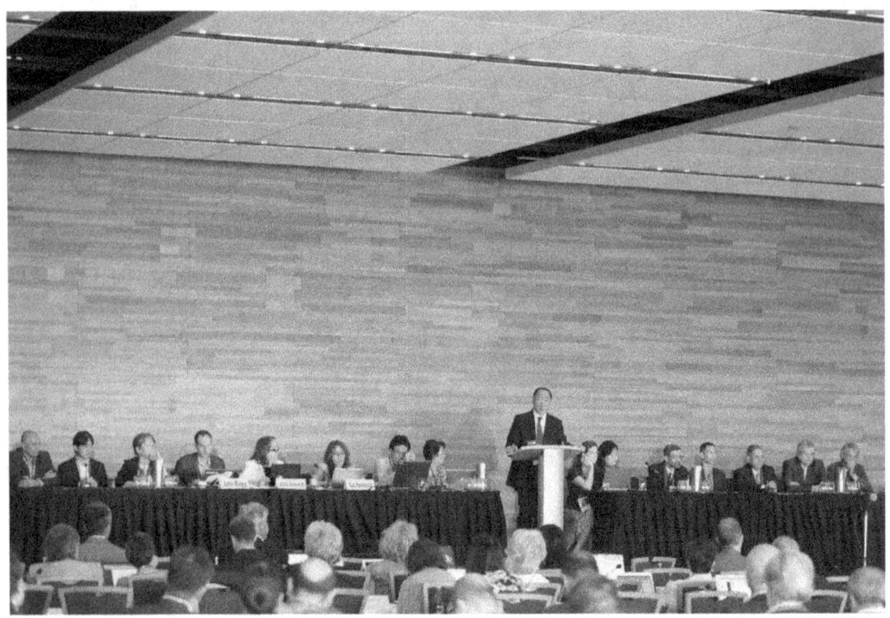

Ahmed Abdelrahman, Mark Chiang, Elizabeth Hodapp, John Grigg, Alana L. Grajewski, Maria Papadopoulos, Robert N. Weinreb, Karen Joos, Peng T. Khaw, Beth Edmunds, Tam Dang, Anil Mandal, Ta Chen Peter Chang, Tanuj Dada, Stefano Gandolfi, Giorgio Marchini (L-R)

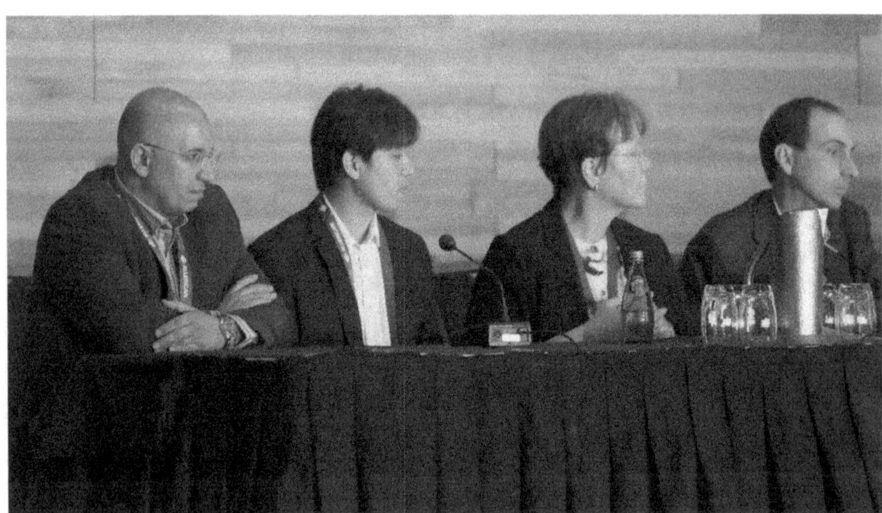

Ahmed Abdelrahman, Mark Chiang, Elizabeth Hodapp, John Grigg (L-R)

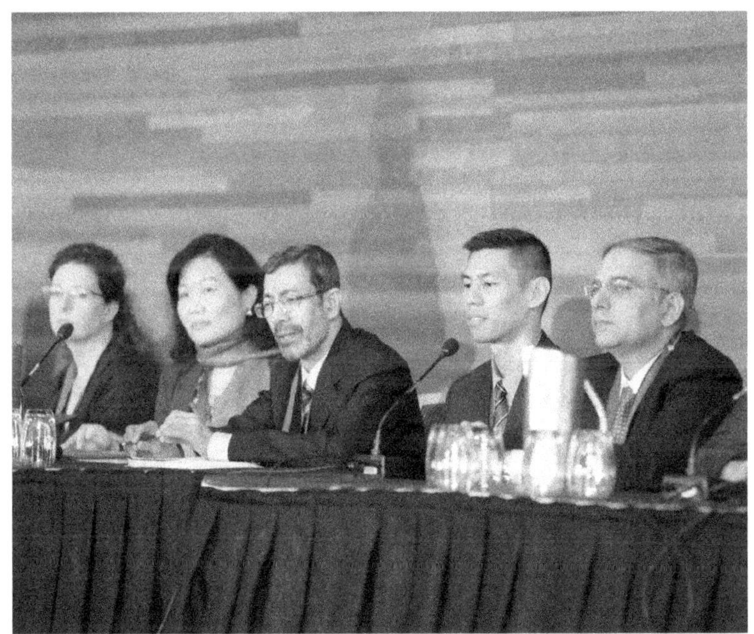

Beth Edmunds, Tam Dang, Anil Mandal, Ta Chen Peter Chang, Tanuj Dada (L-R)

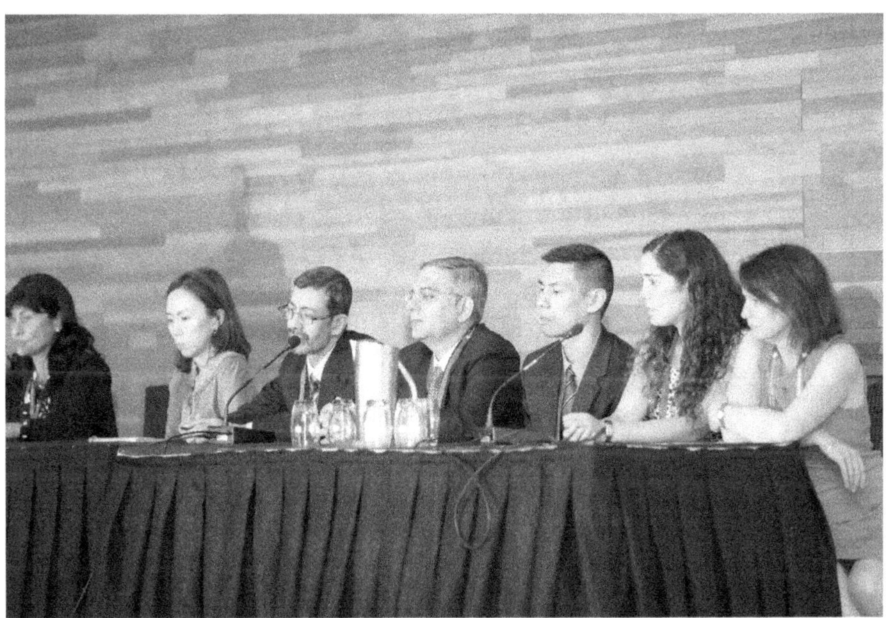

Valeria Coltrivir, Jocelyn Chua, Anil Mandal, Tanuj Dada, Ta Chen Peter Chang, Elena Bitrian, Cecilia Fernerty (L-R)

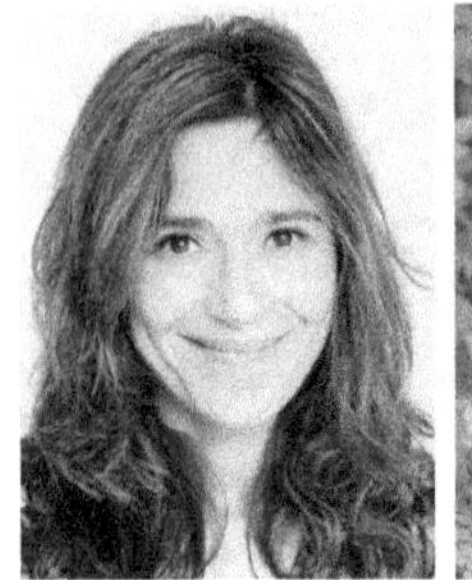

Maria Papadopoulos

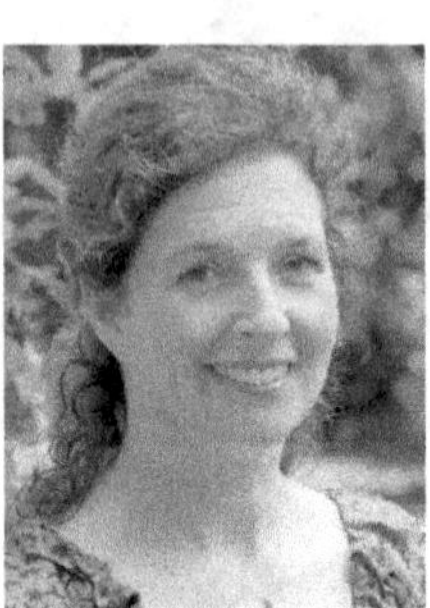

Beth Edmunds

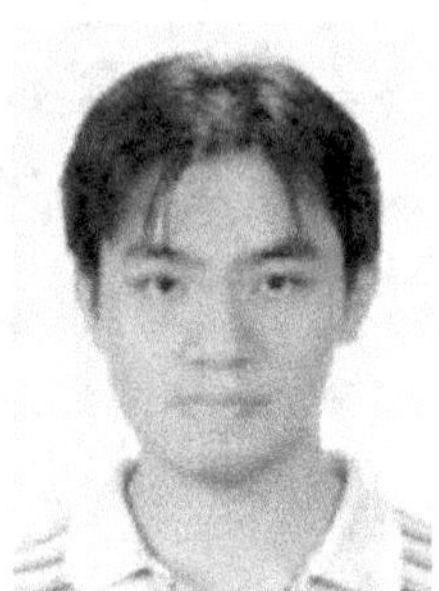

Mark Chiang

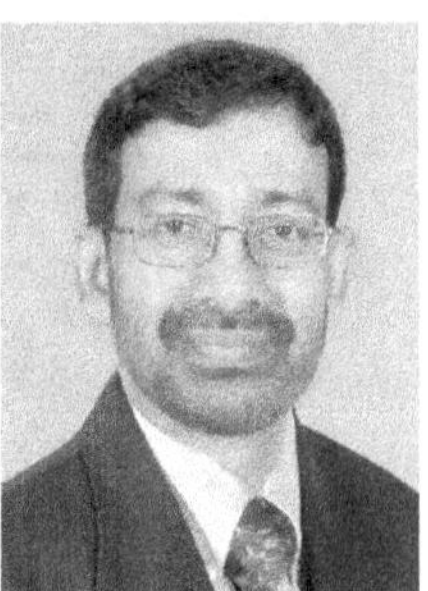

Anil Mandal

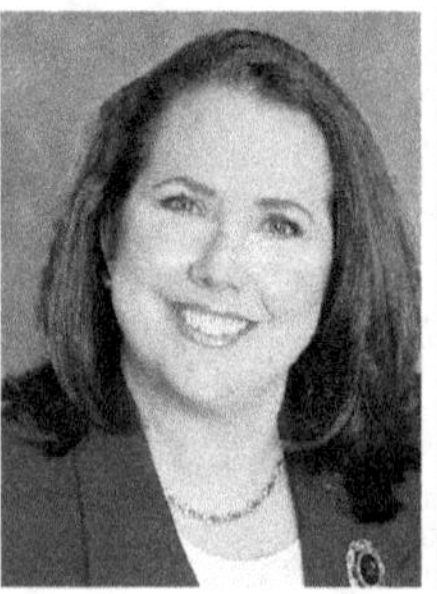

Alana L. Grajewski

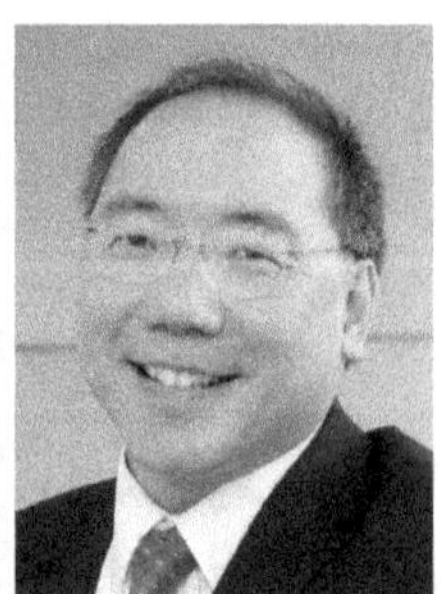

Peng T. Khaw

5. GLAUCOMA SURGERY IN CHILDREN

Maria Papadopoulos, Beth Edmunds, Mark Chiang, Anil Mandal,
Alana L. Grajewski, Peng T. Khaw

Section Leaders: Alana L. Grajewski, Maria Papadopoulos, Peng T. Khaw,
Beth Edmunds, Anil Mandal
Contributors: Karen Joos, Gabor Scharioth, Vera Essuman,
Elizabeth Hodapp, Tam Dang, Jan Erik Jakobsen, S.R. Krishnadas,
Sola Olawoye, David Plager, Luis Silva, Roberto Caputo, Tanuj Dada,
Velota Sung

Consensus statements

1. Surgery is a critical component of the management of childhood glaucoma.
   Comment: It is important to prepare patients and parents or caregivers for lifelong follow-up and possible future surgeries.
2. Glaucoma surgery should preferably be performed by a trained surgeon in centers where there is sufficient volume to ensure surgical experience and skill, and safe anesthesia.
   Comment: A long-term surgical strategy including choice of procedures should be based on training, experience, logistics, and surgeon's preference.
   Comment: The first chance for surgery is often the best chance, and it is important to choose the most appropriate operation.
3. Glaucoma surgery in children is more challenging than in adults with a higher failure and complication rate than in adults.
4. Angle surgery (goniotomy and trabeculotomy – conventional or circumferential) is the procedure of choice for primary congenital glaucoma with the exact choice dictated by corneal clarity and the surgeon's experience and preference.
   Comment: Angle surgery success rates for secondary childhood glaucomas are generally not as good as for primary congenital glaucoma (PCG) with certain exceptions [*e.g.*, glaucoma with acquired condition (uveitis) in juvenile idiopathic arthritis (JIA)].
5. Trabeculectomy, when performed by experienced childhood glaucoma surgeons, can be associated with good outcomes in appropriate cases.

Childhood Glaucoma, pp. 95-134
*Edited by Robert N. Weinreb, Alana L. Grajewski, Maria Papadopoulos, John Grigg,
and Sharon Freedman*
2013 © Kugler Publications, Amsterdam, The Netherlands

Comment: Anti-scarring agents and other adjunctive techniques may be beneficial.

6. Glaucoma drainage devices (GDD) may offer the most effective long-term intraocular pressure (IOP) control in many childhood glaucomas especially those that are refractory to other surgical treatment.
    Comment: There is no prospective evidence that anti-scarring agents influence drainage device outcomes.

7. Cyclophotocoagulation with the diode laser has limited long-term success and often requires re-treatment and the continuation of medications.

8. Other glaucoma procedures advocated in children for the treatment of glaucoma have not been widely adopted either because of the technical challenges in buphthalmic eyes or because they are yet to be proven efficacious or safe in children.

9. Concurrent with glaucoma therapy, visual development needs to be evaluated and optimized with ametropic correction and amblyopia therapy.

10. With childhood glaucoma surgery, one needs carefully to consider the risks and benefits of each intervention, especially in refractory cases when the fellow eye is healthier, and in only eyes.
    Comment: Whenever possible, the assent of the child should be sought when making these difficult decisions.

Introduction

Childhood glaucoma is recognized to be one of the most challenging in the field of glaucoma, especially with regards surgical management.[1] Surgery is the mainstay of treatment and is almost inevitable in the child's lifetime.[2,3] Just as there is variation in the way children can present with glaucoma, there is also variation in the approach to surgical treatment. Considering that multiple surgical interventions are likely, whatever the approach, the need for a long-term surgical strategy, an 'algorithm of action', is essential. The first operation chosen is often the child's best chance of long-term success.[4-7] These highly specialized operations should preferably be performed by a trained surgeon in centers where there is sufficient volume to ensure surgical experience and skill and safe anesthesia. Lastly, glaucoma surgeries in children are at higher risk of failure and complications than in adults. A lack of familiarity with buphthalmic eyes is associated with more complications and so surgical technique must be modified and performed meticulously to keep complications to a minimum.

In this section we aim to provide a general overview of the surgical approach to childhood glaucomas as well as a more detailed discussion of each of the surgical techniques[8-13] with the understanding that approaches can vary. There are very few randomized surgical trials in childhood glaucoma and only a few regarding medical treatment.[14,15] In the absence of these trials, consensus becomes even more important. We have therefore included perspectives from experts of the WGA online consensus forum and from a 'worldwide childhood glaucoma surgical survey'. This survey is the largest ever worldwide survey of childhood glaucoma experts, who manage between them considerable numbers of patients with childhood glaucoma. Although there was no attempt to achieve consensus through the survey, the data provides an informative and important glimpse of current practices among childhood glaucoma surgeons. The practices presented are not intended to replace the judgment of an individual surgeon or serve as guidelines or standards of practice.

Worldwide surgical consensus survey

The survey was conducted using SurveyMonkey with an OpenEyes (open source clinical software) front end to create a comprehensive survey containing 77 questions divided into key sections on childhood glaucoma surgery. The participants were identified by the section leaders from: (1) a list of WGA childhood glaucoma consensus participants known to have an interest in surgery; (2) Pubmed search on the lead authors who have published on childhood glaucoma surgery; and (3) ophthalmologists or trainees from countries in which was otherwise difficult to identify the key ophthalmologists performing childhood glaucoma surgery. The selected participants included both glaucoma specialists and pediatric ophthalmologists with an interest in childhood glaucoma. The participants were sent an email stating the survey objectives, the expected time of survey completion and a link to the SurveyMonkey survey. They were informed that the results of the survey would be reflected in the WGA childhood glaucoma consensus and that their participation in the survey would be acknowledged. If the individual did not respond after the first survey invitation, an email was resent once more.

A total of 116 participants were invited of which 78 responded, resulting in a 67% response rate. Analysis of the survey was performed using a combination of SurveyMonkey outputs and Microsoft Excel. The relevant results, excluding open-ended questions and comments, have been tabulated where possible. The majority of the open-ended answers and comments have also been summarized and amalgamated into the consensus document. More than two thirds of respondents had practiced for over ten years (69%). The majority worked in an academic university practice (74%) and treated both adult and childhood glaucoma (70%).

Survey respondents (78): *Argentina*: Juan R. Sampaolesi; *Australia*: Jonathan Ruddle, John Grigg; *Brazil*: Alberto Jorge Betinjane, Christiane Rolim de Moura; *Canada*: Patrick Hamel, Christopher Lyons; *Chile*: Hernán Iturriaga-Valenzuela; *China*: Jian Ge; *Denmark*: John Thygesen; *Egypt*: Ahmed Abdelrahman; *Germany*: Thomas S. Dietlein, Thomas Klink; *Ghana*: Vera Essuman; *India*: S.R. Krishnadas, Manju Anilkumar, Sirisha Senthil, Sushmita Kaushik, Anil Mandal, Tanuj Dada; *Iran*: Mohammad Pakravan; *Ireland*: Michael O'Keefe; *Israel*: Shlomo Melamed, Itay Ben Zion, Orna Geyer; *Italy*: Stefano Gandolfi, Giorgio Marchini, Roberto Caputo; *Japan*: Tomomi Higashide, Akira Negi, Kazuhisa Sugiyama, Yoshiaki

Kiuchi; *Kenya*: Sheila Marco; *Korea*: Ki Ho Park; *Kuwait*: Faisal Alghadhfan; *Malaysia*: Ming-Yueh Lee; *Mexico*: Oscar Albis-Donado; *Nepal*: Suman S. Thapa; *New Zealand*: Justin Mora; *Norway*: Jan Erik Jakobsen; *Portugal*: Cristina Brito; *Romania*: Valeria Coviltir; *Saudi Arabia*: Saleh Alobeidan; *Singapore*: Ching Lin Ho; *South Africa*: Ellen Ancker, Nicola Freeman; *Spain*: Carmen Mendez-Hernandez, Alicia Serra-Castanera, Julian Garcia-Feijoo; *Taiwan*: Da-Wen Lu; *UK*: Velota Sung, Peng Khaw, Chris Lloyd, Maria Papadopoulos, Geoffrey Woodruff, John Brookes, Joseph Abbott, Cecilia Fenerty; *USA*: Simon K. Law, Robert Feldman, Anya Trumler, Teresa Chen, Shira Robbins, Alex Levin, Sayoko E. Moroi, Janet Serle, Mohamad S. Jaafar, Albert S. Khouri, Pradeep Ramulu, Sharon F. Freedman, Beth Edmunds, Allen Beck, Elizabeth Hodapp, James D. Brandt, Dale Heuer, Karen Joos; *Venezuela*: Luis Silva; *Vietnam*: Dang Tam Mai (Fig. 1).

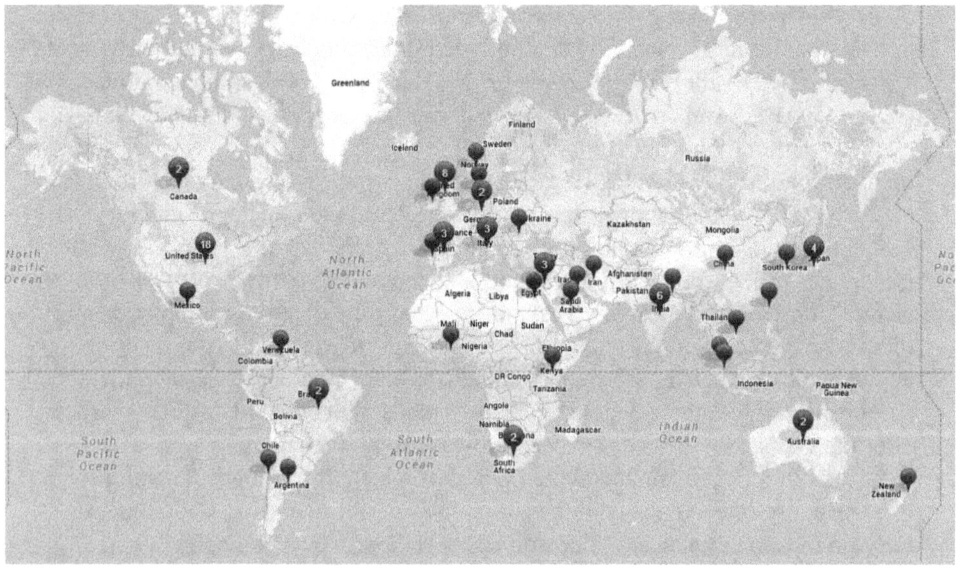

Fig. 1. Geographical distribution of 78 respondents by country.

Challenges

Glaucoma surgery in children is more challenging than in adults for a number of reasons, but mostly due to anatomical factors related to ocular enlargement and aggressive healing. These factors result in a higher risk of both complications and failure of glaucoma surgery in children when compared to adults.

Firstly, there are reasons related to the anatomy of buphthalmic eyes. The wide limbus with distorted limbal anatomy makes surgery different, for example the posterior edge of the scleral flap in a trabeculectomy is often more posterior from the cornea than usual due to the wide limbus. Thin, elastic sclera predisposes to leakage around a tube and makes it difficult to fashion a sclera flap through which sutures will not cheese-wire. There can also be distortion due to previous surgeries or concomitant pathology that further add to the challenge. The orbital space is often limited with difficult access. However, what plays the greatest role is the thin elastic sclera with low rigidity of the buphthalmic, pediatric eye that increases the tendency of the anterior chamber (AC) to collapse and the posterior chamber to move forward, potentially leading to iris prolapse and vitreous loss. It is these features that make these eyes prone to complications, especially hypotony. Finally, the enlarged eye is also associated with lens subluxation from stretched zonules and with synergetic vitreous which is more likely to prolapse.

Children generally have lower surgical success rates than adults[16] except for angle surgery, where the opposite is true. An aggressive inflammatory and healing response in children is thought to account for this fact. The thick Tenon capsule impedes filtration and contains a large reservoir of fibrocytes and fibroblasts involved in the inflammatory response and scarring. Furthermore, complications and failure are much more likely in an inflamed eye. So ideally it is important to wait for a 'quiet eye' before performing glaucoma surgery. This is especially so in children with uveitic glaucoma, who often need additional topical and systemic immunosuppression peri-operatively.

Significant intra- and postoperative complications are reported in the literature especially with the use of anti-scarring agents in trabeculectomy surgery[17-19] and with GDD surgery relating to hypotony and tube specific complications requiring revision.[20-27] Subsequently, modifications to techniques are mandatory in pediatric surgery to minimise these complications. Anesthetic risks are potentially higher in children than in adults.

Lastly, lack of co-operation affects the degree of monitoring and post-op follow-up, which can compromise surgical results. Multiple examinations under anesthesia (EUA) may be required which may lead to a delay in implementation of adjunctive measures such as suture removal and anti-scarring agents. Furthermore, regional, socioeconomic and logistic differences play an important role in the ability to closely follow up patients after surgery.[28,29] There is also the critical dependence on the caregiver's commitment to post operative regime of anti-inflammatory medications. Children with the most engaged caregivers often have the best outcomes. Concurrent with controlling IOP, ametropia correction and amblyopia management is essential to optimise long term visual outcomes.[30] Not to be forgotten is the consideration of the impact of the diagnosis on the child's life (*i.e.*, school, hobbies) and the caregivers which still needs further research.[31,32]

The above facts were supported by the survey, in which all the respondents felt childhood glaucoma surgery was more demanding than adult surgery and that more research was required to improve outcomes. The majority thought glaucoma surgery in children was associated with more complications (79%) and that surgical success could be improved by meticulous and appropriate surgical technique (96%).

Factors influencing the choice of operation

Planning a course of action to preserve vision is essential because of the long life expectancy of a child and the inevitability of repeat surgery due to the chronic nature of glaucoma. Making the right choice initially is paramount as the first operation has the greatest chance of success. In eyes that have undergone multiple procedures it is important to make the next operation the definitive one. Once the various options have been discussed with the parents, a decision is made regarding the most appropriate operation and discussed in detail with the parents. It is important not to trivialize surgery in children and to set realistic expectations regarding the outcome and the need for regular follow up and possible unplanned surgery. Whichever operation is chosen, the technique must be safe and it must be one that 'works in your hands' for your population.

A number of factors influence the choice of surgery, particularly the type of glaucoma. For example, for PCG, angle surgery is usually the preferred first line treatment and for which it has the best success rates. In glaucoma associated with Axenfeld-Rieger anomaly, access to angle structures may be inhibited by iris attachments to Schwalbe line or by peripheral anterior synechiae (PAS) in uveitic glaucoma making angle surgery impractical. Glaucoma following removal of congenital cataract is usually associated with poor results when treated with trabeculectomy, even when Mitomycin (MMC) is used.[33-35]

Age at onset and/or age at presentation may influence the choice of surgery. PCG presentation within the first three months of birth carries a poor prognosis for angle surgery success,[7,36-39] as does a late presentation over the age of 2-3.[37,40,41] However, given the low rate of complications with angle surgery, it is still typically the first procedure of choice in these children.

There are also anatomical factors, such as corneal clarity required for goniotomy. Corneal edema can be overcome by epithelial debridement in 90% of Caucasian patients.[42] The state of conjunctiva, for example heavily scarred conjunctiva, would indicate GDD surgery as being more appropriate. Occasionally, significant superior conjunctival scarring leads to inferior placement of a GDD. Furthermore, accompanying ocular anomalies and systemic disease often need to be taken into consideration. A significantly disorganised anterior segment as may occur with Peters anomaly, may respond better to GDD surgery than to trabeculectomy.

The severity of glaucoma needs to be considered, as advanced optic nerve damage or a very hazy cornea require an especially low IOP, more likely to be achieved by trabeculectomy with MMC rather than without. On the other hand, limited visual potential or the altered structural integrity of a severely buphthalmic eye may influence the surgical choice to be less aggressive.

Previous surgical history and anticipated future surgical interventions – for example, the presence of a cataract needing future removal – may sway the decision towards GDD surgery rather than trabeculectomy, the latter being less likely to survive subsequent lensectomy. The fate of the fellow eye with prior surgery is also important, because if the fellow eye has done badly with one type of operation despite its being well executed, then an alternative procedure may need to be considered. Lastly, the surgeon's training and experience significantly influence their choice of surgery, as does geographic location, access to tertiary care, likelihood of follow-up and the availability of facilities/equipment.

Surgical procedures

There are a number of surgical procedures to choose from with varying indications as well as advantages and disadvantages. Potentially good success rates are possible, especially when surgical procedures are performed at referral centers with sufficient volume to ensure skillful surgery and safe anesthesia. The aim of surgery is to eliminate or bypass aqueous flow obstruction. The challenge of surgery is to balance increased success with decreased complications. This fine balance is achieved by having the surgeon modify and develop a technique that is safe and 'works in the surgeon's hands'. All operations can be technically challenging and potentially complicated if meticulous attention is not to detail.

Angle surgery

The prognosis for childhood glaucoma at the beginning of the twentieth century was very poor up until Otto Barkan, under direct gonioscopy with a specially designed lens, resurrected a technique that incised the angle,[43] which he called *goniotomy*. Results of angle surgery in adults previously published by De Vincentiis and Barkan were very disappointing.[44] In 1942, Barkan reported the successful reduction of IOP in 16 out of 17 eyes with congenital glaucoma and the preservation of vision in 14 eyes.[45] This seminal work was to have a major impact on the prognosis of this condition, as evidenced by the fact that the technique of goniotomy, performed essentially unchanged, is still the procedure of choice for many children with PCG. However, the problem with goniotomy was that it was unsuitable for cases with hazy corneas in which the angle structures were not clearly visible even after epithelial stripping.

The next major advance in angle surgery came in 1960 with *trabeculotomy*. It was simultaneously and independently described in 1960 by Redmond Smith,[46] who ruptured the trabecular meshwork with a nylon suture ('nylon filament trabeculotomy') and by Hermann Burian[47] who instead used a specially designed instrument called a *trabeculotome* and named the operation *'trabeculotomy ab externo'*. In 1962, Allen and Burian described its role in childhood glaucoma.[48] Harms and Dannheim subsequently modified the technique by dissecting a superficial scleral flap[49] and then identifying and entering Schlemm canal with a modified *trabeculotome* (Harms trabeculotome). The advantage of trabeculotomy was that it could be used in all cases of glaucoma in children regardless of corneal clarity.

Subsequently, endoscopic goniotomy was described to enable goniotomy in the presence of a hazy cornea.[50-53]

With time it became obvious that repeating conventional (probe) trabeculotomy or goniotomy, which only incise a limited extent of the angle (90-120°) each time, improved outcomes, suggesting that the extent of angle incised was important in some cases. So to achieve a circumferential incision with one procedure alone and to minimize anesthetic exposure, in 1995 Beck and Lynch proposed circumferential suture trabeculotomy with a blunted 6-0 prolene.[54] The more recent introduction of an illuminated microcatheter[55] as a substitute for the suture, allowing continuous visualization of the filament tip and early detection of misdirection, has potentially improved the safety and technical ease of the procedure. Circumferential trabeculotomy is advocated by some authors as the entire angle is treated in one session and the surgery therefore does not have to be repeated.[56,57]

Others have tried to also improve the results of trabeculotomy by combining it with other procedures. In 1980, Maul and colleagues described combined trabeculotomy-trabeculectomy (CTT) in an infant with severe bilateral primary congenital glaucoma who had failed goniotomy.[58] Although in theory, combining these two procedures should provide two major outflow pathways and so improve results, there are no prospective comparisons to support this assertion. Combined trabeculotomy-trabeculectomy is argued to be more successful than either procedure performed alone and is the primary procedure of choice, in populations who are thought to be at greater risk of failure because of more severe or advanced presentations, such as in the Middle East and India.

The indications for angle surgery (goniotomy, trabeculotomy [conventional and circumferential], CCT) along with advantages, disadvantages and poor prognostic factors are summarized in Table 1. Each operation will be discussed in turn with regards preoperative considerations, surgical highlights,[12,13] complications, outcomes and consensus survey results.

General anesthesia and an operating microscope (angled 45 degrees for goniotomy) are required for all operations. If there has been a reasonable but suboptimal lowering of IOP after the first goniotomy or conventional trabeculotomy, they can be repeated in the non-operated part of the angle.

Goniotomy

To perform goniotomy safely, clear visibility of intraocular and angle structures is crucial so that the exact location of the knife within the AC is always obvious. Hence, preoperative medications to maximally reduce the IOP and so improve corneal clarity and the view of the angle are recommended. Furthermore, pilocarpine (1-2%) preoperatively is advisable to achieve adequate miosis and protect the lens against trauma. If miosis is poor, it can be further augmented with the use of acetylcholine chloride 1:100 (Miochol, Novartis Ophthalmics) intra-operatively.

The keys to successfully performing goniotomy are adequate access, visualization of the angle and the maintenance of the AC. Exposure and access to the peripheral cornea is very important and may not always be possible in buphthalmic eyes, in which case consider performing a lateral canthotomy. To improve angle visualization, corneal haziness from epithelial oedema can be reduced by debriding the corneal epithelium following the use of absolute alcohol. Glycerine can also be used to improve corneal clarity but is less effective. Hypertonic sodium chloride (5%) is also helpful. Stromal haze and Haab striae may still obscure the view. Angle details are improved with the use of a goniolens (Barkan lens, traditional or modified Swan-Jacobs goniolens or a wide angle Khaw goniotomy lens) coupled with viscoelastic to minimise air bubble formation or with irrigation. Maintenance of the AC is achieved by using a tapered knife, viscoelastic or an AC maintainer. Furthermore, the assistant should be instructed not push or pull on the eye while holding the eye securely in position with fixating forceps as it may cause loss of aqueous and AC depth and also distort the cornea. If the AC shallows or collapses at any stage there is significant risk of damage to intraocular structures, especially the lens.

A blade (Barraquer knife, Worst knife, Swan spade) or needle (23G/25G needle on a viscoelastic syringe or infusion tubing) is introduced in the temporal cornea avoiding a short tunnel to prevent iris prolapse. Once inside the eye, the blade or needle must be visible at all times, and directed in a slightly upward direction to avoid the iris and lens. The angle is gently engaged by the blade tip halfway between the root of the iris and Schwalbe line and is swept across the angle circumferentially resulting in a superficial incision of the nasal angle over 90-120 degrees. The end point of the operation is a falling back of the peripheral iris and widening of the angle. The incision can be extended by requesting the assistant to gently intort or extort the eye. The knife is slowly withdrawn and followed by a shallowing of the AC, which is quickly reformed with balance salt solution or kept formed with sterile air while suturing. The corneal incision may then be sutured to prevent leakage (often seen in buphthalmic eyes) and AC shallowing, particularly in the periphery, potentially compromising the result of surgery. A mild hyphema on withdrawal of the blade from the AC is typical and thought to be a favorable sign indicating a correctly placed incision. If viscoelastic has been used it must be thoroughly removed as it may cause an IOP spike resulting in further splits in Descemet membrane and nerve damage. Overfilling the AC can drive fluid into the suprachoroidal space, and using sterile air in the AC rather than just fluid can reduce then chance of this happening. Pilocarpine can be applied topically to keep the angle open and theoretically reduce PAS formation. Subconjunctival steroid and antibiotic are injected, the eye is patched and a shield placed at the conclusion of surgery. The patient is examined the first day following surgery. Postoperatively, topical antibiotics are typically continued until review. Topical steroid may also be used and tapered over a few weeks to avoid an IOP rise.

Table 1. Angle surgery

	Indications	Advantages	Disadvantages	Poor prognostic factors
Goniotomy	• Primary congenital glaucoma (PCG) where the cornea allows satisfactory visualization of angle ▪ most effective between 3 to 12 months, with diminishing efficacy with age • Secondary childhood glaucomas but usually less successful than PCG with the exceptions of: ▪ Uveitic and steroid-induced glaucoma with open angles ▪ Conditions with 'PCG-like angles', *e.g.*, congenital rubella and Sturge-Weber Syndrome may also respond well	• Does not violate conjunctiva and prejudice success of future surgery • Visualisation of angle allows precise incision • Less traumatic and safer compared to other procedures • Shorter operating time • Repeatable in other areas of angle • Avoids long term-risk of bleb-related complications • Minimal risk of significant hypotony	• Technically demanding with considerable surgical experience necessary • Requires adequate angle visualization and maintenance of anterior chamber (AC) depth • Special instrumentation and patient or microscope positioning required • Discomfort associated with epithelium debridement • Need for an assistant to fixate the eye • Often has to be repeated to achieve control	• Onset at or within 3 months of birth[36-38] • Late presentation PCG over the age of 2-3[37,40,41] • Enlarged ocular dimensions as a measure of structural damage over time • Corneal diameter $\geq$ 14 mm[36,37,161,162] • Positive family history[37]
Trabeculotomy (conventional & circumferential)	• Same as for goniotomy	• Can be performed in the presence of an opaque cornea and so more applicable especially in populations where this is a common finding • Does not require patient or microscope positioning • Many components of technique similar to trabeculectomy • 360° angle treatment in single session is possible with a blunted suture or an illuminated microcatheter (circumferential	• Damages conjunctiva and prejudices success of future filtering surgery – temporal or inferior site are preferable • Angle not directly visualized which may increase the risk of trauma • Usually requires special instrumentation (trabeculotome or illuminated microcatheter) • Schlemm canal is not found in 4-20% of cases • Longer procedure	• Onset < 3 months of age[39,163] • Late presentation[93] • Enlarged ocular dimensions ▪ Axial length > 24 mm[163] ▪ Corneal diameter $\geq$ 14 mm[93]

		trabeculotomy) • In some populations, a higher success rate may be possible when combined with trabeculectomy • Can be converted to trabeculectomy if Schlemm canal is not found with superior incision • Repeatable in other areas of the angle	• Converting a trabeculotomy entry site into trabeculectomy places sclerostomy very close to iris root, predisposing to iris incarceration • If trabeculotomy is performed temporally or inferiorly and cannot be completed, conversion to trabeculectomy is not possible • Undesirable external filtration is possible if scleral flap closure is not watertight • Often has to be repeated to achieve IOP control	
Combined trabeculotomy-trabeculectomy	• Same as for goniotomy • Especially severe disease with marked corneal edema	• Can be performed with opaque cornea • Single surgery with quicker rehabilitation than separate surgeries • Argued to be more successful in populations at high risk of failure but there are no prospective studies comparing the three procedures	• Longer anesthetic time than either trabeculotomy alone or trabeculectomy alone • May be technically more difficult than each procedure alone • It is possible that the two operations are incompatible, as a functioning trabeculectomy may result in the closure of the trabeculotomy cleft due to inadequate flow of aqueous through the trabecular meshwork or synechial closure secondary to hypotony from an overfiltering bleb • May prejudice future trabeculectomy outcome	• Same as for trabeculotomy and trabeculectomy

After surgery, the child is re-examined again four to six weeks later as it can take take this long for a response to be seen. Gonioscopy usually reveals the site of the incision as an area of widened angle. Peripheral anterior synechiae are very often seen in the region of the incision even with a successful outcome.[59] There is no obvious correlation between post-operative angle appearance and pressure control.[60]

The safety of goniotomy depends on the surgeon's experience with the technique, perfect equipment and careful attention to detail. When meticulously performed by skilled surgeon it has minimal operative complications. Shaffer reviewed 577 consecutive goniotomies over a forty-year period and reported only 13 surgical complications (2%). There were no episodes of corneal or lens injury nor endophthalmitis despite simultaneous goniotomies.[61] A low complication rate (4%), was similarly reported by Rice in his series of 246 goniotomies, with retinal detachment (1.6%) and iris incarceration (1.2%) being the most common problems.[62] Other complications include: inadvertent iridodialysis, cyclodialysis, hypotony, scleral perforation and epithelial ingrowth.[63]

Goniotomy is a very effective operation with success usually ranging from 75-90% in large series (110-335 eyes) after multiple goniotomies.[36,40-42,64-66] But after a second operation, it becomes technically more difficult to incise any remaining angle and the success rate decreases with subsequent goniotomies.[62] Response in children from an African or African Caribbean background has been reported to be as good as Caucasian.[4,62,67,68] However, success may be reduced in other racial groups.[69,70] Failure of goniotomy is thought to be due to failure to obtain a gaping incision at the time of surgery or due to fibrous proliferation of tissue especially if the incision is deep into the sclera.[71]

CONSENSUS SURVEY: Goniotomy was selected as the procedure of choice for PCG by 28% of experts. Goniotomy was preferred as first-line surgery for Sturge Weber syndrome by 26% and for uveitic glaucoma by 14%. Almost all specialists perform goniotomy using the conventional approach with direct visualization.

Trabeculotomy

Similar to the preparations for goniotomy, topical miotics (pilocarpine 1-2%) can be given preoperatively to achieve miosis and to protect lens from intra-operative damage or alternatively intracameral miotics (such as acetylcholine chloride 1:100 (Miochol, Novartis Ophthalmics)) can be given intra-operatively.

Conventional trabeculotomy (probe)
As conjunctival dissection and scleral flap incision is required, a temporal or inferior approach leaves the superior position unscarred for future surgery. The use of an operating microscope allows high magnification for the more delicate parts of the surgery (identification and dissection of Schlemm canal). An initial paracentesis is made to allow reformation of the AC during the procedure. Specific instruments required for the conventional approach include a metal trabeculotome probe.

Accurate localization of Schlemm canal is key: the external landmark is the junction between the trabecular band and sclera. A partial thickness scleral flap is fashioned and Schlemm canal is located under high magnification by slowly and carefully deepening while spreading the incision walls of a small radial incision at the limbus near the grey zone. Care is taken to avoid perforation of the inner wall of Schlemm and inadvertent entry into the anterior chamber. Successful entry into Schlemm canal is often accompanied by a reflux of blood and/or aqueous from the cut ends of the canal. This ostium can be probed gently with a 6/0 nylon or polypropylene suture tip to confirm its patency, before introducing the trabeculotome probe. If the probe cannot be passed easily into the canal, it should be withdrawn and dissection of the outer wall continued until all fibers are cut. Confirmation of correct probe positioning may be determined by moving the probe gently forward and backward with small motions: if when swept towards the AC, bubbles appear in limbal corneal stroma, or the iris base is seen to move then it is likely the trabeculotome is not in the canal but in the cornea or anterior chamber; if while making a small motion with the probe posteriorly it moves easily posteriorly, it is likely the trabeculotome is not in the canal but in the suprachoroidal space.

There are several more recent modifications of this traditional technique. One is the viscotrabeculotomy in which a Grieshaber cannula is introduced into each opening of Schlemm canal and a small amount of Healon GV injected to dilate approximately 5 mm of the canal on either side, before inserting the trabeculotome.[72] A small amount of viscoelastic can also be injected and left between the lips of the trabecular incision once the Harms trabeculotome incisions have been completed, to theoretically keep them separated in the early postoperative period. More extensive viscodissection and viscodilation of the canal can also be performed using the iScience microcatheter.

If Schlemm canal cannot be identified, the procedure can be converted to trabeculectomy, provided the approach has been superior. The anterior segment structures and lens can be protected from probe damage by deepening the AC with sterile air or viscoelastic before rupturing trabecular meshwork. A mild to moderate hyphema can occur but is usually transitory. The scleral flap should be sutured tightly to prevent inadvertent bleb formation or the site of future staphyloma. The paracentesis incisions are sutured to avoid leakage. The conjunctiva is closed and subconjunctival steroid and antibiotic are injected, the eye is patched and a shield placed at the conclusion of surgery. The patient is examined the first day following surgery. Postoperatively, typically topical antibiotics are continued until review. Topical steroid may also be used and tapered over a few weeks to avoid an intraocular pressure rise. After surgery, the child is re-examined four to six weeks later.

Circumferential trabeculotomy (suture or catheter)
An alternative to the traditional metal trabeculotome approach, which incises up to one third of Schlemm canal, is to use a blunted suture (*e.g.*, 6/0 prolene) or an illuminated microcatheter to incise 360 degrees (iTrack, iCath, iScience, Glaucolight). Either the suture or the catheter is threaded into one of the cut ends of the

canal, and advanced through 360 degrees until it presents again in the ostium. This is then gently pulled to cheese-wire through the trabecular meshwork into the AC and then removed from the eye. However, the suture or catheter may meet obstruction in the canal and fail to cannulate the full circumference and/or can be misdirected to create false passages into the suprachoriodal space, under Descemet membrane or into the anterior chamber. The illuminated tip of the microcatheter makes monitoring its position much easier than when using the suture approach, which requires a gonioscopic view for its identification in Schlemm canal to avoid misdirection.[73] If the suture or catheter meets obstruction, there are several maneuvers that may be attempted to bypass it. Entering the opposite opening in Schlemm canal may allow a smoother passage in the opposite direction. Withdrawing slightly from the site of obstruction and giving a small bolus of viscoelastic through the catheter may open the lumen to allow it to pass. Decompressing or re-inflating the eye a little may change the tension across the canal and allow easier passage. If the catheter has reached close to 180 degrees or further along the canal before meeting obstruction, it is possible to cut down at the catheter tip to externalize it. Pulling on both ends of the catheter simultaneously will incise the trabecular meshwork for the extent that the catheter was able to pass. In the case of misdirection, withdrawing the suture or catheter and cannulating from the opposite side may be useful. If collector channels may be diverting the catheter out of Schlemm canal, applying external pressure with forceps over presumed collector channel openings in the canal when trying to re-direct the suture or catheter, may allow the catheter to remain in the canal. If all attempts fail, a conventional trabeculotomy can be performed with a trabeculotome, or a trabeculectomy can be performed if the incision is superior.

The majority of conventional trabeculotomy complications are related to the positioning and manipulation of the probe. There may be a higher risk of anterior segment trauma since the procedure is performed without direct visualization of the angle, often in the presence of distorted limbal anatomy and corneal haze or opacification. False passages can lead to stripping of Descemet membrane, iris prolapse, iridodialysis, cyclodialysis and lens subluxation.[4,39,49,74] Reflux of blood through Schlemm canal can lead to hyphema, which is usually limited. Hypotony may be transient but can be persistent if there is inadvertent bleb formation or a cyclodialysis cleft. Blebs are subject to similar risks as trabeculectomy blebs, especially if not well covered by the upper lid. Cataract formation may also follow surgical trauma or hypotony. Regarding circumferential trabeculotomy, other reported complications apart from misdirection of the suture include severe hypotony[75] and significant persistent hyphema in children with Sturge-Weber syndrome.[56]

Conventional trabeculotomy success rates following multiple surgeries are similar to those of goniotomy.[4,7,39,67] In studies comparing goniotomy to conventional trabeculotomy, success is thought to be determined more by the severity and duration of the disease rather than the technique.[76] Circumferential trabeculotomy has a reported overall success of around 90% after 1-4 years.[54,57,77] Mendicino *et al.* suggested it may be more successful than goniotomy in a retrospective comparison but the mean follow up for the goniotomy group was over twice as long (nine versus four years).[77] Success of trabeculotomy may be reduced in certain racial groups for example, India[78] and Middle East[69,79] which has led to the adoption of CTT in these areas. Modifications such as the viscotrabeculotomy have been reported to enjoy superior results compared to traditional trabeculotomy in a Turkish population.[72,80] Failure of trabeculotomy is thought to be due to scar tissue covering the trabeculotomy site, which has been shown in monkeys.[81]

The decision to perform one angle procedure in preference to the other is influenced largely by corneal transparency and the surgeon's experience and preference. Trabeculotomy is possible in the presence of both a clear and hazy cornea, it may be more useful for surgeons comfortable with trabeculectomy who have not had much exposure to goniotomy, and the circumferential approach also offers the possibility of 360 degrees of angle treatment in one procedure. However, trabeculotomy is more invasive, causes conjunctival scarring and even with experience, may be technically difficult at times due to the inability to find Schlemm canal.

CONSENSUS SURVEY: The preferred trabeculotomy approach of experts was conventional trabeculotomy with probe in 68% and circumferential trabeculotomy in 21% with more favouring an illuminated microcatheter (15%) to suture (6%). A superior approach for trabeculotomy was used by 37%, temporal by 19%, while 8% adopted an inferior approach.

Trabeculotomy was selected as the procedure of choice for PCG by 41% of experts (conventional probe 28% and circumferential trabeculotomy 13%). Trabeculotomy was preferred as first-line surgery for: Sturge Weber syndrome by 22% (conventional probe 17% and circumferential trabeculotomy 5%); for aniridic glaucoma by 18% (conventional probe 15% and circumferential trabeculotomy 3%) and uveitic glaucoma by 8% (conventional probe 8% and circumferential trabeculotomy 0%).

Combined trabeculotomy-trabeculectomy (CTT)
The preoperative considerations when preparing for CTT surgery are similar to those for the other angle surgeries and trabeculectomy. As with trabeculectomy, this surgery may be performed with or without MMC. The surgical points made in the trabeculotomy and trabeculectomy sections hold for this combined procedure as well. After performing the trabeculotomy, the initial Schlemm canal incision is extended so that a block of sclera is removed at the limbus by scissors or punch. This places the sclerostomy more posteriorly than is usual for trabeculectomy which predisposes the iris incarceration and hemorrhage. An option is to make a separate more anterior incision under the hinge of the scleral flap for the sclerostomy. One study suggests that combining deep sclerectomy with CTT may facilitate finding Schlemm canal.[82] The complications mentioned in the trabeculotomy and trabeculectomy sections apply here, in addition to the potential complications of a more extensive procedure and longer surgical time, than when each is performed alone.

The argument in favor of primary CTT in some ethnic populations is a higher incidence of successful IOP control with a single operative procedure, as has been reported from India[78,83-86] and the Middle East.[70,87,88] In the largest Indian series of 624 eyes of 360 consecutive Indian children with PCG undergoing CCT without MMC, IOP control was achieved in 85% of children after one year reducing to 58% after six years. Forty two per cent of patients achieved vision of $\geq$ 20/60.[86]

Elder reported poor long term success (IOP $\leq$ 21 mmHg and no medication) in a Palestinian Arab population with predominantly PCG undergoing multiple angle surgery as compared to primary trabeculectomy without anti-scarring agents.[69] In a subsequent study by the same author comparing retrospective trabeculectomy data to prospectively collected CTT data, both without anti-scarring agents, the cumulative chance of success for CTT was 93.5% compared to trabeculectomy which was 72% after a 24-month follow-up.[87] For a similar follow up in the same population, trabeculotomy only had a 51% cumulative chance of success.[69]

Similar poor results for trabeculotomy of 54% were reported retrospectively by Debnath *et al.* in Saudi Arabian children with 'congenital glaucoma' and a short mean follow up of only 11 months. In the same study, trabeculectomy without anti-scarring agent achieved a 67% success rate (IOP $\leq$ 16 mmHg under general anesthesia and no medication).[79] The difference was not statistically significant. In a similar Saudi-Arabian population and with a comparable short mean follow-up (ten months), CTT augmented with MMC achieved 78% success rate (IOP $\leq$ 21 mmHg) for children with PCG but only 45% success for secondary glaucomas.[88] It was this higher success rate of CTT with anti-scarring agents, over both trabeculotomy and trabeculectomy in a similar population to Debnath[79] that prompted Mullaney *et al.* to suggest 'CTT is superior to trabeculotomy or trabeculectomy alone', however, they did use MMC. In the largest reported series, Al-Hazmi *et al.* in a retrospective review of 820 eyes of Saudi-Arabian patients with PCG, found CTT with MMC resulted in significantly better IOP control than trabeculotomy alone in moderate to severe forms of the condition, *e.g.*, trabeculotomy success was 40% compared to 80% for CCT with MMC in moderate disease. However, there was a significant learning curve for trabeculotomy with success increasing from 29% to 82% over the ten-year period studied. There was a clear correlation between success rate of procedures and severity of the disease.[70]

A retrospective study of largely Caucasian patients with PCG (Caucasian 71%, Turkish and Arabian 29%) comparing trabeculotomy, trabeculectomy and CTT without anti-scarring agents, showed no statistical difference in success between the three procedures after a median follow-up of three years. The authors argued that success was determined more by the severity of the disease than by the type of surgery.[7]

A recent series of West African children with PCG described poor results from CCT, with probability of success falling from 83% at six months to 44% at one year, possibly due to severe disease at presentation, racial influences and no anti-scarring agent use.[89] When primary CTT fails to control glaucoma, trabeculectomy with MMC can be performed as the second surgical procedure.[90,91] Alternatively, GDD surgery may also be performed.

CONSENSUS SURVEY: CTT was selected as the procedure of choice for treating PCG by 14% of experts. CTT was the procedure of choice for aniridia and Sturge-Weber syndrome for 19% of experts. Of those experts performing CTT, 41% would use MMC and the majority a fornix based conjunctival flap (51%).

In summary, angle surgery (goniotomy and trabeculotomy – conventional or circumferential) is the first line for PCG with the procedure of choice dictated by corneal clarity and the surgeon's experience and preference. When angle surgery is possible but unlikely to succeed due to numerous poor prognostic factors, especially advanced disease or late presentation, then consideration should be given to combining angle surgery with trabeculectomy or performing another type of operation. Angle surgery success rates in the literature for secondary childhood glaucomas are generally not as good as for PCG.[62,92-96] Angle surgery can be considered in cases of Sturge-Weber syndrome with an element of goniodysgenesis (infantile presentations)[97] and for uveitis (*e.g.*, JIA) where the literature suggests satisfactory long term IOP control on medications.[98,99] For other secondary glaucomas, angle surgery can be performed but may be unsuccessful in the long term even after multiple attempts.

Trabeculectomy (filtering surgery)

Trabeculectomy was introduced by Cairns in 1968 for the treatment of adult glaucoma[100] but came to be performed also in children who had repeatedly failed angle or other types of surgery. As a secondary procedure after previous multiple failed surgeries, these initial results were poor and associated with high complication rates.[101] But more encouraging reports of primary unenhanced trabeculectomy surgery followed [102,103] with fewer serious complications. The main indications for trabeculectomy are repeated failed angle surgery and most secondary childhood glaucomas. For further indications, advantages, disadvantages and poor prognostic factors for trabeculectomy refer to Table 2.

Trabeculectomy as a primary or secondary procedure was still associated with failure in some cases due to excessive scarring. In 1991, Miller and Rice showed that beta radiation as an anti-scarring agent at the time of surgery prolonged trabeculectomy survival with lower IOP and was associated with elevated diffuse blebs.[104] The subsequent introduction of further anti-scarring agents in the 1990s was found to be useful in children to counteract the vigorous wound healing response and the success rates appeared to improve in some series but so did the complications, especially those related to hypotony. However, recent modifications to the intra-operative application of MMC and to the surgical technique have resulted in more favorable bleb morphology and reduced complication rates.[105,106] The use of an anti-scarring agent is recommended in the refractory glaucomas with the more potent MMC generally preferred over 5-FU. Although there are many

Table 2. Trabeculectomy

	Indications	Advantages	Disadvantages	Poor prognostic indicators
Trabeculectomy	• Failed angle surgery • Surgeon has limited experience with angle surgery • Patient unlikely to respond to angle surgery (very early or late presentation of PCG or known racial groups with lower success) • Very low target IOP required due to advanced disc damage or for improved corneal clarity • Most secondary glaucomas	• 'Titratable' post-op IOP with the use of: • releasable sutures, which can be adjusted or removed • post-op subconjunctival 5FU (0.2-0.3 ml of 5FU 50 mg/ml) and steroids can be injected adjacent to the bleb during an EUA • Lower IOP achievable with anti-scarring agents which may significantly clear cloudy corneas, and therefore avoid corneal surgery • Many surgeons have experience performing trabeculectomy in adults	• More invasive procedure with greater risk of hypotony with choroidal effusion and hemorrhage than angle surgery especially with the use of Mitomycin C (MMC) • Greater risk of endophthalmitis in the presence of a thin, avascular bleb • Poor results in aphakic glaucoma even with MMC	• Aphakia[33-35] • Less than 1 year of age[17,164,165]

ways of performing trabeculectomy in children, refer to Table 3 for surgical tips on a trabeculectomy technique. Postoperative topical steroids, on a weaning regime for up to three to four months are important to maximize success.

Complications associated with trabeculectomy usually relate to hypotony in the early stages (shallow or flat AC, hypotony maculopathy, choroidal effusion, suprachoroidal hemorrhage) and to progressive bleb thinning and the formation of

Table 3. Trabeculectomy (technique is aimed towards minimizing intra-/early postoperative hypotony, encouraging posterior flow and the formation of a diffuse bleb).

Surgical steps	Surgical points/rationale
Corneal traction suture	• Allows adequate exposure • Avoids hemorrhage from superior rectus muscle suture
Fornix-based conjunctival flap	• Allows better visualization of limbal anatomy • Easier placement of scleral flap sutures • Less likely to form a scar limiting posterior flow
Wet field cautery	• Hemostasis • Avoids scleral shrinkage
Anti-scarring agents	• Diffuse large treatment to minimize risk of a focal, avascular bleb
Scleral flap	• Consider fashioning scleral flap first before anti-scarring treatment to enable treatment under the flap • Dissection forward into cornea avoids iris, ciliary body and vitreous incarceration • Posterior edge must be well beyond limbus • Large and thick (5x3-4 mm) • Sutures less likely to cheese-wire • Greater resistance to aqueous outflow • Short radial cuts enough to allow reflection of scleral flap for the sclerostomy • Directs aqueous flow posteriorly to prevent cystic blebs • Valve effect to prevent hypotony
Preplaced scleral flap sutures before sclerostomy	• Easier to place with formed globe • Reduces duration of intraoperative hypotony after sclerostomy and peripheral iridotomy performed • Releasable along posterior borders of scleral flap, and fixed sutures at apices • Releasable loop buried in cornea so suture can be left indefinitely and reduces risk of endophthalmitis • Can be adjusted or removed under anesthetic without laser
Paracentesis for AC maintainer	• Oblique, peripheral long tunnel (21G needle) minimizes risks of inadvertent lens damage, avoids wound leak and stabilizes infusion cannula • Allows anterior chamber reformation and maintenance of IOP intra-operatively preventing formation of intra-operative choroidal effusion, suprachoroidal hemorrhage and minimizes risk of vitreous prolapse with PI • Must be turned off when tying scleral flap sutures tight to prevent cheese-wiring • Can be used to gauge flow through sclera flap and ensure adequate flap closure

Table 3. Cont.

Surgical steps	Surgical points/rationale
Sclerostomy	• Small sclerostomy punch (500μm diameter) allows increased control of aqueous outflow both intra- and postoperatively and is quicker to perform • As anterior as possible prevents iris, ciliary body, and vitreous incarceration
Scleral flap closure	• Tight closure vital with anti-scarring agent use • Add additional sutures as required to reduce flow
Fornix-based conjunctival closure (or limbal-based if preferred)	• 10-0 nylon retains tension longer than dissolvable sutures with minimal inflammation • Purse string at edges, with limbal vertical mattress sutures, or modified Wise technique,[166] for watertight closure • Ends of nylon buried under conjunctiva to minimize discomfort
Prevention of post-op hypotony	• Short radial cuts create valve effect and minimize leakage from the sides of scleral flap • Tight scleral flap sutures with option to adjust/release at later stage • Watertight conjunctival closure • Suture paracentesis • May leave viscoelastic in anterior chamber if flow rate too high despite maximal suturing; or if ciliary body shut down anticipated (uveitic cases) • Air bubble in AC

cystic blebs, 'blebs at risk', (blebitis, endophthalmitis, chronic bleb leak) in the later stages.[17-19] Patients and their caregivers must be educated and warned about potential complications especially with 'blebs at risk'. They should be instructed to report immediately to an ophthalmologist should symptoms or signs of bleb-related infection occur. Other complications include: hyphema, iris incarceration, lens dislocation, lens trauma, cataract, vitreous loss, vitreous hemorrhage, retinal detachment and staphyloma.

Early results of trabeculectomy without anti-scarring agents had poor long-term success rates of only 30-40% especially when performed after multiple failed surgeries.[101] As a primary surgical procedure (*i.e.*, first surgery on a virgin eye) the results were found to be better.[102,103] With MMC, cumulative success rates of 59-90% at two years and 51% at five years have been reported.[19,33,107]

CONSENSUS SURVEY: Of the experts surveyed, 81% would use anti-scarring agents, 65% a fornix-based conjunctival flap and 27% would use adjustable/releasable sutures when performing trabeculectomy. Seventeen percent also use an intra-operative AC maintainer.

In PCG after failed repeat angle surgery, 62% experts would perform trabeculectomy as their next surgery. Trabeculectomy was reported as the first line option for JOAG by 68%; for AR anomaly and Peters anomaly by 45%.

Glaucoma drainage device (GDD)

Glaucoma drainage device surgery (also known as glaucoma implant/tube and aqueous shunt) is an important part of the therapeutic repertoire in childhood glaucoma, especially for those children with refractory glaucoma whose disease relentlessly progresses or as the first surgical procedure in certain secondary childhood glaucomas. Since their introduction it appears that the threshold for performing GDD surgery in childhood glaucoma has lowered. The indications, advantages and disadvantages of GDDs are summarized in Table 4.

The use of a GDD in children was first described by Molteno in 1973.[108] The design of all GDDs is similar in that a tube is connected to a reservoir (plate) that shunts aqueous from the AC to the equator but they differ largely according to the implant material, surface area of the plate and whether there is restriction to aqueous flow. The Ahmed implant is a popular flow-restricted device with a built-in 'valve' designed to regulate aqueous outflow and reduce the risk of hypotony. The Baerveldt and the Molteno implants are not flow-restricted and so measures are required to prevent hypotony. Both Molteno and Ahmed implants are available in smaller pediatric versions (Ahmed Model S3 and FP8 [96 mm^2] and Molteno M1 implant [8 mm diameter plate]).

The most commonly used GDDs worldwide in children are the Ahmed (184 mm^2) and Baerveldt (250 mm^2 and 350 mm^2) depending on surgeon preference and case circumstances. The use of adult size implants is recommended where possible to take advantage of the larger surface area. The Ahmed implant plate is also available as either polypropylene or silicone. Studies comparing the polypropylene against silicone Ahmed implant in children, have shown better long-term IOP control with the silicone Ahmed (model FP7 or FP8). It has been suggested that the implant material and design of an Ahmed implant may be more important than plate area in providing IOP control.[109,110]

The most commonly used GDDs have single-quadrant placement. For Baerveldt implants, it is advisable to place the plate behind the rectus muscles to prevent anterior plate migration. Avoiding a limbal conjunctival incision may be considered in aniridia due to the underlying limbal stem cell deficiency. Depending on the clinical scenario, the location of the tube can be in the anterior chamber, sulcus or pars plana. The location of the tube and certain diagnoses will influence the length of the tube. For sulcus and pars plana approaches, it is preferable to leave the tube long enough to allow tip visualization when assessing for tube occlusion with either iris or vitreous. In aniridia, a short tube with oblique AC orientation directed away from lens can be used both to avoid lens trauma and minimize corneal endothelial cell loss.[111] In uveitis, longer tubes may be used to allow easier occlusion in cases of post-operative hypotony. This also reduces the risk of tube occlusion or incarceration from advancing PAS.

Plate encapsulation is a major cause of GDD failure requiring the majority of patients to recommence topical medications. In the adult literature, prospective randomized control trials have suggested that after a mean follow-up of just one

Table 4. Glaucoma drainage devices

	Indications	Advantages	Disadvantages
Glaucoma drainage devices	• Following failed surgery (angle surgery or trabeculectomy) • As initial surgery when: • Surgeon has limited experience with angle surgery and/or trabeculectomy • Patient unlikely to respond to angle surgery (very early or late presentation, or racial groups known with lower success) • Secondary glaucomas such as Axenfeld Rieger Anomaly, Peters anomaly, Sturge-Weber, aniridia and especially aphakia and uveitic glaucoma • Future intraocular surgery particularly cataract surgery is contemplated as it is more likely to control IOP postoperatively than trabeculectomy	• Effective in long term IOP reduction even after failed trabeculectomy with anti-scarring agents • Most likely to survive future intraocular surgery (*e.g.*, penetrating keratoplasty, lensectomy, vitrectomy), therefore best drainage option in these circumstances • Contact lens wear possible in aphakic glaucoma	• Higher complication rates regardless of implant used • Longest rehabilitation period if tube is totally occluded with extraluminal and intraluminal sutures to prevent hypotony • Needs competent accessible vitreo-retinal surgeon in preparation for pars plana placed tubes

year, there was no advantage to augmenting GDD surgery with MMC in terms of IOP control, medication use or complications, supporting the evidence from retrospective studies.[112-114] However, the role of MMC is yet to be established in pediatric patients. A retrospective study in 31 infant eyes suggested that MMC use with Ahmed implants was associated with worse outcomes after a two-year follow-up. However, there appeared to be selection bias with differences between the MMC group and the non-MMC group in underlying diagnoses and previous numbers of interventions (surgery and diode).[25] Another smaller retrospective, non-randomized study involving 19 eyes showed no difference in IOP control with MMC or without MMC using Ahmed implants in aphakic glaucoma.[115] A prospective randomized study comparing Bevacizumab 1.25 mg to either high dose MMC 0.4 mg/ml for three minutes or no treatment with Ahmed implant (20 eyes in each group) suggested improved success with treatment (80% overall success for Bevacizumab vs. 90% MMC vs. 60% no treatment) at one year.[116] Two eyes developed tube exposure (10%) in the Ahmed group with no adjuvant treatment, no eyes (0%) in the Bevacizumab group, compared to four eyes (20%) in the Ahmed group with MMC, one of which resulted in perception of light and phthisis. The other eye which developed light perception vision in the MMC group, was due to 'optic atrophy'.

GDDs offer the most effective long-term IOP control in many childhood glaucomas, but they have a significant complication profile, even more so than adults, related commonly to either hypotony or the tube itself.[20,22,25,27,117-120] Complications due to hypotony include shallow or flat AC, hypotony maculopathy, choroidal effusion, suprachoroidal hemorrhage and phthisis. Lens and corneal touch may lead to cataract and corneal decompensation. Buphthalmic eyes are especially prone to hypotony-related complications because of the reduced scleral rigidity allowing leakage around the tube at its entry site; making subsequent problems such as choroidal effusions and suprachoroidal hemorrhage more likely, even with the use of valved implants.[24,121-123] Modifications in surgical technique to protect from intra- and postoperative hypotony are mandatory (*see* Table 5). Tube related complications include tube erosion, occlusion, migration, corneal touch, iris touch and lens touch. When these occur, a high revision rate has been reported in children under two years of age.[22] Anterior tube migration may occur with normalization of IOP or inadequate fixation of the plate. Posterior migration may take place because of uncontrolled IOP with globe enlargement, as well as an aggressive healing/scarring response causing retraction. Corneal touch may lead to corneal decompensation[124] and iris touch (chaffing) may cause iritis and corectopia. Motility issues and strabismus should also be considered in children.[125]

Several studies have reported the success rates of GDDs to be around 80% with a mean follow-up of two years or less.[20,110,126,127] This falls to approximately 50% with longer-term follow-up.[22,23,128,129] Success does not appear to be influenced by the type of implant used.[130] The choice of implant is determined by availability, the surgeon's experience and the special circumstances of the case. The ongoing attrition in success rate with follow up and the requirement for adjunctive medication are common to all studies.

Table 5. Preventing complications in glaucoma drainage device surgery

Complications	Preventative strategies
Anterior tube migration	• Secure plate and tube well to minimize migration • Place Baerveldt plate behind rectus muscles
Posterior tube migration	• Secure plate and tube well • Avoid very short tube
Corneal decompensation	• Place tube away from cornea and as posterior as possible in anterior chamber • Avoid long tube
Intra or postoperative hypotony	• AC maintainer • Relatively long, snug limbal tunnel incision (eg. 25G needle usually adequate for tube entry as sclera is elastic) • Intraluminal stent in non-valved GDDs (e.g., 3/0 Supramid suture) • Extraluminal ligating vicryl suture in non-valved GDDs (e.g., 6/0 vicryl) with venting 'Sherwood' slit anterior to the suture[167] • Viscoelastic or gas in AC at end of surgery • Two stage implantation[117,122,168]
Tube obstruction	• In aphakic cases with AC or sulcus placed tubes, ensure no vitreous present or likely to prolapse into AC otherwise consider vitrectomy • For pars plana tube placement extensive posterior vitrectomy required • Treat inflammation aggressively • Leave tube long in uveitics – reduces risk of iris related obstruction from peripheral anterior synechiae
Tube erosion	• Intrascleral tunnel with entry into AC at or as posterior to limbus as possible – avoid corneal tunnel which is more likely to erode • Oblique entry into eye rather than 90 degree which may produce knuckle of tube at entry point • Patch graft: sclera or cornea, other tissue (e.g., pericardium) along whole of tube length • Avoiding conjunctival tension over limbal area with closure; may require conjunctival relieving incisions and advancement • Tube entry when inferiorly placed should be covered by lower lid

CONSENSUS SURVEY: Most experts use the Ahmed implant (63%) followed by the Baerveldt impant (41%) with 15% favoring the adjunctive use of anti-scarring agents, although 92% thought that better drainage devices were needed for childhood glaucoma. Most surgeons prefer anterior chamber tube placement, except under special circumstances where the cornea has failed or is at risk of failing, there is an extremely shallow or obliterated AC or when a simultaneous vitreoretinal procedure is required.

GDD surgery was the preferred primary operation chosen by 44% of experts for glaucoma following removal of childhood cataract and by 30% for uveitic glaucoma. After failed trabeculectomy, 82% of experts would opt next for GDD surgery whereas after failed angle surgery 53% of experts preferred it as the next surgical option.

Cyclodestruction

Cyclodestruction was traditionally reserved for challenging, refractory cases with poor surgical prognoses because of significant complications, especially with cyclocryotherapy.[131] This has now largely been replaced with laser cyclophotocoagulation, which is less destructive. Transscleral diode laser (810 nm) has become increasingly more popular than Nd:YAG laser[132,133] because it is better tolerated and associated with fewer complications. Transscleral diode laser requires transillumination of the eye to ensure accurate laser placement (buphthalmic eyes often have distorted landmarks). Furthermore, it is important to avoid areas of pigmentation, hemorrhage and scleral thinning to prevent scleral perforation, which has been described in a buphthalmic eye.[134] A further refinement has been endoscopic diode laser, which allows precise treatment of the ciliary processes, however it requires an intraocular approach.[135] For indications, advantages and disadvantages of cyclodestruction refer to Table 6.

Complications associated with transscleral diode laser include: hypotony, significant uveitis, phthisis, conjunctival burns, uveitis, scleromalacia, cataract, retinal detachment and loss of vision with up to 18% reported mostly in eyes with ≥ 2 treatments or in eyes with pre-existing poor vision. [133,136-138]

Short-to-medium term outcomes of transscleral diode laser quote over 50% success with medical therapy[137,138] achieved with total energy doses of between 74 and 113 J and a variable retreatment rate of 33-70%.[136,137] Similar results are achieved with endoscopic diode but with a lower re-treatment rate.[135,139] In the largest reported series, Kirwan *et al.* found aphakic eyes to have a more sustained lowering of IOP compared to the other secondary glaucomas, however, 9% (3/34) aphakic eyes developed a retinal detachment,[137] a similar figure to that of endoscopic diode (6%).[139]

In summary, diode laser cyclophotocoagulation is difficult to titrate with a transscleral approach, has limited long term success rates, often requires re-treatment and continuation of medications, and lastly may be associated with vision-threatening complications. Most clinicians reserve cyclodestruction until other treatments have failed but some advocate it early in the treatment regimen, moving on to GDD surgery if it fails.

CONSENSUS SURVEY: Transscleral diode laser was preferred by 78% of specialists (31% advocated transillumination) and 21% preferred an endoscopic approach. Ninety-five percent of experts would move to cyclodestruction when other surgeries have failed.

Cyclodestruction as an initial procedure would be performed by 15% of experts for blind and painful eyes, as temporizing measure before surgery and when the risk/consequence of hypotony is high such as in Sturge-Weber syndrome and aphakia.

Table 6. Cyclodestruction

	Indications	Advantages	Disadvantages

Cyclodestruction	• Blind, painful eye
	• Poor visual potential
	• Poor prognosis with surgery
	• Other surgeries technically difficult/impossible, *e.g.*, severely scarred conjunctiva or significant ocular abnormalities
	• As adjunct to other surgery – *i.e.*, in hypertensive phase of tube; after failed tube; at time of vitrectomy/lens extraction with endoscopic approach; after graft surgery
	• As temporizing measure, *e.g.*, an acute presentation of significantly elevated IOP or if cannot proceed with more definitive procedure, *e.g.*, fellow eye has undergone major surgery
		• Short surgical time and rapid rehabilitation
		• Good short-term response
		• Technically easier
		• Useful when surgery is high risk especially in only eyes
		• Endoscopic diode allows precise treatment and avoids risk of scleral perforation
			• Often needs to be repeated in > 50% of cases due to ciliary body recovery
			• Most patients remain on medical therapy
			• Pressure control is worse than filtering surgery
			• Risk of phthisis with multiple recurrent treatments
			• Endoscopic diode requires intraocular approach with risk of infection and cataract formation
			• May affect future glaucoma drainage device surgery
			  • Possible chronic hypotony due to hyposecretion or fibrotic failure due to effect on blood-aqueous barrier
			  • scleral thinning at burn sites may make future suture and tube positioning difficult
			• Pro-inflammatory and may accelerate cataract formation

Other glaucoma procedures

There are reports of non-penetrating surgery in children with glaucoma or adult patients with CG. This has been suggested as an alternative to trabeculectomy surgery, on the basis that it is potentially associated with less overfiltration and early postoperative hypotony and avoids the complications of thin avascular blebs. Despite this advantageous risk profile it has not been widely adopted because it is technically challenging in buphthalmic eyes with thin sclera.

Initial results from a small series of 12 eyes in which deep sclerectomy was performed as primary surgery in nine eyes, reported a 75% success rate but with a short follow-up of only ten months and no significant complications.[140] In contrast to this study, Lüke et al. highlighted in their series the risks of deep sclerectomy in the buphthalmic eye with thin sclera, abnormal limbus and location of Schlemm canal.[141] A more recent study of 43 eyes with a mean follow up of almost two years, reported 30% (13 eyes) requiring conversion to trabeculectomy. In this series, the overall success rate (including medications) for the entire group of cases treated by single non-penetrating surgery (without anti-scarring agents) was 58% (25 of 43 eyes).[142] A larger series from Saudi Arabia with 143 eyes undergoing primary deep sclerectomy with MMC (0.2 mg/ml) showed better success rates without major complications. The overall success rate for the group was 86% at 35.8 months, but nearly 50% had macroperforation and required conversion to 'penetrating deep sclerectomy'. For the 74 eyes without macroperforations, the overall success rate was 82.4%.[143]

In an attempt to modify deep sclerectomy to make it safer and more effective in such eyes, Feusier et al.[144] proposed a combined deep sclerectomy and trabeculectomy approach to create an intrascleral bleb that might be less affected by postoperative fibrosis and so increase long term success. In a single surgeon series of 35 eyes, combined deep sclerectomy and trabeculectomy resulted in the cumulative chance of complete and qualified success, of 52.3% and 70.6% respectively, after nine years. This was a mixed cohort of PCG, secondary and juvenile glaucomas and also showed that those eyes that had undergone previous surgeries or which had advanced glaucoma, had a higher risk of sight-threatening complications.

Another series from the Middle East compared viscocanalostomy to conventional trabeculotomy in a small group of children with PCG and found them to be equally efficacious after a mean follow-up of one year.[145] Certainly the learning curve is steep and longer-term results are necessary.

Numerous other glaucoma procedures have been described in adults in the literature, and include suprachoroidal shunts (SOLX, Cypass), canaloplasty and trabecular removal (e.g., Trabectome). Trabectome, 'ab interno trabeculotomy', is a disposable, high frequency electrocautery hand piece that removes the inner wall of Schlemm canal. Like a goniotomy, the hand piece is introduced in the temporal cornea, passed over the lens to treat the opposite angle, and a clear view of the angle is thus required. Although there are studies that include pediatric cases, there are no published results that specifically detail the outcomes in children.[146] Further research into these and the newer minimally invasive glaucoma procedures: tra-becular meshwork bypass shunts (*e.g.*, iStent, Hydrus) and trans-scleral shunt (Aquesys Xen) are required with regards to efficacy and safety before they can be recommended for use in children.

Visual rehabilitation

Concurrent to controlling IOP, it is essential to correct ametropia and commence amblyopia therapy if indicated, in order to maximise the visual potential. Children with significant visual impairment can be helped by low visual aids and should be referred for assessment.

Follow up

It is important to remember that even with long term well controlled IOP, relapse can occur at any stage. Following successful goniotomy, approximately 2-3% of eyes each year and 20% over a 30-year period were found to relapse.[42] Children who required multiple goniotomies in infancy were more likely to relapse than those controlled by a single procedure. Furthermore, sight threatening complica-tions may occur at any time, even after years of stability.[147] This emphasizes the need for lifelong follow-up.

Combining glaucoma surgery with other surgery

Performing simultaneous glaucoma and other ocular surgery potentially increases the risks of surgery and renders the outcomes less certain. The surgical requirements and success must be balanced with repeated or prolonged anesthetic time. Careful planning is essential with the impact of each surgery on the other meriting careful consideration. A cohesive approach requires good relationships and access to skil-ful colleagues with pediatric cataract, corneal or vitreoretinal expertise.

In a retrospective study of simultaneous combined Ahmed implants and penetrat-ing keratoplasty in 20 infant eyes (mean age at surgery 11.7 months) the long-term success was low and complication rate high. At 48 months, only 33% of eyes achieved an IOP $\leq$ 21 mmHg and the graft survival rate was 17%. There was a significant risk of infection in the series, six eyes had infective corneal ulceration (30%) and two eyes endophthalmitis (10%), one from a corneal ulcer and another due to tube erosion.[148]

Most consensus specialists (86%) preferred consecutive rather than combined simultaneous surgeries when more than one procedure was required.

Lens surgery and glaucoma

When contemplating glaucoma surgery, the status of the lens, and the likelihood of any lens-related surgery, should also be considered. The underlying disease mechanism is also relevant as cataracts and glaucoma may be part of the same disease phenotype such as in Lowe syndrome, congenital rubella, aniridia, and persistent fetal vasculature. Glaucoma may also follow cataract extraction or be secondary to lens subluxation (*see* Sections 8 and 10). The variations in presentation will dictate when or if lens extraction and/or glaucoma surgery are required, but both should be performed with consideration of the other, generally favoring isolated glaucoma surgery, rather than combined procedures, to minimize risks.

Role of corneal surgery in childhood glaucoma

As with the lens, there is an intimate relationship between corneal pathology and glaucoma in pediatric cases. Both corneal pathology and glaucoma may co-exist as part of the primary disease phenotype, or each can arise secondary to the other, or as a complication of surgery for either. As corneal clarity is profoundly affected by IOP, reducing IOP before turning to corneal surgery is advocated. Successful glaucoma surgery may eliminate or delay the need for corneal grafting. If corneal surgery is contemplated, IOP should be addressed first, if possible.

Penetrating keratoplasty generally has poor results in childhood glaucoma, especially in the very young.[149-152] Descemet stripping endothelial keratoplasty (DSEK), Descemet stripping automated endothelial keratoplasty (DSAEK) and Descemet membrane endothelial keratoplasty (DMEK) may be safer procedures but more studies are required.[153-155] These more modern surgeries are probably best avoided in eyes with a previous trabeculectomy as air is injected into the AC under pressure to tamponade the back of the graft; in eyes with a trabeculectomy the air may pass through the sclerostomy and result in bleb rupture. Tubes positioned in the AC may also compromise DSEK outcome because of proximity of tube to graft, particularly in a small eye. In such cases a pars plana approach would have the advantage of protecting the cornea or corneal graft from tube touch, however, this also requires lensectomy and thorough vitrectomy to prevent tube occlusion by vitreous. Intensive steroids are required in the short term if any surgery, including transscleral diode laser, is performed in the presence of a corneal graft to reduce high risk of rejection.

Options following failed surgery

Failed angle surgery (goniotomy and conventional trabeculotomy)

Options:

1. Repeat angle surgery
   - if some response from initial surgery
   - may repeat up to three times in promising cases
   - may repeat and combine with trabeculectomy (CTT)
   - performing circumferential trabeculotomy after goniotomy or conventional trabeculotomy is not advised as the suture or the microcatheter may enter the AC.
2. Trabeculectomy (± anti-scarring agent).
3. Glaucoma drainage device.

CONSENSUS SURVEY: After failed angle surgery, 51% of experts would repeat angle surgery (depending on initial response, age, severity of glaucoma), 22% would perform trabeculectomy and 15% would proceed with a GDD.

Failed combined trabeculotomy-trabeculectomy

Options:
1. Bleb needling.
2. Trabeculectomy (+ anti-scarring agent).
3. Glaucoma drainage device.

CONSENSUS SURVEY: Forty-two percent of experts would move onto GDD surgery, 18% would perform trabeculectomy with anti-scarring agent and 13% would perform bleb needing.

Failed trabeculectomy

Options:
1. Bleb needling with anti-scarring agent if bleb architecture allows and sclerostomy patent.
2. Repeat trabeculectomy with anti-scarring agent.
3. Glaucoma drainage device.

CONSENSUS SURVEY: Forty-seven percent of experts would move onto GDD surgery, 12% would repeat trabeculectomy surgery with anti-scarring agent and 28% would perform bleb needling.

Failed glaucoma drainage device (GDD)

Plate fibrosis, scarring, encapsulation

Options:
1. Second GDD (± anti-scarring agent) without removing the first implant.[26,156,157]
2. Bleb needling + anti-scarring agent.

3. Capsule excision ± anti-scarring agent.
4. Cyclodestruction.[156]

CONSENSUS SURVEY: The experts were fairly evenly split with regards the next procedure following a failed GDD: 26% of experts would proceed with cyclodestruction, 26% would revise the GDD (capsule excision ± anti-scarring agent) and 23% would insert a second GDD. Only 9% would perform bleb needling.

Tube occlusion

Options depend on the cause of the occlusion:
1. Flushing the tube.
2. AC washout.
3. Vitrectomy.
4. Iridectomy.
5. Fracture of leaflets in Ahmed.

Tube retraction

Options:
1. Tube repositioning.
2. Tube extension using angiocatheter material[158] or a commercial tube extender, however, it must be fixated well as they have been reported to migrate[159] or spontaneously disconnect[160]
3. Second GDD (± anti-scarring agent).
4. Cyclodestruction.

Surgery in childhood glaucomas

The surgical management of the following conditions have been discussed in the relevant sections of this WGA consensus. We present here the first-line surgical preference of the international experts surveyed according to type of glaucoma.

Surgery in primary congenital glaucoma

CONSENSUS SURVEY:
- Goniotomy   28%
- Trabeculotomy (probe)   28%
- Circumferential trabeculotomy   13%
- CTT   14%
- Trabeculectomy   1%
- GDD   1%
- Other   15%

There was no significant difference between pediatric ophthalmologists and glaucoma specialists.

The factors that influenced the choice of procedures were complex, some of which included surgical training, geographical location, severity of glaucoma on presentation and whether the procedure violated the conjunctiva or not.

Surgery in secondary glaucomas

Uveitic Glaucoma

CONSENSUS SURVEY:
- GDD   30%
- Trabeculectomy   26%
- Angle surgery   22%   (goniotomy (14%) > trabeculotomy (8%))
- CTT   9%
- Other   13%

Thirty-three percent would perform goniosynechialysis and 85% would use perioperative systemic immunosuppressive drugs.

Glaucoma following cataract surgery

CONSENSUS SURVEY:
- GDD   44%
- Trabeculectomy   21%
- Angle surgery   19%   (trabeculotomy > goniotomy > circumferential trabeculotomy)
- CTT   6%
- Other   10%

Sturge-Weber syndrome

CONSENSUS SURVEY:
For children < 3 years of age:
- Angle surgery   48%   (goniotomy (26%) > trabeculotomy (17%) > circumferential trabeculotomy (5%))
- CTT   19%
- Trabeculectomy   8%
- GDD   8%
- Other   17%

For children > 3 years of age:
- GDD   32%
- Trabeculectomy   24%

- Angle surgery   15%   (trabeculotomy (9%) > goniotomy (3%) = circumferential trabeculotomy)
- CTT   15%
- Other   14%

Eighty-one percent would take specific precautions to minimize complications with surgery in patients with Sturge-Weber syndrome.

Aniridia with glaucoma

CONSENSUS SURVEY:

For open angles:
- Angle surgery   31%   (trabeculotomy (15%) > goniotomy (13%) > circumferential trabeculotomy (3%))
- GDD   26%
- CTT   19%
- Trabeculectomy   12%
- Other   12%

For closed angles:
- GDD   37%
- Trabeculectomy   28%
- Angle surgery   14%   (goniotomy (7%) = trabeculotomy (7%) > circumferential trabeculotomy (0%))
- CTT   13%
- Other   8%

Fifty-four percent would take specific precautions to minimize complications with surgery in aniridic patients. The main concern of the consensus group was lens damage. Many surgeons use either viscoelastic or an anterior chamber maintainer during surgery.

GDD surgery needs precise placement (oblique placement advocated by several surgeons), both to avoid lens trauma and minimize corneal endothelial cell loss.

References

1. Khaw PT, Freedman S, Gandolfi S. Management of congenital glaucoma. J Glaucoma 1999; 8: 81-85.
2. Aponte EP, Diehl N, Mohney BG. Medical and surgical outcomes in childhood glaucoma: a population-based study. J AAPOS 2011; 15: 263-267.
3. Ou Y, Caprioli J. Surgical management of pediatric glaucoma. Dev Ophthalmol 2012; 50: 157-172.

4.   McPherson SD, Jr., McFarland D. External trabeculotomy for developmental glaucoma. Ophthalmology 1980; 87: 302-305.
5.   Inaba Z. Long-term results of trabeculectomy in the Japanese: an analysis by life-table method. Jpn J Ophthalmol 1982; 26: 361-373.
6.   Broadway DC, Grierson I, Hitchings RA. Local effects of previous conjunctival incisional surgery and the subsequent outcome of filtration surgery. Am J Ophthalmol 1998; 125: 805-818.
7.   Dietlein TS, Jacobi PC, Krieglstein GK. Prognosis of primary ab externo surgery for primary congenital glaucoma. Br J Ophthalmol 1999; 83: 317-322.
8.   Khaw PT, Narita A, Rice N. The developmental glaucomas. In: Easty DL, Sparrow JM (Eds.), Oxford textbook of ophthalmology, Oxford: Oxford University Press 1999, pp. 92-110.
9.   Khaw PT, Fraser S, Papadopoulos M, et al. The childhood glaucomas: assessment. In: Hitchings RA (Ed.), Glaucoma. London: BMJ Books 2000: 171-182.
10. Khaw PT, Fraser S, Papadopoulos M, et al. The childhood glaucomas: management. In: Hitchings RA (Ed.), Glaucoma. London: BMJ Books 2000, pp. 183-195.
11. Papadopoulos M, Khaw PT. Childhood glaucoma. In: Taylor D, Hoyt CS (Eds.), Pediatric ophthalmology and strabismus. 3rd ed. London/New York: Elsevier Saunders 2005, pp. 458-471.
12. Papadopoulos M, Khaw PT. Goniotomy and Trabeculectomy. In: Shaarawy T, Sherwood MB, Hitchings RA, Crowston JG (Eds.), Glaucoma. Philadelphia: Saunders/Elsevier 2009, pp. 493-499.
13. Mandal AK, Netland PA. Initial surgical treatment of congenital glaucoma. In: Mandal AK, Netland PA (Eds.), The pediatric glaucomas. Philadelphia, PA: Elsevier Butterworth Heinemann 2006, pp. 65-75.
14. Maeda-Chubachi T, Chi-Burris K, Simons BD, et al. Comparison of latanoprost and timolol in pediatric glaucoma: a phase 3, 12-week, randomized, double-masked multicenter study. Ophthalmology 2011; 118: 2014-2021.
15. Maeda-Chubachi T, Chi-Burris K, Simons B, et al. Impact of Age, Diagnosis, and History of Glaucoma Surgery on Outcomes in Pediatric Patients Treated With Latanoprost. J Glaucoma 2013 Mar 20; doi: 10.1097/IJG.0b013e31824d4fb9. [Advanced online publication].
16. Gressel MG, Heuer DK, Parrish RK, 2nd. Trabeculectomy in young patients. Ophthalmology 1984; 91: 1242-1246.
17. Susanna R Jr, Oltrogge EW, Carani JC, Nicolela MT. Mitomycin as adjunct chemotherapy with trabeculectomy in congenital and developmental glaucomas. J Glaucoma 1995; 4: 151-157.
18. Freedman SF, McCormick K, Cox TA. Mitomycin C-augumented trabeculectomy with postoperative wound modulation in pediatric glaucoma. J AAPOS 1999; 3: 117-124.
19. Sidoti PA, Belmonte SJ, Liebmann JM, Ritch R. Trabeculectomy with mitomycin-C in the treatment of pediatric glaucomas. Ophthalmology 2000; 107: 422-429.
20. Fellenbaum PS, Sidoti PA, Heuer DK, et al. Experience with the Baerveldt implant in young patients with complicated glaucomas. J Glaucoma 1995; 4: 91-97.
21. Cunliffe IA, Molteno AC. Long-term follow-up of Molteno drains used in the treatment of glaucoma presenting in childhood. Eye (Lond) 1998; 12 (Pt 3a):379-385.
22. Beck AD, Freedman S, Kammer J, Jin J. Aqueous shunt devices compared with trabeculectomy with Mitomycin-C for children in the first two years of life. Am J Ophthalmol 2003; 136: 994-1000.
23. van Overdam KA, de Faber JT, Lemij HG, de Waard PW. Baerveldt glaucoma implant in paediatric patients. Br J Ophthalmol 2006; 90: 328-332.
24. O'Malley Schotthoefer E, Yanovitch TL, Freedman SF. Aqueous drainage device surgery in refractory pediatric glaucomas: I. Long-term outcomes. J AAPOS 2008; 12: 33-39.
25. Al-Mobarak F, Khan AO. Two-year survival of Ahmed valve implantation in the first 2 years of life with and without intraoperative mitomycin-C. Ophthalmology 2009; 116: 1862-1865.

26. Ou Y, Yu F, Law SK, et al. Outcomes of Ahmed glaucoma valve implantation in children with primary congenital glaucoma. Arch Ophthalmol 2009; 127: 1436-1441.
27. Nassiri N, Nouri-Mahdavi K, Coleman A. Ahmed glaucoma valve in children: A review. Saudi Journal of Ophthalmology 2011; 25: 317-327.
28. Beck AD. Primary congenital glaucoma in the developing world. Ophthalmology 2011; 118: 229-230.
29. Moore DB, Tomkins O, Ben-Zion I. A review of primary congenital glaucoma in the developing world. Surv Ophthalmol 2013; 58: 278-285.
30. Khitri MR, Mills MD, Ying GS, et al. Visual acuity outcomes in pediatric glaucomas. J AAPOS 2012; 16: 376-381.
31. Zhang XL, Du SL, Ge J, et al. [Quality of life in patients with primary congenital glaucoma following antiglaucoma surgical management]. Zhonghua Yan Ke Za Zhi 2009; 45: 514-521.
32. Dada T, Aggarwal A, Bali SJ, et al. Caregiver burden assessment in primary congenital glaucoma. Eur J Ophthalmol 2013; 23: 324-328.
33. Beck AD, Wilson WR, Lynch MG, et al. Trabeculectomy with adjunctive mitomycin C in pediatric glaucoma. Am J Ophthalmol 1998; 126: 648-657.
34. Azuara-Blanco A, Wilson RP, Spaeth GL, et al. Filtration procedures supplemented with mitomycin C in the management of childhood glaucoma. Br J Ophthalmol 1999; 83: 151-156.
35. Mandal AK, Bagga H, Nutheti R, et al. Trabeculectomy with or without mitomycin-C for paediatric glaucoma in aphakia and pseudophakia following congenital cataract surgery. Eye (Lond) 2003; 17: 53-62.
36. Haas JS. End results of treatment. Trans Am Acad Ophthalmol Otolaryngol 1955; 59: 333-341.
37. Lister A. The prognosis in congenital glaucoma. Trans Ophthalmol Soc U K 1966; 86: 5-18.
38. Walton DS. Primary congenital open-angle glaucoma. In: Chandler PA, Grant WM, Epstein DL (Eds.), Chandler and Grant's Glaucoma. 2nd ed. Philadelphia: Lea & Febiger 1979, pp. 329-343.
39. Akimoto M, Tanihara H, Negi A, Nagata M. Surgical results of trabeculotomy ab externo for developmental glaucoma. Arch Ophthalmol 1994; 112: 1540-1544.
40. Morin JD, Merin S, Sheppard RW. Primary congenital glaucoma – a survey. Can J Ophthalmol 1974; 9: 17-28.
41. Shaffer RN. Prognosis of goniotomy in primary infantile glaucoma (trabeculodysgenesis). Trans Am Ophthalmol Soc 1982; 80: 321-325.
42. Russell-Eggitt IM, Rice NS, Jay B, Wyse RK. Relapse following goniotomy for congenital glaucoma due to trabecular dysgenesis. Eye (Lond) 1992; 6: 197-200.
43. De Vincentiis C. Incisione dell'angolo irideo nel glaucoma. Ann di Ottal 1893; 22: 540-542.
44. Barkan O. A new operation for chronic glaucoma. Am J Ophthalmol 1936; 19: 951-966.
45. Barkan O. Operation for congenital glaucoma. Am J Ophthalmol 1942; 25: 552-568.
46. Smith R. A new technique for opening the canal of Schlemm. Preliminary report. Br J Ophthalmol 1960; 44: 370-373.
47. Burian HM. A case of Marfan's syndrome with bilateral glaucoma. With description of a new type of operation for developmental glaucoma (trabeculotomy ab externo). Am J Ophthalmol 1960; 50: 1187-1192.
48. Allen L, Burian HM. Trabeculotomy ab externo. A new glaucoma operation: technique and results of experimental surgery. Am J Ophthalmol 1962; 53: 19-26.
49. Harms H, Dannheim R. Epicritical consideration of 300 cases of trabeculotomy 'ab externo'. Trans Ophthalmol Soc U K 1969; 89: 491-499.
50. Joos KM, Alward WL, Folberg R. Experimental endoscopic goniotomy. A potential treatment for primary infantile glaucoma. Ophthalmology 1993; 100: 1066-1070.
51. Medow NB, Sauer HL. Endoscopic goniotomy for congenital glaucoma. J Pediatr Ophthalmol Strabismus 1997; 34: 258-259.

52. Joos KM, Shen JH. An ocular endoscope enables a goniotomy despite a cloudy cornea. Arch Ophthalmol 2001; 119: 134-135.

53. Kulkarni SV, Damji KF, Fournier AV, et al. Endoscopic goniotomy: early clinical experience in congenital glaucoma. J Glaucoma 2010; 19: 264-269.

54. Beck AD, Lynch MG. 360 degrees trabeculotomy for primary congenital glaucoma. Arch Ophthalmol 1995; 113: 1200-1202.

55. Sarkisian SR, Jr. An illuminated microcatheter for 360-degree trabeculotomy [corrected] in congenital glaucoma: a retrospective case series. J AAPOS 2010; 14: 412-416.

56. Beck AD, Lynn MJ, Crandall J, Mobin-Uddin O. Surgical outcomes with 360-degree suture trabeculotomy in poor-prognosis primary congenital glaucoma and glaucoma associated with congenital anomalies or cataract surgery. J AAPOS 2011; 15: 54-58.

57. Girkin CA, Rhodes L, McGwin G, et al. Goniotomy versus circumferential trabeculotomy with an illuminated microcatheter in congenital glaucoma. J AAPOS 2012; 16: 424-427.

58. Maul E, Strozzi L, Munoz C, Reyes C. The outflow pathway in congenital glaucoma. Am J Ophthalmol 1980; 89: 667-673.

59. Litinsky SM, Shaffer RN, Hetherington J, Hoskins HD. Operative complications of goniotomy. Trans Sect Ophthalmol Am Acad Ophthalmol Otolaryngol 1977; 83: 78-79.

60. Senft SH, Tomey KF, Traverso CE. Neodymium-YAG laser goniotomy vs surgical goniotomy. A preliminary study in paired eyes. Arch Ophthalmol 1989; 107: 1773-1776.

61. Shaffer RN. Prognosis of Goniotomy in Primary Infantile Glaucoma (Trabeculodysgenesis). In: Krieglstein GK, Leydhecker W (Eds.), Glaucoma update II. Berlin: Springer-Verlag 1983, pp. 185-188.

62. Rice NSC. The surgical management of congenital glaucomas. Aust J Ophthalmol. 1977; 5: 174-179.

63. Rummelt V, Naumann GO. Cystic epithelial ingrowth after goniotomy for congenital glaucoma. A clinicopathologic report. J Glaucoma 1997; 6: 353-356.

64. Barkan O. Surgery of congenital glaucoma; review of 196 eyes operated by goniotomy. Am J Ophthalmol 1953; 36: 1523-1534.

65. Bietti GB. Contribution a la connaissance des résultats de la goniotomie dans le glaucome congénital. [Contribution to the knowledge of the results of goniotomy in congenital glaucoma]. Ann Ocul (Paris) 1966; 199: 481-496.

66. Douglas DH. Reflections on buphthalmos and goniotomy. Trans Ophthalmol Soc U K 1970; 90: 931-937.

67. Luntz MH, Livingston DG. Trabeculotomy ab externo and trabeculectomy in congenital and adult-onset glaucoma. Am J Ophthalmol 1977; 83: 174-179.

68. Bowman RJ, Dickerson M, Mwende J, Khaw PT. Outcomes of goniotomy for primary congenital glaucoma in East Africa. Ophthalmology 2011; 118: 236-240.

69. Elder MJ. Congenital glaucoma in the West Bank and Gaza Strip. Br J Ophthalmol 1993; 77: 413-416.

70. al-Hazmi A, Awad A, Zwaan J, et al. Correlation between surgical success rate and severity of congenital glaucoma. Br J Ophthalmol 2005; 89: 449-453.

71. Shaffer RN, Weiss DI. Congenital and pediatric glaucomas. Saint Louis: Mosby 1970.

72. Tamcelik N, Ozkiris A. Long-term results of viscotrabeculotomy in congenital glaucoma: comparison to classical trabeculotomy. Br J Ophthalmol 2008; 92: 36-39.

73. Neely DE. False passage: a complication of 360 degrees suture trabeculotomy. J AAPOS 2005; 9: 396-397.

74. Meyer G, Schwenn O, Pfeiffer N, Grehn F. Trabeculotomy in congenital glaucoma. Graefes Arch Clin Exp Ophthalmol 2000; 238: 207-213.

75. Gloor BR. [Risks of 360 degree suture trabeculotomy]. Ophthalmologe 1998; 95: 100-103. Gefahren der 360 degrees-Fadentrabekulotomie.

76. Anderson DR. Trabeculotomy compared to goniotomy for glaucoma in children. Ophthalmology 1983; 90: 805-806.

77. Mendicino ME, Lynch MG, Drack A, et al. Long-term surgical and visual outcomes in primary congenital glaucoma: 360 degrees trabeculotomy versus goniotomy. J AAPOS 2000; 4: 205-210.
78. Mandal AK, Naduvilath TJ, Jayagandan A. Surgical results of combined trabeculotomy-trabeculectomy for developmental glaucoma. Ophthalmology 1998; 105: 974-982.
79. Debnath SC, Teichmann KD, Salamah K. Trabeculectomy versus trabeculotomy in congenital glaucoma. Br J Ophthalmol 1989; 73: 608-611.
80. Tamcelik N, Ozkiris A, Sarici AM. Long-term results of combined viscotrabeculotomy-trabeculectomy in refractory developmental glaucoma. Eye (Lond) 2010; 24: 613-618.
81. Ito S, Nishikawa M, Tokura T, et al. [Histopathological study of trabecular meshwork after trabeculotomy in monkeys]. Nihon Ganka Gakkai Zasshi 1994; 98: 811-819.
82. Bayoumi NH. Deep sclerectomy in pediatric glaucoma filtering surgery. Eye (Lond) 2012 Oct 12; doi: 10.1038/eye.2012.215. [Advanced online publication].
83. Mandal AK. Primary combined trabeculotomy-trabeculectomy for early-onset glaucoma in Sturge-Weber syndrome. Ophthalmology 1999; 106: 1621-1627.
84. Mandal AK, Bhatia PG, Gothwal VK, et al. Safety and efficacy of simultaneous bilateral primary combined trabeculotomy-trabeculectomy for developmental glaucoma. Indian J Ophthalmol 2002; 50: 13-19.
85. Mandal AK, Matalia JH, Nutheti R, Krishnaiah S. Combined trabeculotomy and trabeculectomy in advanced primary developmental glaucoma with corneal diameter of 14 mm or more. Eye (Lond) 2006; 20: 135-143.
86. Mandal AK, Gothwal VK, Nutheti R. Surgical outcome of primary developmental glaucoma: a single surgeon's long-term experience from a tertiary eye care centre in India. Eye (Lond) 2007; 21: 764-774.
87. Elder MJ. Combined trabeculotomy-trabeculectomy compared with primary trabeculectomy for congenital glaucoma. Br J Ophthalmol 1994; 78: 745-748.
88. Mullaney PB, Selleck C, Al-Awad A, et al. Combined trabeculotomy and trabeculectomy as an initial procedure in uncomplicated congenital glaucoma. Arch Ophthalmol 1999; 117: 457-460.
89. Essuman VA, Braimah IZ, Ndanu TA, Ntim-Amponsah CT. Combined trabeculotomy and trabeculectomy: outcome for primary congenital glaucoma in a West African population. Eye (Lond) 2011; 25: 77-83.
90. Mandal AK, Walton DS, John T, Jayagandan A. Mitomycin C-augmented trabeculectomy in refractory congenital glaucoma. Ophthalmology 1997; 104: 996-1001; discussion 1002-1003.
91. Mandal AK, Prasad K, Naduvilath TJ. Surgical results and complications of mitomycin C-augmented trabeculectomy in refractory developmental glaucoma. Ophthalmic Surg Lasers 1999; 30: 473-480.
92. Luntz MH. Congenital, infantile, and juvenile glaucoma. Ophthalmology 1979; 86: 793-802.
93. Quigley HA. Childhood glaucoma: results with trabeculotomy and study of reversible cupping. Ophthalmology 1982; 89: 219-226.
94. Shields MB, Buckley E, Klintworth GK, Thresher R. Axenfeld-Rieger syndrome. A spectrum of developmental disorders. Surv Ophthalmol 1985; 29: 387-409.
95. Walton DS. Aniridic glaucoma: the results of gonio-surgery to prevent and treat this problem. Trans Am Ophthalmol Soc 1986; 84: 59-70.
96. Chen TC, Walton DS, Bhatia LS. Aphakic glaucoma after congenital cataract surgery. Arch Ophthalmol 2004; 122: 1819-1825.
97. Olsen KE, Huang AS, Wright MM. The efficacy of goniotomy/trabeculotomy in early-onset glaucoma associated with the Sturge-Weber syndrome. J AAPOS 1998; 2: 365-368.
98. Ho CL, Walton DS. Goniosurgery for glaucoma secondary to chronic anterior uveitis: prognostic factors and surgical technique. J Glaucoma 2004; 13: 445-449.
99. Bohnsack BL, Freedman SF. Surgical outcomes in childhood uveitic glaucoma. Am J Ophthalmol 2013; 155: 134-142.

100. Cairns JE. Trabeculectomy. Preliminary report of a new method. Am J Ophthalmol 1968; 66: 673-679.
101. Beauchamp GR, Parks MM. Filtering surgery in children: barriers to success. Ophthalmology 1979; 86: 170-180.
102. Burke JP, Bowell R. Primary trabeculectomy in congenital glaucoma. Br J Ophthalmol 1989; 73: 186-190.
103. Fulcher T, Chan J, Lanigan B, et al. Long-term follow up of primary trabeculectomy for infantile glaucoma. Br J Ophthalmol 1996; 80: 499-502.
104. Miller MH, Rice NS. Trabeculectomy combined with beta irradiation for congenital glaucoma. Br J Ophthalmol 1991; 75: 584-590.
105. Wells AP, Cordeiro MF, Bunce C, Khaw PT. Cystic bleb formation and related complications in limbus- versus fornix-based conjunctival flaps in pediatric and young adult trabeculectomy with mitomycin C. Ophthalmology 2003; 110: 2192-2197.
106. Solus JF, Jampel HD, Tracey PA, et al. Comparison of limbus-based and fornix-based trabeculectomy: success, bleb-related complications, and bleb morphology. Ophthalmology 2012; 119: 703-711.
107. Giampani J, Jr., Borges-Giampani AS, Carani JC, et al. Efficacy and safety of trabeculectomy with mitomycin C for childhood glaucoma: a study of results with long-term follow-up. Clinics (Sao Paulo) 2008; 63: 421-426.
108. Molteno AC. Children with advanced glaucoma treated with drainage implants. S Afr Arch Ophthalmol 1973; 1: 55-61.
109. Khan AO, Al-Mobarak F. Comparison of polypropylene and silicone Ahmed valve survival 2 years following implantation in the first 2 years of life. Br J Ophthalmol 2009; 93: 791-794.
110. El Sayed Y, Awadein A. Polypropylene vs silicone Ahmed valve with adjunctive mitomycin C in paediatric age group: a prospective controlled study. Eye (Lond) 2013 Apr 12; doi: 10.1038/eye.2013.51. [Advanced online publication].
111. Khaw PT. Aniridia. J Glaucoma 2002; 11: 164-168.
112. Cantor L, Burgoyne J, Sanders S, et al. The effect of mitomycin C on Molteno implant surgery: a 1-year randomized, masked, prospective study. J Glaucoma 1998; 7: 240-246.
113. Costa VP, Azuara-Blanco A, Netland PA, et al. Efficacy and safety of adjunctive mitomycin C during Ahmed Glaucoma Valve implantation: a prospective randomized clinical trial. Ophthalmology 2004; 111: 1071-1076.
114. Kurnaz E, Kubaloglu A, Yilmaz Y, et al. The effect of adjunctive Mitomycin C in Ahmed glaucoma valve implantation. Eur J Ophthalmol 2005; 15:27-31.
115. Kirwan C, O'Keefe M, Lanigan B, Mahmood U. Ahmed valve drainage implant surgery in the management of paediatric aphakic glaucoma. Br J Ophthalmol 2005; 89: 855-858.
116. Mahdy RA. Adjunctive use of bevacizumab versus mitomycin C with Ahmed valve implantation in treatment of pediatric glaucoma. J Glaucoma 2011; 20: 458-463.
117. Hill RA, Heuer DK, Baerveldt G, et al. Molteno implantation for glaucoma in young patients. Ophthalmology 1991; 98: 1042-1046.
118. Eid TE, Katz LJ, Spaeth GL, Augsburger JJ. Long-term effects of tube-shunt procedures on management of refractory childhood glaucoma. Ophthalmology 1997; 104: 1011-1016.
119. Djodeyre MR, Peralta Calvo J, Abelairas Gomez J. Clinical evaluation and risk factors of time to failure of Ahmed Glaucoma Valve implant in pediatric patients. Ophthalmology 2001; 108: 614-620.
120. Al-Torbak AA, Al-Shahwan S, Al-Jadaan I, et al. Endophthalmitis associated with the Ahmed glaucoma valve implant. Br J Ophthalmol 2005; 89: 454-458.
121. Coleman AL, Smyth RJ, Wilson MR, Tam M. Initial clinical experience with the Ahmed Glaucoma Valve implant in pediatric patients. Arch Ophthalmol 1997; 115: 186-191.
122. Englert JA, Freedman SF, Cox TA. The Ahmed valve in refractory pediatric glaucoma. Am J Ophthalmol 1999; 127: 34-42.

123. Morales J, Al Shahwan S, Al Odhayb S, et al. Current surgical options for the management of pediatric glaucoma. J Ophthalmol 2013; 2013: 763735.
124. Kalinina Ayuso V, Scheerlinck LM, de Boer JH. The effect of an Ahmed glaucoma valve implant on corneal endothelial cell density in children with glaucoma secondary to uveitis. Am J Ophthalmol. 2013; 155: 530-535.
125. O'Malley Schotthoefer E, Yanovitch TL, Freedman SF. Aqueous drainage device surgery in refractory pediatric glaucoma: II. Ocular motility consequences. J AAPOS 2008; 12: 40-45.
126. Morad Y, Donaldson CE, Kim YM, et al. The Ahmed drainage implant in the treatment of pediatric glaucoma. Am J Ophthalmol 2003; 135: 821-829.
127. Ishida K, Mandal AK, Netland PA. Glaucoma drainage implants in pediatric patients. Ophthalmol Clin North Am 2005; 18: 431-442, vii.
128. Budenz DL, Gedde SJ, Brandt JD, et al. Baerveldt glaucoma implant in the management of refractory childhood glaucomas. Ophthalmology 2004; 111: 2204-2210.
129. Rolim de Moura C, Fraser-Bell S, Stout A, et al. Experience with the Baerveldt glaucoma implant in the management of pediatric glaucoma. Am J Ophthalmol 2005; 139: 847-854.
130. Tanimoto SA, Brandt JD. Options in pediatric glaucoma after angle surgery has failed. Curr Opin Ophthalmol 2006; 17: 132-137.
131. Wagle NS, Freedman SF, Buckley EG, et al. Long-term outcome of cyclocryotherapy for refractory pediatric glaucoma. Ophthalmology 1998; 105: 1921-1926; discussion 1926-1927.
132. Phelan MJ, Higginbotham EJ. Contact transscleral Nd:YAG laser cyclophotocoagulation for the treatment of refractory pediatric glaucoma. Ophthalmic Surg Lasers 1995; 26: 401-403.
133. Bock CJ, Freedman SF, Buckley EG, Shields MB. Transscleral diode laser cyclophotocoagulation for refractory pediatric glaucomas. J Pediatr Ophthalmol Strabismus 1997; 34: 235-239.
134. Sabri K, Vernon SA. Scleral perforation following trans-scleral cyclodiode. Br J Ophthalmol 1999; 83: 502-503.
135. Plager DA, Neely DE. Intermediate-term results of endoscopic diode laser cyclophotocoagulation for pediatric glaucoma. J AAPOS 1999; 3: 131-137.
136. Hamard P, May F, Quesnot S, Hamard H. La cyclophotocoagulation transsclérale au laser diode dans le traitement des glaucomes réfractaires du sujet jeune. [Trans-scleral diode laser cyclophotocoagulation for the treatment of refractory pediatric glaucoma]. J Fr Ophtalmol 2000; 23: 773-780.
137. Kirwan JF, Shah P, Khaw PT. Diode laser cyclophotocoagulation: role in the management of refractory pediatric glaucomas. Ophthalmology 2002; 109: 316-323.
138. Autrata R, Rehurek J. Long-term results of transscleral cyclophotocoagulation in refractory pediatric glaucoma patients. Ophthalmologica 2003; 217: 393-400.
139. Carter BC, Plager DA, Neely DE, et al. Endoscopic diode laser cyclophotocoagulation in the management of aphakic and pseudophakic glaucoma in children. J AAPOS 2007; 11: 34-40.
140. Tixier J, Dureau P, Becquet F, Dufier JL. Sclérectomie profonde dans le glaucome congénital. Résultats préliminaires. [Deep sclerectomy in congenital glaucoma. Preliminary results]. J Fr Ophtalmol 1999; 22: 545-548.
141. Luke C, Dietlein TS, Jacobi PC, et al. Risk profile of deep sclerectomy for treatment of refractory congenital glaucomas. Ophthalmology 2002; 109: 1066-1071.
142. Roche O, Beby F, Parsa A, et al. Nonpenetrating external trabeculectomy for congenital glaucoma: a retrospective study. Ophthalmology 2007; 114: 1994-1999.
143. Al-Obeidan SA, Osman EE, Dewedar AS, et al. Efficacy and safety of deep sclerectomy in childhood glaucoma in Saudi Arabia. Acta Ophthalmol 2012 Dec 15; doi: 10.1111/j.1755-3768.2012.02558.x. [Advanced online publication].
144. Feusier M, Roy S, Mermoud A. Deep sclerectomy combined with trabeculectomy in pediatric glaucoma. Ophthalmology 2009; 116: 30-38.
145. Noureddin BN, El-Haibi CP, Cheikha A, Bashshur ZF. Viscocanalostomy versus trabeculotomy ab externo in primary congenital glaucoma: 1-year follow-up of a prospective controlled pilot study. Br J Ophthalmol 2006; 90: 1281-1285.

146. Minckler D, Baerveldt G, Ramirez MA, et al. Clinical results with the Trabectome, a novel surgical device for treatment of open-angle glaucoma. Trans Am Ophthalmol Soc 2006; 104: 40-50.

147. de Silva DJ, Khaw PT, Brookes JL. Long-term outcome of primary congenital glaucoma. J AAPOS 2011; 15: 148-152.

148. Al-Torbak AA. Outcome of combined Ahmed glaucoma valve implant and penetrating keratoplasty in refractory congenital glaucoma with corneal opacity. Cornea 2004; 23: 554-559.

149. Erlich CM, Rootman DS, Morin JD. Corneal transplantation in infants, children and young adults: experience of the Toronto Hospital for Sick Children, 1979-88. Can J Ophthalmol 1991; 26: 206-210.

150. McClellan K, Lai T, Grigg J, Billson F. Penetrating keratoplasty in children: visual and graft outcome. Br J Ophthalmol 2003; 87: 1212-1214.

151. Yang LL, Lambert SR, Lynn MJ, Stulting RD. Surgical management of glaucoma in infants and children with Peters anomaly: long-term structural and functional outcome. Ophthalmology 2004; 111: 112-117.

152. Lowe MT, Keane MC, Coster DJ, Williams KA. The outcome of corneal transplantation in infants, children, and adolescents. Ophthalmology 2011; 118:492-497.

153. Unterlauft JD, Weller K, Geerling G. A 10.0-mm posterior lamellar graft for bullous keratopathy in a buphthalmic eye. Cornea 2010; 29: 1195-1198.

154. Hashemi H, Ghaffari R, Mohebi M. Posterior lamellar keratoplasty (DSAEK) in Peters anomaly. Cornea 2012; 31: 1201-1205.

155. Quilendrino R, Yeh RY, Dapena I, et al. Large diameter descemet membrane endothelial keratoplasty in buphthalmic eyes. Cornea 2013; 32:e74-78.

156. Sood S, Beck AD. Cyclophotocoagulation versus sequential tube shunt as a secondary intervention following primary tube shunt failure in pediatric glaucoma. J AAPOS 2009; 13: 379-383.

157. Yang HK, Park KH. Clinical outcomes after Ahmed valve implantation in refractory paediatric glaucoma. Eye (Lond) 2009; 23: 1427-1435.

158. Smith MF, Doyle JW. Results of another modality for extending glaucoma drainage tubes. J Glaucoma 1999; 8: 310-314.

159. Sheets CW, Ramjattan TK, Smith MF, Doyle JW. Migration of glaucoma drainage device extender into anterior chamber after trauma. J Glaucoma 2006; 15: 559-561.

160. Dawodu O, Levin AV. Spontaneous disconnection of glaucoma tube shunt extenders. J AAPOS 2010; 14: 361-363.

161. Barkan O. Surgery of congenital glaucoma; review of 196 eyes operated by goniotomy. Am J Ophthalmol 1953; 36: 1523-1534.

162. Scheie HG. The management of infantile glaucoma. AMA Arch Ophthalmol 1959; 62: 35-54.

163. Dietlein TS, Jacobi PC, Krieglstein GK. Prognosis of primary ab externo surgery for primary congenital glaucoma. Br J Ophthalmol 1999; 83: 317-322.

164. al-Hazmi A, Zwaan J, Awad A, et al. Effectiveness and complications of mitomycin C use during pediatric glaucoma surgery. Ophthalmology 1998; 105: 1915-1920.

165. Freedman SF, McCormick K, Cox TA. Mitomycin C-augumented trabeculectomy with postoperative wound modulation in pediatric glaucoma. J AAPOS 1999; 3: 117-124.

166. Wise JB. Mitomycin-compatible suture technique for fornix-based conjunctival flaps in glaucoma filtration surgery. Arch Ophthalmol 1993; 111: 992-997.

167. Sherwood MB, Smith MF. Prevention of early hypotony associated with Molteno implants by a new occluding stent technique. Ophthalmology 1993; 100: 85-90.

168. Molteno AC, Ancker E, Van Biljon G. Surgical technique for advanced juvenile glaucoma. Arch Ophthalmol 1984; 102: 51-57.

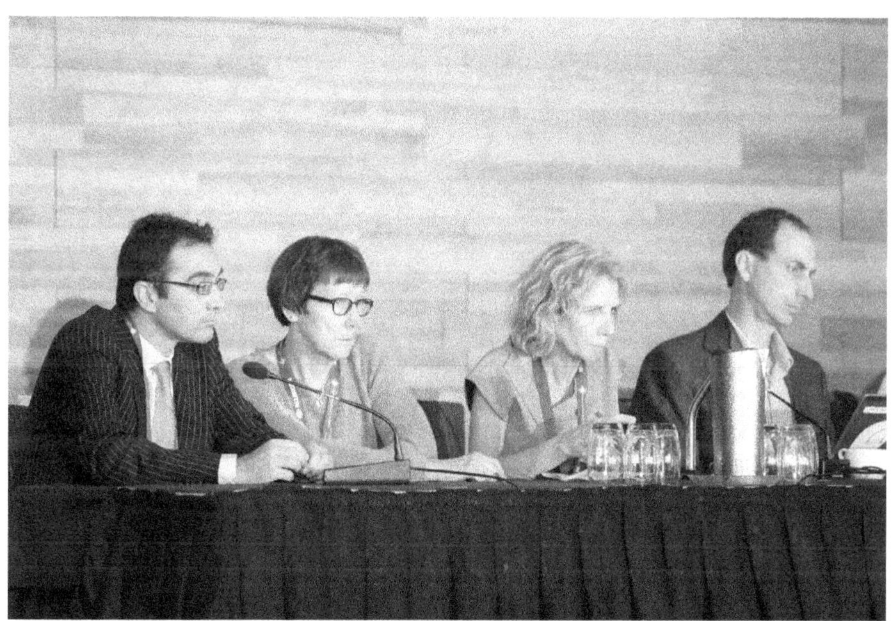

Julian Garcia Feijoo, Barbara Cvenkel, Orna Geyer, John Grigg (L-R)

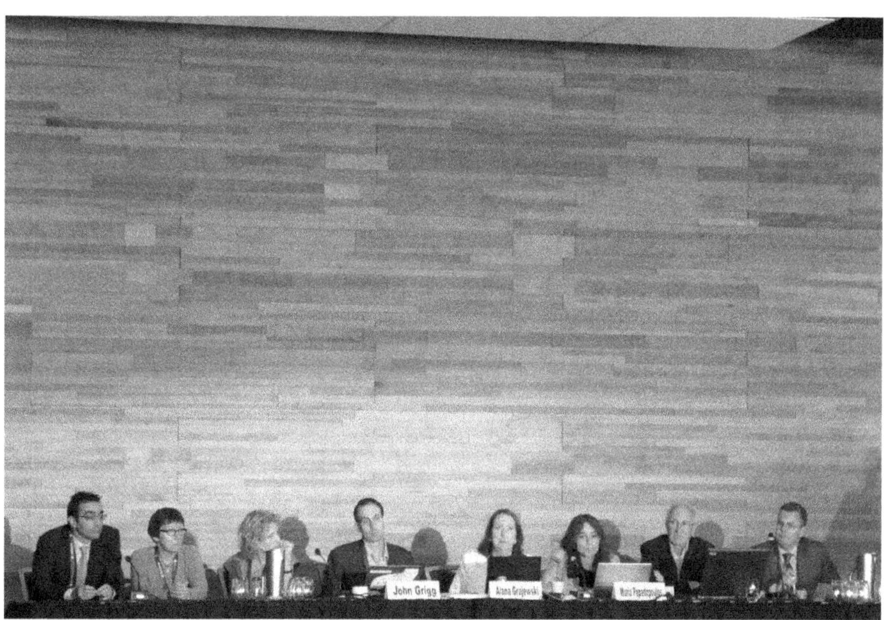

Julian Garcia Feijoo , Barbara Cvenkel, Orna Geyer, John Grigg, Alana L. Grajewski, Maria Papadopoulos, Franz Grehn, John Brookes (L-R)

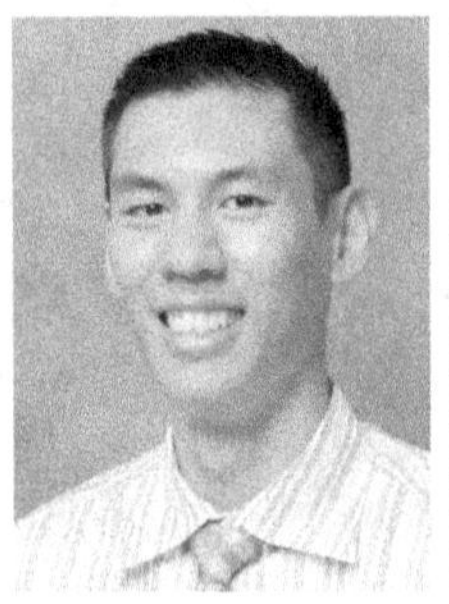

Ta Chen Peter Chang

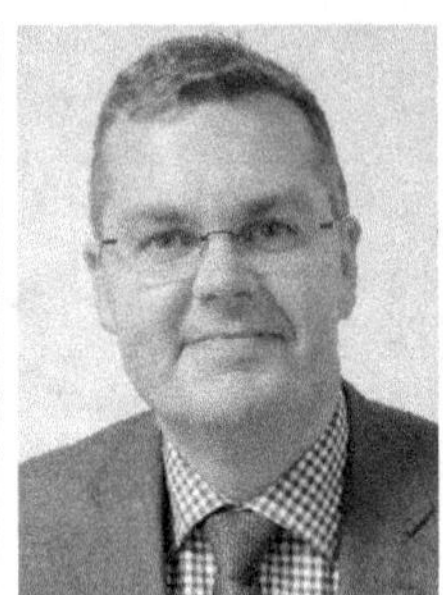

John Brookes

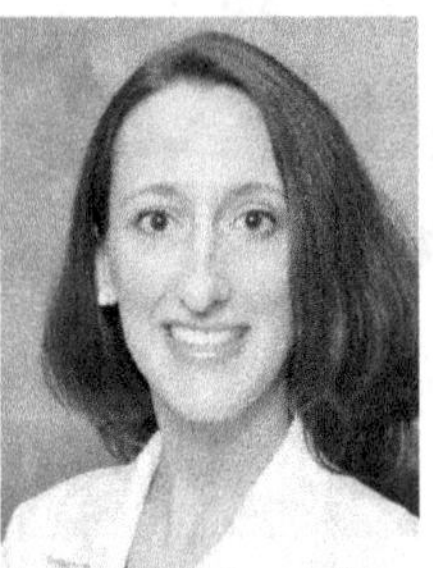

Kara Cavuoto

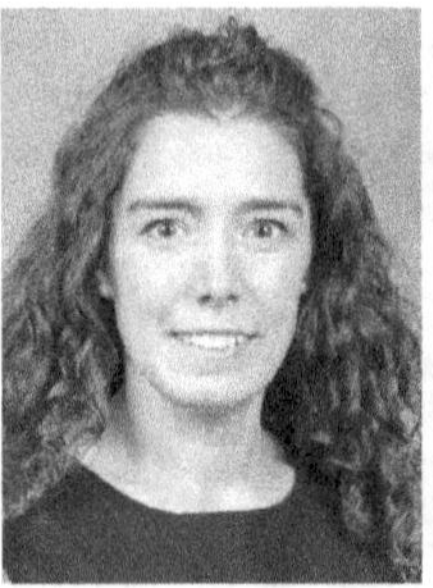

Elena Bitrian

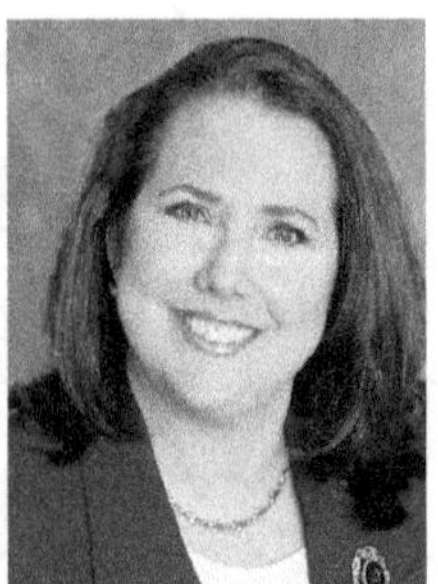

Alana L. Grajewski

6. PRIMARY CONGENITAL GLAUCOMA AND JUVENILE OPEN-ANGLE GLAUCOMA

Ta Chen Peter Chang, John Brookes, Kara Cavuoto, Elena Bitrian, Alana L. Grajewski

Section Leaders: Alana L. Grajewski, John Brookes, Ta Chen Peter Chang
Contributors: Joseph Abbott, Ahmed Abdelrahman, Jocelyn Chua, Valeria Coviltir, Barbara Cvenkel, Julian Garcia Feijoo , Cecilia Fenerty, Simone Finzi, Orna Geyer, Faisal Ghadhfan, Franz Grehn, Arif Khan, S.R. Krishnadas, Anil Mandal, Sheila Marco, Gabor Scharioth, Tanuj Dada

Consensus statements

1. Primary congenital glaucoma (PCG) is the most common non-sydromic glaucoma in infancy and is classified according to onset of signs. Its worldwide incidence is variable and influenced by consanguinity.
2. PCG is usually inherited in an autosomal recessive manner, with a family history reported in 10-40% of cases and is more common in consanguineous populations.
   Comment: Mutations in the *CYP1B1* gene have been identified and show variable expressivity and phenotypes.
   Comment: Clinical screening of current and future siblings is essential if there is parental consanguinity.
3. The pathogenesis of PCG remains uncertain but the immature angle appearance seen clinically is thought to result from the arrested maturation of tissues derived from cranial neural crest cells.
4. PCG is a surgical condition and the surgical procedure of choice is usually angle surgery (goniotomy or trabeculotomy) with high rates of success reported for both in favorable cases and after multiple procedures.
   Comment: Combined trabeculotomy with trabeculectomy as an initial procedure is suggested by some to be more successful than either procedure performed alone in certain populations. There are no supporting prospective comparisons in the literature.
5. Once angle surgery fails, the next procedure of choice is either trabeculectomy or a glaucoma drainage device.

Childhood Glaucoma, pp. 137-153
Edited by Robert N. Weinreb, Alana L. Grajewski, Maria Papadopoulos, John Grigg,
and Sharon Freedman
2013 © Kugler Publications, Amsterdam, The Netherlands

6. Juvenile open-angle glaucoma (JOAG) is a relatively rare form of childhood glaucoma usually presenting after the age of four years, with a normal angle appearance and no signs of other ocular anomalies or systemic disease.
7. Depending on age, medical therapy is the first-line treatment for JOAG, although surgery is often required.
8. Evidence remains weak for the optimum first-line surgical intervention for JOAG.

Primary congenital glaucoma

Introduction

Primary congenital glaucoma (PCG) usually presents in neonates and infants characteristically with symptoms of photophobia and tearing, and physical signs of corneal edema, ocular enlargement and optic disc cupping. It occurs in eyes with a developmental abnormality of the angle, resulting in decreased aqueous outflow. This is a non-syndromic abnormality of the trabecular meshwork and the diagnosis is made after finding isolated trabeculodysgenesis with no other ocular anomalies. The more severe the angle anomaly, the earlier the presentation is thought to be and the worse the prognosis. The pathogenesis of PCG is disputed and the anatomical basis of outflow obstruction remains unclear, although good evidence suggests that the trabeculodysgenesis relates to embryologic arrest of angle formation. Identification of numerous *CYP1B1* gene mutations in various populations have been associated with the pathogenesis of PCG. The management of PCG is primarily surgical with medical therapy playing a supportive role.

Classification

PCG is classified according to age of onset of signs into (1) neonatal or newborn onset (0-1 month); (2) Infantile onset (> 1-24 months); (3) Late onset or late-recognized (> 2 years). Cases with normal intraocular pressure (IOP) and optic disc but typical signs of PCG, such as buphthalmos and Haab striae are classified as spontaneously arrested PCG (*see* Section 1).

Epidemiology

Primary congenital glaucoma is the most common non-sydromic glaucoma in infancy,[1,2] but it has a variable reported incidence worldwide. A higher prevalence has been observed in those cultures and groups with an increased rate of consanguinity, especially in those groups in which cousin-cousin marriage is common.[3-5] PCG occurs in one of 10,000-20,000 live births in Western countries.[2,6,7] The incidence rises in the Middle East to 1:8,200 live births in Palestinian Arabs[3] to 1;2,500 live births in Saudi Arabians.[8] The highest reported incidence is 1:1,1250 in Slovakian Gypsies.[4]

PCG is usually bilateral (70%) with the severity of involvement frequently asymmetrical. The male gender has a slightly higher prevalence[6,9,10] but familial cases tend to have an equal sex distribution.[5,11]

Genetics

PCG is usually inherited in an autosomal recessive manner. In many cases there is no family history (sporadic) whereas a family history is more common in consanguineous populations. A family history of glaucoma is reported in 10-40% of cases with variable penetrance ranging from 40-100%.[11,12] To date, three primary congenital glaucoma loci have been identified (GLC3A, GLC3B, GLC3C). The GCL3A locus maps to the short arm of chromosome 2p22-p21 and is the major locus for PCG accounting for 85-90% of all familial cases. Mutations of the GLC3A locus affect the gene *CYP1B1* which encodes for the enzyme cytochrome P450, family 1, subfamily B, polypeptide 1, which has been postulated to participate in the development and function of the eye. Variable expressivity and varied phenotypes are known to be associated with *CYP1B1* mutations. Attempts at genotype-phenotype correlations have been inconclusive. The GLC3B locus maps to chromosome 1p36.2-p36.1 and GLC3C locus to chromosome 14q24.3. No gene has been identified yet for these loci.

The risk of PCG in siblings and offspring, in Caucasian patients (low parental consanguinity), is low (< 5%) but it is prudent to examine the siblings and offspring of patients, especially in the first 6 months of life. If there is a history of consanguinity the risk is higher and screening siblings and offspring is essential (*see* Section 3).

Pathogenesis

The mature corneal endothelial and stromal layers, the mesenchymal layer of the limbus, and the trabecular meshwork in mammals each consist of two mature cell lineages, one derived from the neural crest and the other from the mesoderm.[13] Trabecular meshwork formation begins around the fourth month of gestation.[14] The mesenchymal cells of the trabecular meshwork form a wedge-shaped structure that lies between the corneal endothelium and the deeper stroma. Schlemm canal forms from a venous plexus anterior to the trabecular anlage which becomes visible in the 16th week of gestation.[15] By 36 weeks the Schlemm canal and outer collecting channels are clearly defined and connected by inter-canalicular links. The development of this system continues post-natally mostly in the first year, until an adult-like configuration is achieved by eight years.[15]

The pathogenesis of PCG remains uncertain. Following the association of PCG with elevated IOP in the 19th century it was thought that either corneal enlargement or intraocular inflammation were the primary defects. However, pathology studies in the late 19th and early 20th century described congenital angle anomalies that were later verified gonioscopically. Furthermore, the defect was isolated to the filtration angle by perfusion and facility of outflow studies. Over the years, many theories have been proposed to explain both the angle changes and the mechanism of raised IOP.

The immature angle appearance is now thought to result from the developmental arrest of tissues derived from cranial neural crest cells in the third trimester of gestation. The severity of the angle abnormality depends on the stage at which angle development is arrested. Obstruction to outflow was popularly thought to be due to the presence of an impermeable membrane, Barkan membrane,[16,17] but this has never been verified histopathologically. With time, the site of obstruction was found to be trabecular rather than pretrabecular.[18,19] It is now thought to be due to thick, compacted trabecular sheets which coalesce preventing the posterior 'sliding' of the iris which occurs during the development of the anterior segment.[19] These trabecular sheets suspend the iris more anteriorly which results in the typical appearance of the 'high' insertion of iris in these children.[19,20]

Presentation

PCG usually presents in neonates or infants, with the majority presenting less than the age of six months.[2] Clinically, PCG is characterized by elevation of IOP, which causes stretching of the tissues of the eye and enlargement of the globe (buphthalmos). The enlargement of the globe and stretching of the cornea can produce breaks in Descemet membrane, known as Haab striae. The elevated IOP also causes corneal edema, which manifests with epiphora and photophobia. Blepharospasm is likely a result of the photophobia. Children with PCG usually present for evaluation because their parents notice something unusual about the appearance (corneal haze/ opacification or enlargement of the eye) of the patient's eyes or their behavior (photophobia and blepharospasm). The severity of the signs and symptoms varies depending on the duration and magnitude of the IOP elevation. Furthermore, the timing of IOP elevation also affects the signs, as a child with late onset PCG after the age of around three, will not present with corneal enlargement.

In PCG, gonioscopy reveals a flat and high iris insertion and the absence of an angle recess. A thin and hypopigmented iris stroma might be detected as well as peripheral scalloping of the posterior pigmented iris layer and easily visible, hyperemic iris vessels with circumferential vessels running tortuously in the peripheral iris.[21] In cases of 'unilateral' disease, the fellow eye usually shows typical gonioscopic findings of PCG with a large corneal diameter and axial length but the disc is normal and this may represent drainage angles that have opened late leading to *spontaneous arrest* of the disease.[22] These fellow eyes of 'unilateral' cases must be followed as closely as the affected eye as arrested disease may relapse at any stage.

Management

Comprehensive office examination is often difficult in this population of young children. When the clinical suspicion for PCG is high, an examination under anesthesia (EUA) is performed to confirm the diagnosis and document baseline findings, followed by surgery at the same anesthetic event if possible. Although PCG is a surgical condition, topical and/or systemic IOP lowering medications may be used prior to the scheduled surgical date to temporize and, in those with corneal edema, to improve the visualization of the intraocular anatomy during the EUA and surgery. The primary surgical goal is to lower the IOP, which allows for a clear visual axis to promote visual development within the critical period and the stabilization of ocular dimensions.

When the diagnosis of PCG is confirmed, angle surgery (goniotomy or trabeculotomy) is usually the procedure of choice. By incising angle tissue, both goniotomy and trabeculotomy aim to eliminate the obstruction to aqueous outflow created by structural abnormalities in the angle found in PCG and to restore a pathway for aqueous outflow. The exact mechanism of action of these procedures remains unknown. However, tonographic studies demonstrate that successful goniotomy increases the facility of outflow.[23,24] However, Maumenee found this to be the case only when Schlemm canal was present, which may explain its reduced success in advanced cases.[25]

Goniotomy was first described by Carlo de Vincentiis in 1893, who performed it in adults without direct visualization of the angle, with poor outcomes.[26] Otto Barkan refined the procedure in 1936 with direct gonioscopic visualization of the angle in adults[27] and in 1942, published unprecedented results in children with glaucoma.[28] However, goniotomy is not possible in the presence of a hazy cornea which obscures the detail of the angle features. With these cases in mind, Redmond Smith described a technique which ruptured the internal wall of Schlemm canal and the trabecular meshwork using a nylon filament,[29] a technique revisited by Beck and Lynch to achieve circumferential suture trabeculotomy.[30] In the same year as Smith, Hermann Burian independently described an alternative operation to achieve the same result with the use of a rigid probe (trabeculotome), which he termed *'trabeculotomy ab externo'*.[31] In 1962, Allen and Burian described its role in childhood glaucoma.[32] The surgical technique was subsequently further refined and popularised by Harms, Dannheim, Luntz and McPherson.

There are no prospective studies comparing goniotomy to trabeculotomy, although both are thought to be associated with similar high rates of success (70-90%) after multiple procedures especially in favorable cases (onset of PCG signs between 3-12 months of age).[35-43] Success is thought to be determined more by the severity and duration of the disease rather than the surgical technique.[44] In other words, failure of either technique is thought to be associated with an immature angle resulting in more aggressive disease or when structural damage to the angle has occurred through excessive enlargement of the anterior segment.

The decision to perform one angle procedure in preference to the other is influenced largely by corneal transparency and the surgeon's experience and preference. Trabeculotomy is possible in the presence of both a clear and hazy cornea hence its popularity in populations where corneal opacification on presentation is a common finding. Additionally, it may be more useful for surgeons more familiar with the surgical approach for trabeculectomy rather than the technique of goniotomy. However, trabeculotomy is more invasive, causes conjunctival scarring and even with experience, may be technically difficult at times due to the inability to find Schlemm canal. By using a temporal or inferotemporal approach, the conjunctival scarring resulting from trabeculotomy is less likely to impact the success of future filtering or shunting procedures.

Over time, a number of modifications to conventional trabeculotomy have been described to improve its success. The fact that IOP control often improves in some cases with additional angle surgery, suggests that the extent of angle incised may be important. In light of this and to minimize anesthetic exposure, Beck and Lynch proposed circumferential suture trabeculotomy with a blunted 6-0 prolene.[30] Its reported overall success in eyes with PCG varies from 77-92% after one to four years.[30,45-47] Mendicino *et al.* suggested it may be more successful than goniotomy in a retrospective comparison but the mean follow-up for the goniotomy group was over twice as long (nine versus four years). Despite its advantages, success may not always be possible with a single incision and the suture may not advance all the way around Schlemm canal, in which case a conventional trabeculotomy can be performed with a trabectome. Furthermore, misdirection of the suture into the anterior chamber and/or suprachoroidal space remains a potentially serious complication. The potential for misdirection lends itself to the recommendation for the suture to be viewed gonioscopically as it is advanced.[48] However, this is not necessary with the recent introduction of an illuminated microcatheter in circumferential trabeculotomy as a substitute for the suture, because it allows continuous visualization of the filament tip and early detection of misdirection.[49]

Theoretically, combining trabeculotomy with trabeculectomy (with or without anti-scarring agents) as an initial procedure provides two major outflow pathways and should improve the results for PCG. However, in practice the clinical benefit is unclear and there are no prospective comparisons. Dietlein *et al.*[43] retrospectively compared trabeculectomy, rigid-probe trabeculotomy and combined trabeculotomy/trabeculectomy (all without the intraoperative use of anti-scarring agents) in 36 PCG patients (Caucasian 71%, Turkish and Arabian 29%). They noted that the surgical outcome in the combined procedure did not differ from either rigid-probe trabeculotomy alone or trabeculectomy alone. They argued that success was determined more by the severity of the disease rather than the type of surgery. In a retrospective series of patients who had undergone combined rigid-probe trabeculotomy and trabeculectomy augmented with mitomycin C (MMC) by Mullaney *et al.*,[50] the Saudi Arabian PCG subset had 78% success rate over ten months, which compares well with the other series with rigid-probe trabeculotomy alone. Despite these results, combined trabeculotomy-trabeculectomy is argued to be more successful than either procedure performed alone in populations thought to be at greater risk of failure such as in the Middle East[3,51] and India,[52,53] especially with the use antiscarring agents such as MMC.[54] Al-Hazmi *et al.* in a retrospective review of 532 cases (820 eyes) of Saudi Arabian patients with PCG who presented less than one year of age, found combined trabeculotomy-trabeculectomy with MMC resulted in better IOP control than trabeculotomy alone in moderate to severe forms of the condition.[54] However, there was a significant learning curve for trabeculotomy with success increasing from 29% to 82% over the ten-year period studied. A recent report from a series of West African children with primary congenital glaucoma suggests poor results from combined trabeculotomy-trabeculectomy possibly due to severe disease at presentation, racial influences and no antiscarring agents use.[55]

In summary, angle surgery (goniotomy and trabeculotomy) is first line for PCG with the procedure of choice dictated by corneal clarity and the surgeon's experience and preference. Rigid probe trabeculotomy or goniotomy incise only a limited extent of the angle (90-120°) at each attempt. Trabeculotomy, can be further modified with the use of a suture (viewed gonioscopically) instead of a rigid probe to achieve a circumferential incision with one procedure alone. It is largely for this reason that circumferential suture trabeculotomy has increased in popularity around the world. In developed world centers, circumferential suture trabeculotomy has increasingly been replaced by circumferential, illuminated microcatheter-assisted trabeculotomy as the preferred technique, even in patients with clear corneas, due to its ease of use and perceived safety. It is worth noting that when angle surgery is possible but unlikely to succeed due to numerous poor prognostic factors, (*see* Section 5) then consideration should be given to performing an alternative operation especially in the presence of advanced disease.

If there has been a reasonable but suboptimal lowering of IOP after the first goniotomy or rigid probe trabeculotomy, the procedure can be repeated in the non-operated part of the angle. After a second operation, it becomes technically more difficult to incise any remaining angle and the success rate decreases with subsequent angle surgery. Once angle surgery fails and glaucoma is uncontrolled despite maximal medical therapy, the next procedure of choice is often dictated by the surgeon's experience, either trabeculectomy with or without antiscarring agents or a glaucoma drainage device (GDD). The consensus seems evenly divided between the two approaches.

Outcomes of trabeculectomy as a treatment of PCG vary widely, from extremely poor due to high complication rates in advanced cases with previous operations,[56] to excellent long-term success without serious complications as a primary procedure.[57,58] The long-term success rates of trabeculectomy surgery in children are lower compared to adults.[59] This is thought to be due to a more aggressive healing response in children, therefore most of the recent reports of pediatric trabeculectomies include the use of antiscarring agents. In a retrospective review of 91 post-trabeculectomy eyes with PCG (30 eyes with MMC and 61 eyes without MMC), Rodrigues *et al.*[60] found that long-term surgical success did not differ between the two groups. However, there was selection bias as only 54% of the group without MMC had undergone previous surgery as opposed to 80% of the MMC group, the difference was statistically significant. Hence the two groups are not comparable as previous surgery is a known risk factor for failure. The MMC group had a higher incidence of complications related to hypotony but they were 'mild and did not require further intervention'. All studies of trabeculectomy in children are limited by many factors such as retrospective design and surgeon bias. Overall, the success rate of trabeculectomy in PCG at one year ranges between 50-87%.[60-62] Trabeculectomy complication rates with MMC are higher than without it, especially those related to hypotony.[62-64] However, modifications to the intraoperative application of MMC and to surgical technique can minimise these.[65] Infants less than one year of age tend to do less well with trabeculectomy.[61,63] The outcome data of GDD in children suggest a wide range of success and complication rates, typically dependent on the individual study's definitions. In a retrospective case-control study of 46 eyes that received GDD before the age of 24 months (various glaucoma subtypes) compared to age-matched eyes that underwent trabeculectomy augmented with MMC, Beck *et al.*[66] found that 20.8% of the trabeculectomy group and 71.7% of the aqueous drainage device group were considered successful after a mean follow up of 11.5 months. However, the trabeculectomy group had 8.3% cumulative incidence of endophthalmitis, while 45.7% of the GDD group required additional surgical procedures for tube-related complications (*e.g.*, re-positioning). Ishida *et al.*[67] reviewed the outcomes of 21 studies of GDD in pediatric patients and reported overall success of 54%-95%, with a mean of approximately 75%, after various follow-up lengths. Altogether, GDD have an overall success rates of approximately 75-86.7% over one to two years and severe complication rate of 26.7% to 45.7%.[66-68] Anecdotally, since the safety and success rate of a GDD is the same whether implanted superiorly or inferiorly,[69] while an inferiorly placed trabeculectomy is associated with increased infection rates,[70] an inferiorly placed GDD as a second procedure may allow more subsequent surgical options, including a trabeculectomy under non-cicatrized conjunctiva.

In summary, once PCG is suspected, medical therapy is initiated to temporize until EUA/surgery can be performed. Both goniotomy and trabeculotomy are appropriate initial procedures. Circumferential suture trabeculotomy offers the advantage of incising all the trabecular meshwork in one procedure and the use of an illuminated microcatheter provides greater safety. After angle surgery failure and confirmed glaucoma progression despite maximum medical therapy, both trabeculectomy and GDD may be the appropriate second surgery. Refer to Figure 1 for a suggested management algorithm.

Juvenile open-angle glaucoma

Introduction

Juvenile open-angle glaucoma (JOAG) is a relatively rare form of childhood glaucoma, typically presenting after four years of age and up to 35 years. It is classified as a primary glaucoma of childhood, along with PCG. JOAG differs from primary open-angle glaucoma (POAG) in its age of onset and magnitude of IOP elevation. Typically, patients with JOAG present with extremely high IOP, sometimes greater than 40-50 mmHg. It is not associated with ocular enlargement, or any congenital ocular anomalies or syndromes and patients have a normal angle appearance. It is often inherited as an autosomal dominant trait.

Definition

JOAG appears like POAG with a normal angle appearance without any associated congenital ocular anomalies or syndromes. There is no ocular enlargement.

Genetics

The gene for the disease has been identified as a trabecular meshwork glucocorticoid response gene, otherwise known as the *TIGR* or myocilin (*MYOC*) gene. The gene, located on chromosome 1, produces the myocilin protein. Although it is not well understood how mutations in the myocilin gene cause glaucoma, it appears to do so by affecting trabecular outflow. Not all cases of JOAG are associated with *MYOC* mutations and additionally, *MYOC* mutations have also been reported in POAG. The *CYP1B1* gene has also been shown to play a part in glaucoma. This gene encodes for a mono-oxygenase, which is part of the cytochrome P450 family. Located on chromosome 2, mutations in the *CYP1B1* gene have been associated with primary congenital glaucoma and have been hypothesized to act as a modifier gene for *MYOC* in JOAG.[71]

Presentation

JOAG is typically asymptomatic and is discovered incidentally on routine eye examination, or screening due to a family history. Although JOAG is a bilateral disease, there can often be marked asymmetry between the two eyes. Markedly elevated IOP with optic disc excavation, and normal angles on gonioscopy are the major presenting signs of the disease. As the disease presents after the age of four years, there are no signs typically seen in PCG, such as corneal oedema and enlargement, Haab striae, or any of the symptoms usually associated with neonatal or infantile onset glaucoma. Typical glaucomatous visual field defects can be documented and are often advanced at presentation. Other forms of glaucoma in childhood should be excluded prior to making the diagnosis of JOAG, such as steroid-induced glaucoma, traumatic and inflammatory glaucomas.

JOAG is a relatively uncommon cause of primary glaucoma in childhood. The British Infantile and Childhood Glaucoma (BIG) Eye Study reported only two cases of 47 primary childhood glaucomas in a prospective, national surveillance study.[2] Other reports have identified JOAG accounting for only 0.2% of glaucoma cases.[72]

Treatment

Medical therapy

Evidence in the literature is lacking regarding the outcomes of medical treatment in JOAG, although most authors suggest that most patients with JOAG eventually require surgical intervention. Gupta *et al.* compared structural and functional changes of the optic nerve head in 42 patients with JOAG, treated either medically or surgically. The mean age of the patients was 26.8 years, with a mean baseline IOP of 35.3 mmHg. Eighty-four percent of eyes that underwent filtering surgery achieved an IOP less than 18 mmHg, compared with 63% on medical treatment alone. Progression was more common in the medically treated group.[73]

A randomized, double-masked multi-center study compared the efficacy and safety of latanoprost and timolol in childhood glaucoma, stratified according to age, diagnosis and IOP level. All patients were under 19 years old. Patients in both groups (PCG versus non-PCG) showed clinically relevant IOP reductions, with no significant differences between the two agents. The responder rates for latanoprost versus timolol in the non-PCG group was 72% versus 57%, although this was a heterogeneous group of glaucomas, not restricted to JOAG. However, the duration of effect of the agents is not known.[74]

Black *et al.* reported in a long term retrospective review of the use of latanoprost in childhood glaucoma. One of the predictors of a favorable IOP response was JOAG, suggesting its efficacy in this group of patients.[75]

Surgical therapy

Goniotomy

Goniotomy surgery was first described in children by Barkan in 1942,[28] based on the earlier work by de Vincentiis in 1893. It is still considered first-line therapy, along with trabeculotomy in PCG and enjoys good success rates.[35] Yeung and Walton reported the surgical results of goniotomy for JOAG, based on the medical records of ten patients with JOAG. The mean age at surgery was 16 years, with a mean follow up interval of 7.8 years. Overall success was achieved in 77% of the eyes (17 eyes); the average IOP for complete success (nine eyes) was 14.7 mmHg, qualified success (four eyes) 16.5 mmHg and failure (four eyes) 33.5 mmHg. No significant surgical complications occurred and the authors suggest that goniotomy is a potentially effective initial surgical treatment in JOAG, using a standard goniotomy technique.[76]

Trabeculotomy

Beck and Lynch[30] described 360^0 suture trabeculotomy, based on the work of Redmond Smith's original work.[29] Their results suggested it may be more successful than goniotomy in a retrospective comparison. More recent modifications have involved the use of an illuminated microcatheter to track its progress through Schlemm canal.[46] Girkin *et al.* reported a retrospective study of the safety and efficacy of circumferential trabeculotomy for congenital glaucomas using an illuminated microcatheter. Cases were both primary (including JOAG) and secondary childhood glaucomas. Although the number of cases was small and heterogeneous with a mean follow-up of 11 months, the qualified and unqualified success rates were 90.1% and 81.8% respectively.[46]

A study reported by Dao and colleagues examined the results of a microcatheter-facilitated 360-degree trabeculotomy for refractory aphakic and JOAG.[77] In the JOAG group (ten eyes), complete cannulation was achieved in all cases and success was reported in 90%, with the mean IOP reducing from 30.7 mmHg to 13.4 mmHg after a short mean follow-up of ten months.

Trabeculectomy

Trabeculectomy is the mainstay of surgical therapy for children with JOAG, although there are few reports in the literature. Some authors have examined the role of antiscarring agents as adjunctive treatment in trabeculectomy. Tsai and colleagues compared the intermediate-term outcomes of initial trabeculectomy with adjunctive MMC versus trabeculectomy alone for JOAG. In a retrospective study, 44 eyes were included, showing a cumulative success probability of 73% for the MMC group and 68% for the control group. Although the group treated with adjunctive MMC achieved lower IOP control, there was a greater incidence of hypotony maculopathy, in the three years following surgery.[78]

Pathania and colleagues reported the outcomes of trabeculectomy in JOAG, involving 60 eyes, who underwent primary trabeculectomy without MMC.[79] The mean age at presentation was 24.1 years (range 12-35 years), with a mean follow-up of 67 months. Complete success was achieved in 80% at five years and qualified success 96% at the end of five years, with the mean IOP reducing from 35 mmHg to 13 mmHg. Younger age at surgery was, however, associated with a higher risk of failure.

Glaucoma drainage devices

There is limited information in the literature looking at the use of glaucoma drainage devices in the management of JOAG. Donahue and colleagues reported the use of the Baerveldt implant in advanced childhood glaucomas, although only three cases had a diagnosis of JOAG.[80] Overall, phakic eyes had a much better short-term outcome but the results in cases of JOAG is not yet known.

Non-penetrating glaucoma surgery: Viscocanalostomy
Twenty consecutive patients were reported by Stangos *et al.*, evaluating primary viscocanalostomy in JOAG.[81] Although 80% of cases were considered an overall success, the age distribution was much greater, with a mean age of 33.7 years. Whether these results reflect the situation in younger patients is debatable.

Optic disc topography before and after treatment in JOAG
Elgin *et al.* compared optic disc topography parameters before and after antiglaucoma treatment in JOAG, using Heidelberg Retinal Tomography (HRT II). Twenty-one eyes with a mean age of 13 years with JOAG were assessed. At the sixth month of treatment, mean cup area and cup-to-disc ratio were significantly smaller than the values at baseline. The mean retinal nerve fiber layer at baseline was also significantly smaller than the value after treatment, suggesting that, as in PCG, glaucomatous changes of optic disc topography may be reversible after antiglaucoma treatment in JOAG.[82]

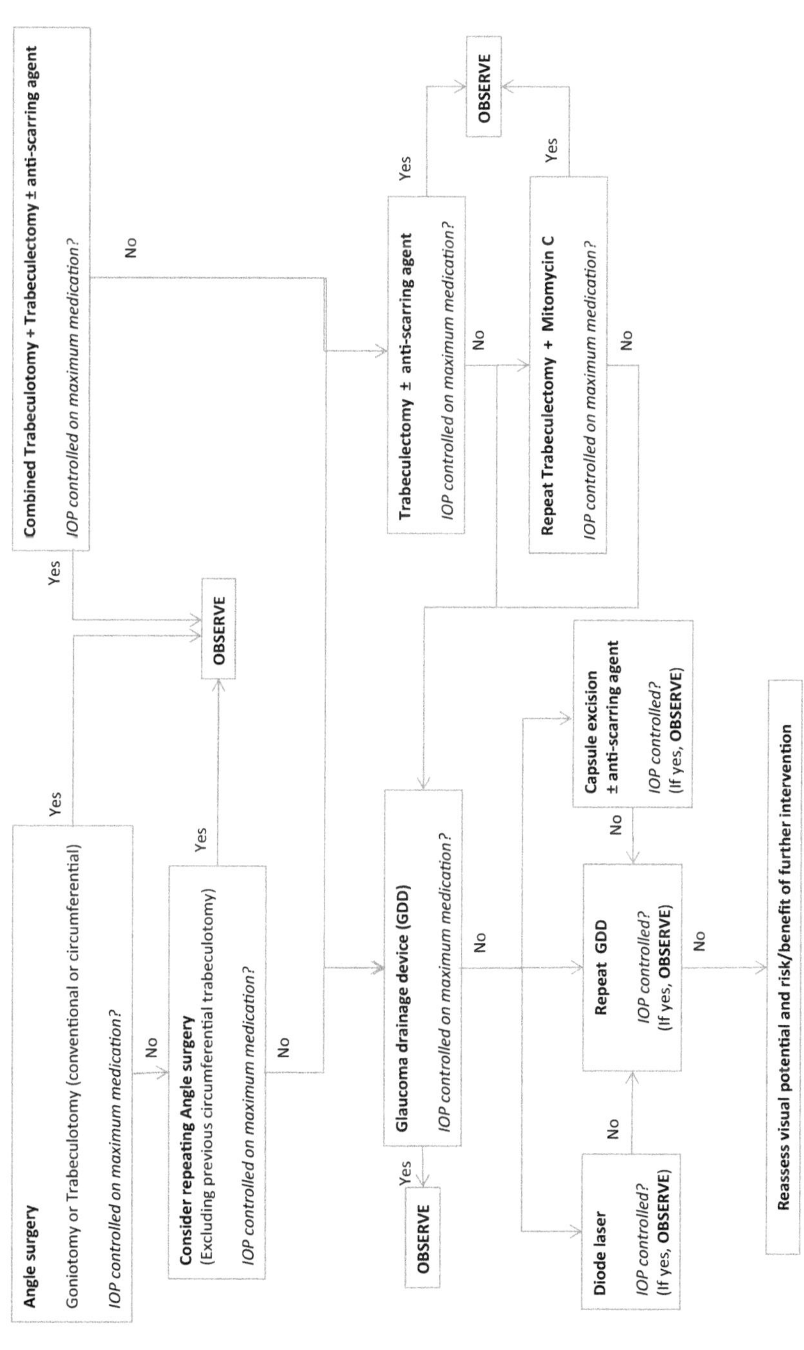

Fig. 1. A suggested approach to the management of primary congenital glaucoma. (It will be influenced by surgeon preference/experience and local facilities/equipment availability.)

References

1. Taylor RH, Ainsworth JR, Evans AR, Levin AV. The epidemiology of pediatric glaucoma: the Toronto experience. J AAPOS 1999; 3: 308-315.
2. Papadopoulos M, Cable N, Rahi J, Khaw PT; BIG Eye Investigators. The British Infantile and Childhood Glaucoma (BIG) Eye Study. Invest Ophthalmol Vis Sci 2007; 48: 4100-4106.
3. Elder MJ. Congenital glaucoma in the West Bank and Gaza Strip. Br J Ophthalmol 1993; 77: 413-416.
4. Gencik A. Epidemiology and genetics of primary congenital glaucoma in Slovakia: description of a form of primary congenital glaucoma in gypsies with autosomal-recessive inheritance and complete penetrance. Dev Ophthalmol 1989; 16: 76-15.
5. Turacli ME, Aktan SG, Sayli BS, Akarsu N. Therapeutic and genetical aspects of congenital glaucomas. Int Ophthalmol 1992; 16: 359-362.
6. McGinnity FG, Page AB, Bryars JH. Primary congenital glaucoma: twenty years experience. IrJ Med Sci 1987; 156: 364-365.
7. François J. Congenital glaucoma and its inheritance. Ophthalmologica. 1980; 181: 61-73.
8. Jaafar MS. Care of the infantile glaucoma patient. In: Reinecke RD (Ed.), Ophthalmology Annual. New York: Raven Press 1988, pp.15-37.
9. Suri F, Chitsazian F, Khoramian-Tusi B, et al. Sex bias in primary congenital glaucoma patients with and without CYP1B1 Mutations. J Ophthalmic Vis Res 2009; 4: 75-78.
10. Walton DS, Nagao K, Yeung HH, Kane SA. Late-recognized primary congenital glaucoma. J Pediatr Ophthalmol Strabismus 2013; 30: 1-5
11. Sarfarazi M, Stoilov I. Molecular genetics of primary congenital glaucoma. Eye 2000; 14: 422-428.
12. Khan AO. Genetics of primary glaucoma. Curr Opin Ophthalmol 2011; 22: 347-355.
13. Gage PJ, Rhoades W, Prucka SK, Hjalt T. Fate maps of neural crest and mesoderm in the mammalian eye. Invest Ophthalmol Vis Sci 2005; 46: 4200-4208.
14. McMenamin PG. A quantitative study of the prenatal development of the aqueous outflow system in the human eye. Exp Eye Res 1991; 53: 507-517.
15. Ramirez JM, Ramirez AI, Salazar JJ, et al. Schlemm's canal and the collector channels at different developmental stages in the human eye. Cells Tissues Organs 2004; 178: 180-185.
16. Barkan O. Pathogenesis of congenital glaucoma. Am J Ophthalmol 1955; 40: 1-40.
17. Worst JGF. Congenital glaucoma. Remarks on the aspect of chamber angle, ontogenetic and pathogenetic background, and mode of action of goniotomy. Invest Ophthalmol 1968; 7: 127-134.
18. Maul E, Strozzi L, Muñoz C, Reyes C. The outflow pathway in congenital glaucoma. Am J Ophthalmol 1980; 89: 667-673.
19. Anderson DR. The development of the trabecular meshwork and its abnormality in primary congenital glaucoma. Trans Am Ophthalmol Soc 1981; 79: 481-485.
20. Hoskins HD, Hetherington J, Shaffer RN, Welling AM. In: Symposium on glaucoma. Transactions of the New Orleans Academy of Ophthalmology. St Louis: CV Mosby 1981, pp.191-202.
21. Perry LP, Jakobiec FA, Zakka FR, Walton DS. Newborn primary congenital glaucoma: histopathologic features of the anterior chamber filtration angle. J AAPOS 2012; 16: 565-568.
22. Shaw M, Handley S, Porooshani H, Papadopoulos M. A case of arrested primary congenital glaucoma. Eye 2013; 27: 100.
23. Shaffer RN. New concepts in infantile glaucoma. Can J Ophthalmol 1967; 2: 243-248.
24. Kupfer C, Ross K. The development of outflow facility in human eyes. Invest Ophthalmol 1971; 10: 513-517.
25. Maumenee AE. Further observations on the pathogenesis of congenital glaucoma. Am J Ophthalmol 1963; 55: 1163-1176.
26. De Vincentiis C. Incisione dell'angolo irideo nel glaucoma. Ann di Ottal 1983; 22: 540-542.

27. Barkan O. A new operation for chronic glaucoma. Am J Ophthalmol 1936; 19: 951-966.
28. Barkan O. Operation for congenital glaucoma. Am J Ophthalmol 1942; 25: 552-568.
29. Smith R. A new technique for opening the canal of Schlemm: Preliminary report. Br J Ophthalmol 1960; 44: 370-373.
30. Beck AD, Lynch MG. 360° trabeculotomy for primary congenital glaucoma. Arch Ophthalmol 1995; 113: 1200-1202.
31. Burian HM. A case of Marfan's syndrome with bilateral glaucoma. With description of a new type of operation for developmental glaucoma (trabeculotomy ab externo). Am J Ophthalmol 1960; 50: 1187-1192.
32. Allen L, Burian HM. Trabeculotomy ab externo. A new glaucoma operation: technique and results of experimental surgery. Am J Ophthalmol 1962; 53: 19-26.
35 Russell-Eggitt IM, Rice NS, Jay B, Wyse RK. Relapse following goniotomy for congenital glaucoma due to trabecular dysgenesis. Eye 1992; 6: 197-200.
36 Shaffer RN. Prognosis of goniotomy in primary infantile glaucoma (trabeculodysgenesis). Trans Am Ophthalmol Soc 1982; 80: 321-325.
37 Morin JD, Merin S, Sheppard RW. Primary congenital glaucoma – a survey. Can J Ophthalmol 1974; 9: 17-28.
38 Lister A. The prognosis in congenital glaucoma. Trans Ophthalmol Soc UK 1966; 86: 5-18.
39 Walton DS. In: Chandler PA, Grant WM (Eds.), Glaucoma. 2nd ed. Philadelphia: Lea & Febiger 1979, pp. 329-343.
40 Luntz MH, Livingston DG. Trabeculotomy ab externo and trabeculectomy in congenital and adult-onset glaucoma. Am J Ophthalmol 1977; 83: 174-179.
41 McPherson SD Jr, McFarland D. External trabeculotomy for developmental glaucoma. Ophthalmol 1980; 87: 302-305.
42 Akimoto M, Tanihara H, Negi A, Negata M. Surgical results of trabeculotomy ab externo for developmental glaucoma. Arch Ophthalmol 1994; 112: 1540-1544.
43 Dietlein TS, Jacobi PC, Krieglstein GK. Prognosis of primary ab externo surgery for primary congenital glaucoma. Br J Ophthalmol 1999; 83: 317-322.
44. Anderson DR. Trabeculotomy compared to goniotomy for glaucoma in children. Ophthalmology 1983; 90: 805-806.
45 Mendicino ME, Lynch MG, Drack A, et al. Long-term surgical and visual outcomes in primary congenital glaucoma: 360 degrees trabeculotomy versus goniotomy. J AAPOS 2000; 4: 205-210.
46. Girkin CA, Rhodes L, McGwin G, et al. Goniotomy versus circumferential trabeculotomy with an illuminated microcatheter in congenital glaucoma. J AAPOS 2012; 16: 424-427.
47. Beck AD, Lynn MJ, Crandall J, Mobin-Uddin O. Surgical outcomes with 360-degree suture trabeculotomy in poor-prognosis primary congenital glaucoma and glaucoma associated with congenital anomalies or cataract surgery. J AAPOS 2011; 15: 54-58.
48. Neely DE. False passage: a complication of 360°suture trabeculotomy. J AAPOS 2005; 9: 396-397.
49. Sarkisian SR Jr. An illuminated microcatheter for 360-degree trabeculotomy [corrected] in congenital glaucoma: a retrospective case series. J AAPOS 2010; 14: 412-416.
50. Mullaney PB, Selleck C, Al-Awad A, et al. Combined trabeculotomy and trabeculectomy as an initial procedure in uncomplicated congenital glaucoma. Arch Ophthalmol 1999; 117: 457-460.
51. Elder MJ. Combined trabeculotomy-trabeculectomy compared with primary trabeculectomy for congenital glaucoma. Br J Ophthalmol 1994; 78: 745-748.
52. Mandal AK, Bhatia PG, Gothwal VK, et al. Safety and efficacy of simultaneous bilateral primary combined trabeculotomy-trabeculectomy for developmental glaucoma. Indian J Ophthalmol 2002; 50: 13-19.
53. Mandal AK, Gothwal VK, Nutheti R. Surgical outcome of primary developmental glaucoma: a single surgeon's long-term experience from a tertiary eye care centre in India. Eye 2007; 21: 764-774.

54. Al-Hazmi A, Awad A, Zwann J, et al. Correlation between surgical success rate and severity of congenital glaucoma. Br J Ophthalmol 2005; 89: 449-453.

55. Essuman VA, Braimah IZ, Ndanu TA, Ntim-Amponsah CT. Combined trabeculotomy and trabeculectomy: outcome for primary congenital glaucoma in a West African population. Eye 2011; 25; 77-83.

56. Beauchamp GR, Parks MM. Filtering surgery in children: barriers to success. Ophthalmology 1979; 86: 170-180.

57. Burke JP, Bowell R. Primary trabeculectomy in congenital glaucoma. Br J Ophthalmol 1989; 73: 186-190.

58. Fulcher T, Chan J, Lanigan B, Bowell R, O'Keefe M. Long-term follow up of primary trabeculectomy for infantile glaucoma. Br J Ophthalmol 1996; 80: 499-502.

59. Gressel MG, Heuer DK, Parrish RK. Trabeculectomy in young patients. Ophthalmology 1984; 91: 1242-1246.

60. Rodrigues AM, Júnior AP, Montezano FT, et al. Comparison between results of trabeculectomy in primary congenital glaucoma with and without the use of mitomycin C. J Glaucoma 2004; 13: 228-232.

61. Al-Hazmi A, Zwaan J, Awad A, et al. Effectiveness and complications of mitomycin C use during pediatric glaucoma surgery. Ophthalmology 1998; 105: 1915-1920.

62. Sidoti PA, Belmonte SJ, Liebmann JM, Ritch R. Trabeculectomy with mitomycin-C in the treatment of pediatric glaucomas. Ophthalmology 2000; 107: 422-429.

63. Freedman SF, McCormick K, Cox TA. Mitomycin C-augmented trabeculectomy with postoperative wound modulation in pediatric glaucoma. J AAPOS 1999; 3: 117-124.

65. Susanna R Jr, Oltrogge EW, Carani JCE, Nicolela MT. Mitomycin as adjunct chemotherapy with trabeculectomy in congenital and developmental glaucomas. J Glaucoma 1995; 4: 151-157.

65. Wells AP, Cordeiro MF, Bunce CV, Khaw PT. Cystic bleb formation and related complications in limbus versus fornix-based conjunctival flaps in pediatric and young adult trabeculectomy with mitomycin C. Ophthalmology 2003; 110: 2192-2197.

66. Beck AD, Freedman S, Kammer J, Jin J. Aqueous shunt devices compared with trabeculectomy with Mitomycin-C for children in the first two years of life. Am J Ophthalmol 2003; 136: 994-1000.

67. Ishida K, Mandal AK, Netland PA. Glaucoma drainage implants in pediatric patients. Ophthalmol Clin North Am 2005; 18: 431-442, vii.

68. Pakravan M, Homayoon N, Shahin Y, Ali Reza BR. Trabeculectomy with mitomycin C versus Ahmed glaucoma implant with mitomycin C for treatment of pediatric aphakic glaucoma. J Glaucoma 2007; 16: 631-636.

69. Martino AZ, Iverson S, Feuer WJ, Greenfield DS. Surgical outcomes of superior versus inferior glaucoma drainage device implantation. J Glaucoma 2013 Feb 19. [Epub ahead of print]

70. Mac I, Soltau JB. Glaucoma-filtering bleb infections. Curr Opin Ophthalmol 2003; 14: 91-94.

71. Su CC, Liu YF, Li SY, et al. Mutations in the CYP1B1 gene may contribute to juvenile-onset open-angle glaucoma. Eye 2012; 26: 1369-1377.

72. Feitl ME, Krupin T, Tanna AP. Juvenile Glaucoma. In: Roy FH, Fraunfelder FW, Fraunfelder FT (Eds.), Current Ocular Therapy. Amsterdam: Elsevier 2008, pp.491-495.

73. Gupta V, Ov M, Rao A, et al. Long-term structural and functional outcomes of therapy in juvenile-onset primary open-angle glaucoma: a five year follow up. Ophthalmologica 2012; 228: 19-25.

74. Maeda-Chubachi T, Chi-Burris K, Simons BD, et al. Comparison of latanoprost and timolol in pediatric glaucoma: a phase 3, 12-week, randomized, double-masked multicenter study. Ophthalmology 2011; 118: 2014-2021.

75. Black AC, Jones S, Yanovitch TL, et al. Latanoprost in pediatric glaucoma – pediatric exposure over a decade. J AAPOS 2009; 13: 558-562.

76. Yeung HH, Walton DS. Goniotomy for juvenile open-angle glaucoma. J Glaucoma 2010; 19: 1-4.
77. Dao JB, Sarkisian SR, Freedman SF. Illuminated microcatheter-facilitated 360-degree trabeculotomy for refractory aphakic and juvenile open-angle glaucoma. J Glaucoma 2013 May (Epub ahead of print).
78. Tsai JC, Chang HW, Kao CN et al. Trabeculectomy with mitomycin C versus trabeculectomy alone for juvenile primary open-angle glaucoma. Ophthalmologica 2003; 217: 24-30.
79. Pathania D, Senthil S, Rao HL, et al. Outcomes of trabeculectomy in juvenile open-angle glaucoma. Indian J Ophthalmol 2013 April (Epub ahead of print).
80. Donahue SP, Keech RV, Munden P, Scott WE. Baerveldt implant surgery in the treatment of advanced childhood glaucoma. J AAPOS 1997; 1: 41-45.
81. Stangos AN, Whatham AR, Sunaric-Megevand G. Primary viscocanalostomy for juvenile open-angle glaucoma. Am J Ophthalmol 2005; 140: 490-496.
82. Elgin U, Ozturk F, Sen E, Serdar K. Comparison of optic disc topography before and after antiglaucoma treatment in juvenile glaucoma. Eur J Ophthalmol 2010; 20: 907-910.

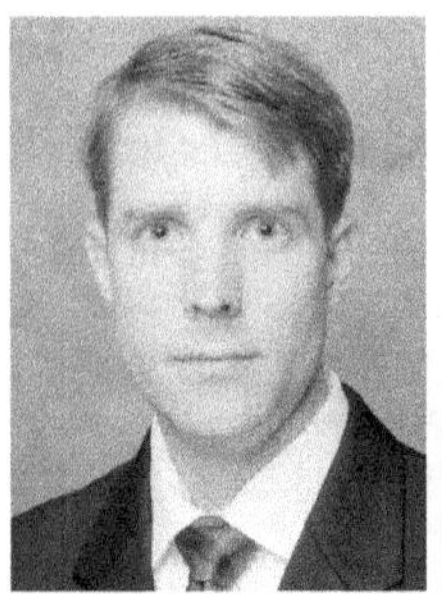
Michael Banitt

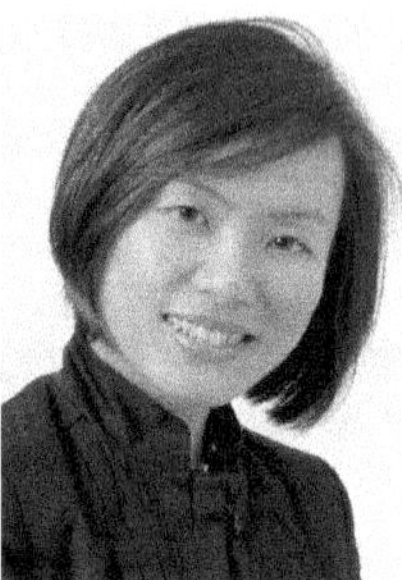
Jocelyn Chua

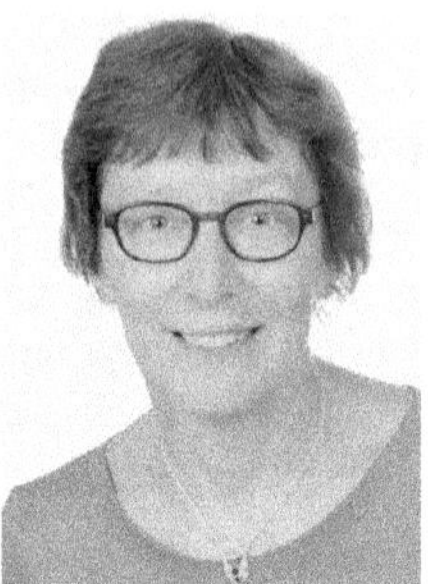
Barbara Cvenkel

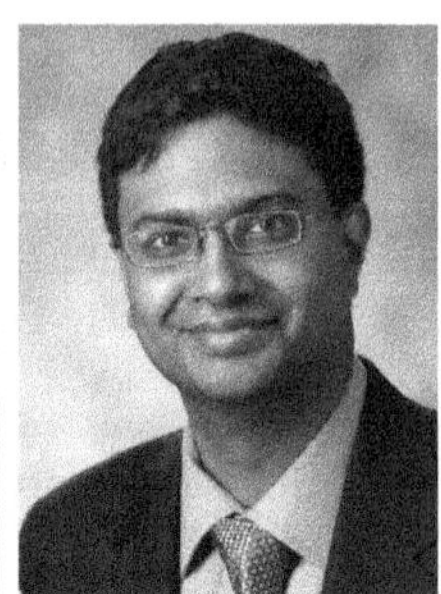
Pradeep Ramula

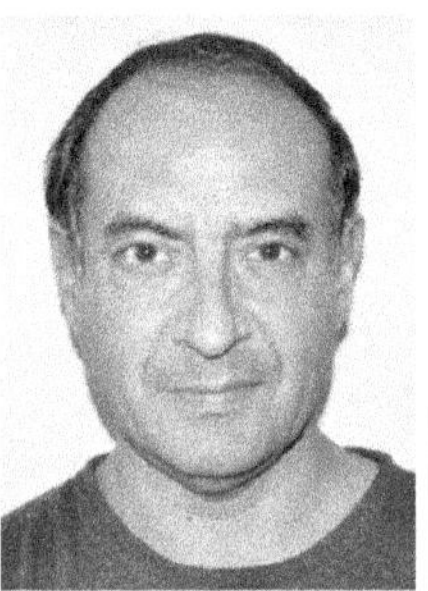
Hernán Iturriaga-Valenzuela

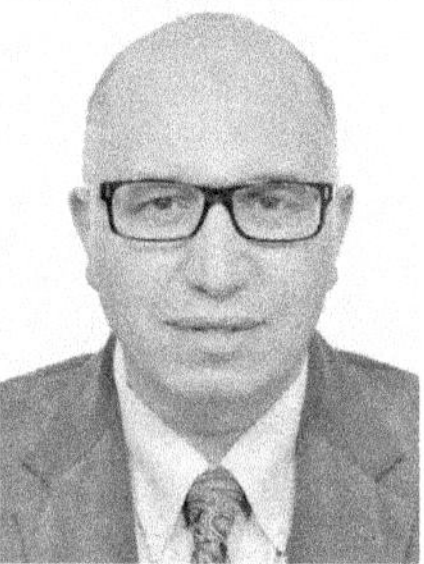
Ahmed Abdelrahman

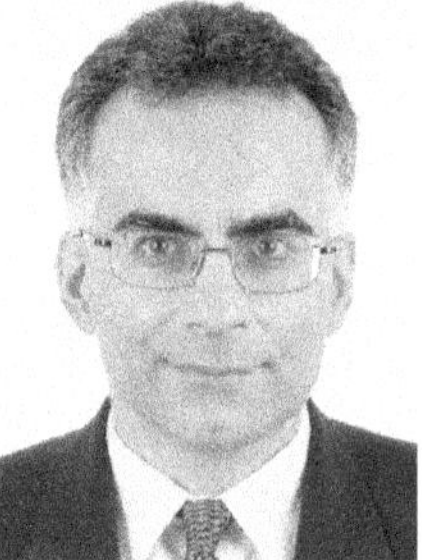
Arif Khan

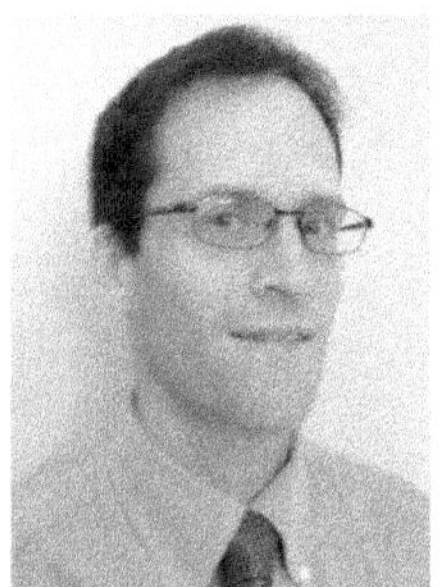
Patrick Hamel

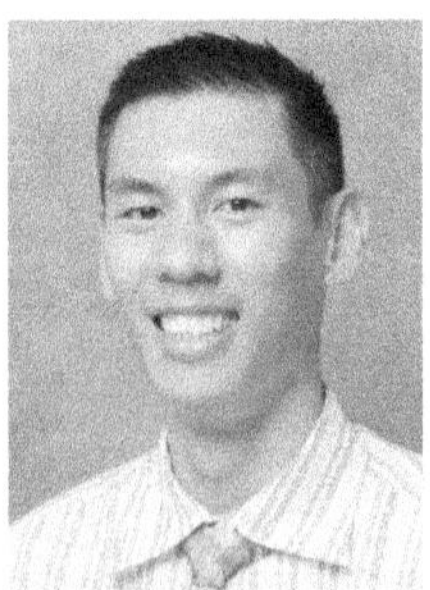
Ta Chen Peter Chang

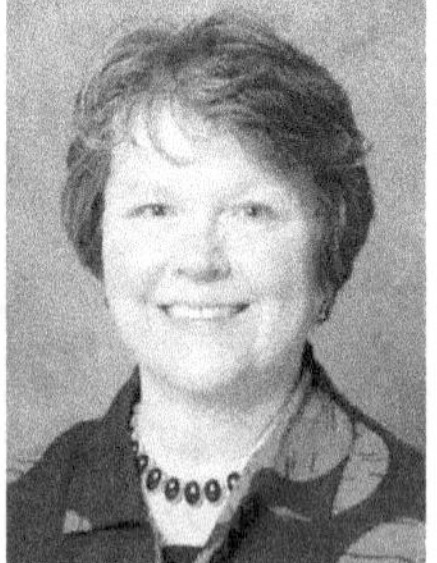
Elizabeth Hodapp

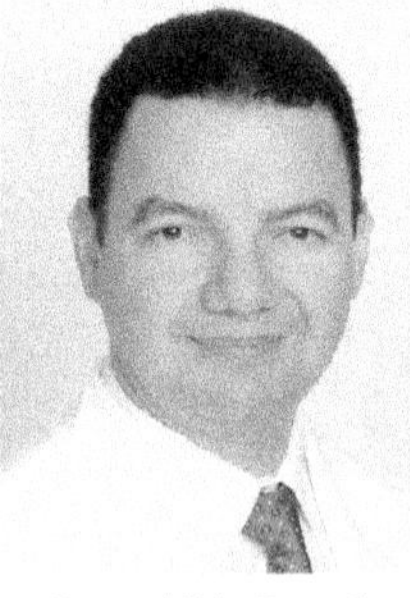
Oscar Albis-Donado

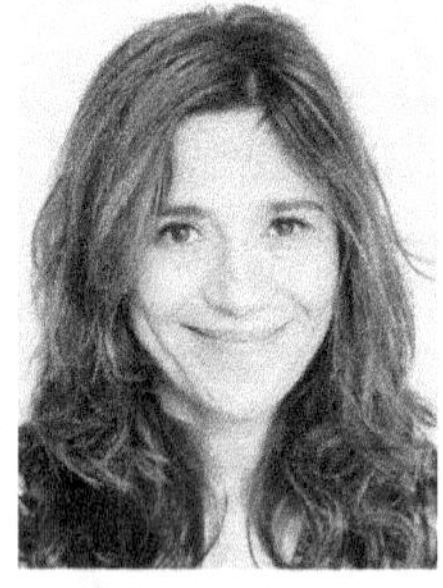
Maria Papadopoulos

7. GLAUCOMA ASSOCIATED WITH NON-ACQUIRED OCULAR ANOMALIES

Michael Banitt, Jocelyn Chua, Barbara Cvenkel, Pradeep Ramula,
Hernán Iturriaga-Valenzuela, Ahmed Abdelrahman, Arif Khan,
Patrick Hamel, Ta Chen Peter Chang, Elizabeth Hodapp, Oscar Albis-Donado,
Maria Papadopoulos

Section Leaders: Maria Papadopoulos, Elizabeth Hodapp, Oscar Albis-Donado
Contributors: Shira Robbins, Akira Negi, Fede Fortunato, Albert Khouri

Consensus statements

1. Children who have non-acquired ocular anomalies often have systemic conditions that require pediatric evaluation and/or treatment.
2. Many non-acquired ocular anomalies are genetic in nature.
   Comment: Screening of family members in such cases and genetic counseling is indicated.
3. Glaucoma related to non-acquired ocular anomalies may be present at birth or may develop over time, so regular lifelong monitoring is necessary.
4. Before glaucoma develops, one should consider treating elevated intraocular pressure (IOP) associated with non-acquired ocular anomalies (secondary ocular hypertension).
5. Infantile onset of glaucoma related to non-acquired ocular anomalies is associated with buphthalmos and the risk of Descemet membrane breaks.
6. Medical treatment is usually first-line, but surgery is often required early for congenital/infantile presentations and should not be delayed.
   Comment: Angle surgery in infants may be effective although the results are usually not as good as for primary congenital glaucoma (PCG).
   Comment: Often trabeculectomy with anti-scarring agents or primary tube surgery is necessary for IOP control.
   Comment: Cyclodestruction may be considered after failed trabeculectomy or tube surgery.
7. There is considerable phenotypic variability associated with genetic mutations recognized in children with non-acquired ocular anomalies.
8. Axenfeld-Rieger (AR) anomaly is recognized now to represent a spectrum of disease previously referred to as Axenfeld anomaly and Rieger anomaly. Axen-

Childhood Glaucoma, pp. 155-177
*Edited by Robert N. Weinreb, Alana L. Grajewski, Maria Papadopoulos, John Grigg,
and Sharon Freedman*
2013 © Kugler Publications, Amsterdam, The Netherlands

feld-Rieger syndrome includes the ocular findings of Axenfeld-Rieger anomaly with the addition of systemic abnormalities.

Comment: Examination of family members including gonioscopy is important to determine whether the patient is part of a larger pedigree or a new case.

9. Peters anomaly is usually seen as an isolated ocular disorder but can be associated with systemic abnormalities of neural crest origin and is referred to as Peters plus syndrome.

Comment: It is important to exclude the presence of systemic involvement and when it is present, to co-manage it with a pediatrician.

Comment: Assessing for glaucoma can be challenging as typical IOP measurement over the central cornea may be inaccurate and the optic discs may not be visible. Measure the IOP in a clear area of cornea if possible.

10. Aniridia is commonly associated with glaucoma and is due to both open- and closed-angle mechanisms.

Comment: Children with sporadic aniridia should be screened for Wilms tumor.

11. Management of persistent fetal vasculature can be challenging because of the heterogeneity of clinical presentation.

Comment: Surgical treatment is aimed towards obtaining useful vision and preventing or treating secondary complications such as glaucoma.

Introduction

A variety of congenital ocular anomalies are associated with glaucoma. Some also have associated systemic conditions. This section deals with conditions commonly associated with glaucoma in which the ocular abnormalities are generally the findings that bring the patient to medical attention. The conditions discussed in this section are associated with a lifelong increased risk of glaucoma necessitating regular intraocular pressure (IOP) review once the anomaly is recognized. Although review intervals have not been studied, some experts suggest review at least four- to six-monthly until puberty and six- to12-monthly thereafter, for conditions with a significant association of glaucoma. Infantile onset of glaucoma from any cause is associated with buphthalmos and the risk of Descemet membrane breaks. In general, consistently elevated IOP should be treated medically if associated with non-acquired ocular anomalies. Medical treatment is usually first-line. Angle surgery in infants may be effective although the results are usually not as good as for primary congenital glaucoma (PCG). Often trabeculectomy with antimetabolites or glaucoma drainage surgery is necessary for IOP control. Following which, ametropia and amblyopia therapy must be addressed as indicated. Patients with conditions known to be associated with systemic findings should be referred for medical evaluation, preferably to a pediatrician. It is important to be mindful that signs can develop with time, warranting vigilance and another referral. Genetic counseling and family screening is definitely indicated for those conditions with a recognized autosomal dominant or recessive inheritance. Furthermore, patients should seek advice when adults as their risk may be different as compared to their parents.

This section will review Axenfeld-Rieger anomaly, Peters anomaly, aniridia, ectropion uveae, persistent fetal vasculature (PFV), microcornea, sclerocornea, and those anterior segment anomalies that do not fit into any recognized category.

Axenfeld-Rieger anomaly

In 1920, Axenfeld described a patient with a deep, linear corneal opacity with adherent iris strands.[1] Later, in 1934, Rieger described patients with similar findings as well as corectopia, iris atrophy and iris holes.[2] Other patients with iridocorneal abnormalities were also noted to have extraocular developmental defects involving the teeth and facial bones. Traditionally, these findings have been referred to by three eponyms: (1) Axenfeld anomaly; (2) Rieger anomaly; and (3) Rieger syndrome. However, many have recognized the overlap between these conditions and have begun to refer to them as one entity: 'anterior chamber cleavage syndrome',[3] 'mesodermal dysgenesis of the cornea and iris',[4] 'neurocristopathy',[5] and 'iridogoniodysgenesis'.

Definition

To minimize confusion, the terms Axenfeld-Rieger anomaly and Axenfeld-Rieger syndrome will be used here. Axenfeld-Rieger anomaly refers to usually bilateral abnormalities of the peripheral cornea, peripheral iris, and angle. Clinically, posterior embryotoxon (prominent Schwalbe line) with iris attachments is seen. These changes may not always be readily visible on the slit lamp but are instead apparent on gonioscopy only (Fig. 1). So the diagnosis of Axenfeld Rieger anomaly can only be excluded when gonioscopy is performed. A prominent Schwalbe line without iris attachments is not considered to be Axenfeld-Rieger anomaly, nor is it considered a risk factor for glaucoma. The corneal findings occur when Schwalbe

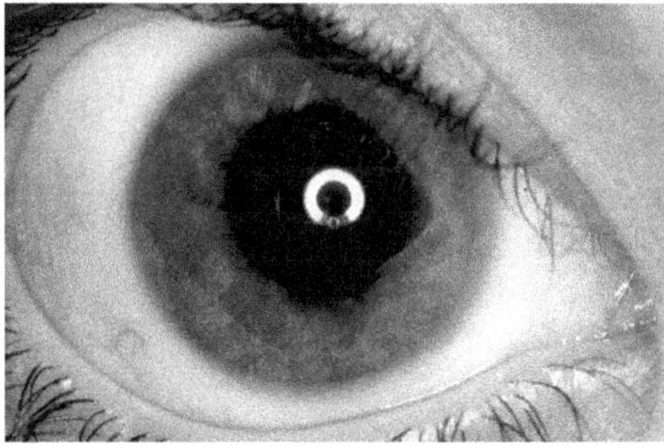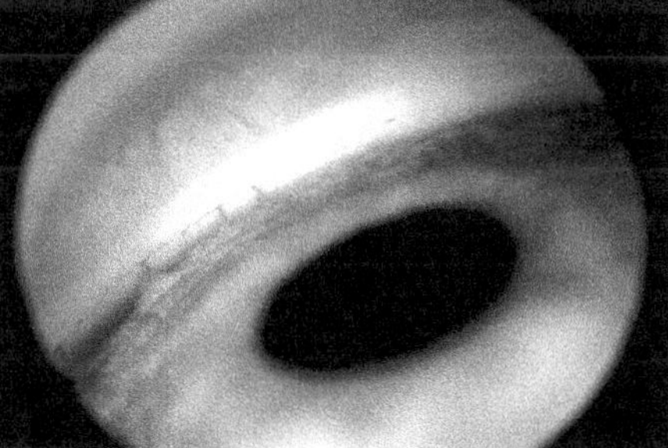

Fig. 1. AR anomaly with typical gonioscopic findings but no posterior embryotoxon evident on slit lamp examination. (Courtesy of Dr. Albert Khouri).

line is anteriorly positioned and appears at or near the limbus as a white line or a ring within the peripheral, posterior cornea. In some cases, it does not exist as a continuous line for the entire circumference of the cornea.

Within the angle, threadlike or broad bands of iris tissue extend from the peripheral iris to both the trabecular meshwork and to the prominent Schwalbe line. In between these attachments, the anterior chamber angle is open, the trabecular meshwork is visible, but the scleral spur may be blurred. The broad bands of attachments obscure the angle structures. Isolated iris bands that only reach the trabecular meshwork are long iris processes, and are not part of the spectrum of Axenfeld-Rieger.

While Axenfeld-Rieger anomaly is defined by the presence of iris attachments to the posterior embryotoxon, other iris findings including generalized stromal thinning or atrophy, corectopia (with the pupil pulled in the direction of the most prominent angle findings), iris hole formation occurring in the quadrant opposite the site of corectopia, and ectropion uveae may be seen. Iris findings do not typically progress but have been demonstrated to worsen over time in some individuals.

Axenfeld-Rieger syndrome includes the ocular findings of Axenfeld-Rieger anomaly with the addition of systemic abnormalities. The most frequent abnormalities seen include developmental anomalies of the face (hypertelorism), teeth (microdontia, hypodontia), heart, umbilicus (periumbilical skin tags), and male genitourinary system (hypospadias). Some other associations include pectum excavatum, empty sella syndrome, growth hormone deficiency and mental retardation.

Inheritance

Axenfeld-Rieger anomaly and syndrome are most commonly inherited in an autosomal dominant fashion and are genetically heterogeneous. Three genetic loci have been identified.[6] These include the chromosomal locus 4q25 and the corresponding gene *PITX2* (MIM number 601542) and the chromosomal locus 6p25 and the corresponding gene *FOXC1* (MIM number 601090). A third locus, 13q14, has been discovered however no gene has been identified (MIM number 601499).[7] Both *PITX2* and *FOXC1* function by regulating the expression of other genes rather than coding for structural proteins. Genotype-phenotype correlations exist as patients with *PITX2* defects and those with *FOXC1* duplication have a more severe glaucoma prognosis than do patients with *FOXC1* mutations.[8] Patients with systemic findings are more likely to have *PITX2* than *FOXC1* defects.[8] Examination of family members including gonioscopy is important to determine whether the patient is part of a larger pedigree or a new case (*see* Section 3).

Incidence of glaucoma

The incidence of glaucoma for an individual affected by Axenfeld-Rieger anomaly is 50%.[9] The onset can be at any time but often occurs in childhood or young adulthood (ten-30 years of age). The IOP is often labile. While the extent of the iris defects and iridocorneal strands does not correlate precisely with the presence or severity of glaucoma, the more anterior the insertion of the iris into the angle the higher the likelihood of developing glaucoma. When the onset of glaucoma occurs in infancy, corneal enlargement, breaks in Descemet membrane (Haab striae), and globe enlargement ensue.

Mechanism of glaucoma

The exact pathogenesis of glaucoma associated with Axenfeld-Rieger anomaly is not known, but is believed to result from maldevelopment of the angle.

Management

If the ocular abnormalities are subtle, a diagnosis may not be made until a routine exam is performed. Signs or symptoms of glaucoma during infancy may prompt an evaluation. Once a diagnosis of Axenfeld-Rieger anomaly has been made, patients should be referred to either a pediatrician or an internist to evaluate for the systemic findings of Axenfeld-Rieger syndrome including cardiac valvular and male genitourinary abnormalities. Since both Axenfeld-Rieger anomaly and syndrome are most commonly transmitted in an autosomal dominant fashion, as already mentioned, family members should undergo a standard ophthalmic examination including gonioscopy.

The most important decision in managing individuals with Axenfeld-Rieger anomaly when the diagnosis is made is to determine if glaucoma exists. If it does not, lifelong monitoring for the development of elevated IOP is necessary. Once consistently elevated IOP is detected, even with normal optic discs (secondary ocular hypertension), it should be treated with medications to delay the onset of glaucoma. Medication is first-line for both secondary ocular hypertension and glaucoma, however, surgery is often required early in congenital or infantile presentations and should not be delayed. Miotics are often ineffective, but all other classes can be utilized. If IOP remains uncontrolled, angle surgery [(goniotomy, trabeculotomy (conventional or circumferential)] can be considered especially in infants but is not thought to be as successful as in PCG.[10-12] Specifically all quadrants of the angle should be mapped out with regard to visible areas of trabecular meshwork and the presence and extent of iris attachments. Care must be taken as angle surgery may be difficult or even damage an eye with a significant amount of iris attachments; for example, performing circumferential trabeculotomy in an area without visible trabecular meshwork may lead to a Descemet membrane detachment and/or iris disinsertion. Goniotomy can cut through smaller iris attachments. If there are no significant areas of visible trabecular meshwork, consider severing iris attachments with a blade or microscissors (that can fit through several paracenteses) to obtain access to the trabecular meshwork. Once the meshwork is both accessible and visible, angle surgery of the surgeon's preference can be performed.

Trabeculectomy surgery with antiscarring agents or glaucoma drainage surgery can be considered first line or if angle surgery is not possible or fails. Transscleral cyclophotocoagulation can be considered after trabeculectomy or glaucoma drainage surgery has failed or if visual potential is limited. After each failed surgery commence medications before considering further surgery.

Management summary (*see* Fig. 2)

1. Refer for medical evaluation to determine presence of systemic involvement.
2. Screen family members.
3. Genetic screening if available.
4. Assess for presence of glaucoma.
   A. If glaucoma is absent: monitor for elevated IOP and treat medically if it develops.
   B. If glaucoma is present or develops:
      a. Medical therapy is indicated, but surgery is often required early for congenital/infantile presentations and should not be delayed.
      b. Surgery.
         i. Angle surgery may be considered in infants if the angle is open and largely unobscured by the peripheral iris attachments. Caution is advised for cases where the angle is significantly obscured by iris attachments. The success rates are poorer than those for PCG.
         ii. Filtering surgery: trabeculectomy with antiscarring agents or glaucoma drainage surgery can be first line or indicated when angle surgery is not possible or fails.
         iii. Transscleral cyclophotocoagulation: considered when trabeculectomy or glaucoma drainage surgery fails or visual potential is limited.
5. Ametropic correction and amblyopic therapy.

Peters anomaly

Definition

Peters anomaly is a mesenchymal dysgenesis of the anterior segment, presenting with a spectrum of disorders that involve ocular structures derived from the embryological mesenchymal layer.[13] This condition is characterized by the presence of a central, corneal opacity present at birth with a corresponding defect in posterior stroma, Descemet membrane and endothelium. The opacity may be variable in size and density and may clear with time. Bilateral involvement occurs in about 80% of cases. Peters anomaly can range in severity from mild with just the corneal opacity being the only abnormality (normal iris and lens) to moderate involving the iris (iridocorneal adhesions, iris defects) and to severe with lenticular abnormalities (corneolenticular adhesions). Peters anomaly is usually seen as an isolated ocular disorder although it can be associated with other ocular abnormalities[13] such as sclerocornea, microphthalmia, aniridia, iris coloboma, posterior embryotoxon, anterior staphyloma, persistent fetal vasculature and cataract.

Peters anomaly can be associated with systemic abnormalities of neural crest origin and is referred to as Peters plus syndrome. Systemic involvement may present with a cleft lip/palate, ear abnormality, dextrocardia, central nervous system abnormality, agenesis of urinary tract, short stature, facial dysmorphism, laryngomalacia and macroglossia. Patients with Peters plus syndrome tend to have more severe ocular disease as well as a higher risk of glaucoma than patients with only Peters anomaly.

Inheritance

The inheritance pattern of Peters anomaly is typically sporadic (new case with no family history) but it can be autosomal dominant or recessive. Peters anomaly may result from abnormalities of the *PITX2*, *FOXC1* and *CYP1B1* gene. Mutations involving the *PAX6* gene on chromosome 11p13 have also been associated with this condition. Dominant *PAX6* gene, recessive *B3GALTL* (Peters plus syndrome), and recessive *CYP1B1* mutations (often in the context of glaucoma) can also cause the phenotype (*see* Section 3).

Incidence of glaucoma

The incidence of glaucoma is about 50% over the lifetime of an individual with Peters anomaly so lifelong IOP surveillance is indicated. Raised intraocular pressure tends to occur during infancy but it can also occur later in childhood.

Mechanism of glaucoma

Several pathogenic mechanisms are known to contribute to the development of glaucoma[14] and these include trabeculodysgenesis, malformation of the Schlemm canal and/or formation of peripheral anterior synechiae. Secondary glaucoma may also occur after surgical intervention for corneal disease and/or after a long-term course of topical steroid post corneal transplant.

Management

It is important to exclude the presence of systemic involvement and when present, to co-manage it with a pediatrician. The extent of ocular involvement determines the visual prognosis[15] as well as the risk of development of glaucoma. Where appropriate and possible, investigation tools such as the ultrasound B-scan, anterior segment optical coherence tomography (AS OCT) or ultrasound biomicroscopy (UBM) may be useful in delineating the anatomical relationship of intraocular structures within the anterior and posterior segments.

Visual rehabilitation is a challenge as the vision may be affected from deprivational amblyopia (due to corneal opacity and/or cataract), uncorrected refractive error, retinal abnormality, neurological deficit or glaucomatous optic neuropathy. In the presence of a dense central corneal opacity and a clear lens, pupillary dilatation or a broad optical iridectomy at the site of maximum corneal clarity may be useful in creating a visual axis.[16] Consider a scleral incision for the optical iridectomy so as to prevent further corneal scarring. Penetrating keratoplasty (PK) may be considered in bilateral dense corneal opacities so as to clear the visual axis in at least one eye. The timing of this surgery is controversial. Early surgery provides the best opportunity for visual development. However, surgery within the first year of life has high rate of rejection, and requires a dedicated caregiver to deal with the postoperative management. Glaucoma is a common complication in these young children following penetrating keratoplasty and requires specific monitoring for its development. In cases of unilateral disease, the pros and cons of corneal transplant need to be carefully discussed with the parents. Lens extraction may also be necessary to clear the visual axis and can be considered in combination with the corneal transplant surgery. IOP control is essential for subsequent corneal graft survival. Published results of corneal transplant surgery for Peters anomaly are disappointing, especially in infants.[17-19] The cumulative probability of a clear graft was 22-44% at two years[19,20] and the predicted mean graft survival of 20 months (95% CI: 4.9-36.3) in one study.[19] Furthermore, there is a significant likelihood of repeating graft surgery with decreased chance of survival for each repeat graft.[20] The main causes of graft failure have been reported to be allograft rejection followed by graft infection.[20] Factors associated with poor prognosis include: young age at surgery (less than six months of age), associated lensectomy or vitrectomy, severity of disease, preoperative glaucoma, peripheral anterior synechiae, poor compliance and running suture closure technique. Descemet stripping automated endothelial keratoplasty (DSAEK) has been reported in two children with Peters anomaly, with prominent corneal opacity localized posteriorly.[21] Both patients had reduction in the density of corneal opacity and improved vision postoperatively. The grafts remained clear up to one year after surgery. However, peripheral graft detachment necessitated repositioning with air in both cases. Descemet membrane endothelial keratoplasty (DMEK) has also been described in adult buphthalmic eyes.[22] The potential advantages of this surgery would be reduced risk of allograft rejection, and avoidance of suture-related and open-globe complications. It is important to remember that lowering IOP medically in the absence of glaucoma may improve corneal clarity. Successful glaucoma surgery can also significantly reduce corneal opacification.

Children with Peters anomaly need to be monitored regularly for elevated IOP as uncontrolled IOP can result in irreversible glaucomatous optic neuropathy as well as corneal graft failure. Assessing these children for glaucoma can be challenging as typical IOP measurement over the central cornea will be inaccurate and the optic discs may not be visible. Therefore measure IOP in clear cornea periphery if possible and ballot the eyes to confirm the accuracy of the measurement. In neonates and infants monitor biometric parameters such as corneal diameter and axial length to assess for the development or progression of glaucoma. Management of elevated IOP is usually difficult in Peters anomaly and more than one surgical intervention is often necessary[18] when medical treatment has failed. Despite all these measures, only one third of cases that require surgery manage to achieve good postoperative IOP control.[18] Angle surgery (trabeculotomy) may be considered in the presence of a deep anterior segment, an open anterior chamber angle of at least 120 degrees and in the absence of irido/lenticular-corneal adhesions. If the angle cannot be visualized or if there are lenticulocorneal adhesions, circumferential trabeculotomy should not be attempted, unless iridocorneal adherences are first cut with microscissors. Blunt dissection of the latter should not be done as detachment of the Descemet membrane may occur. Glaucoma drainage surgery is often the primary filtration surgery of choice to control IOP especially in the moderate to severe forms of Peters anomaly. Trabeculectomy with antiscarring agents may be considered in mild Peters anomaly. Transscleral cyclophotocoagulation is useful in the reduction of IOP in cases of very advanced refractory glaucoma and / or those with poor visual potential. After each failed surgery commence medications before considering further surgery.

Management summary (*see* Fig. 2)

1. Refer for medical evaluation to determine presence of systemic involvement.
2. Genetic screening if available.
3. Ascertain the extent of ocular involvement if not obvious clinically.
4. Assess for presence of glaucoma.
   A. If glaucoma is absent: monitor for elevated IOP and treat medically if it develops.
   B. If glaucoma is present or develops:
      a. Medical therapy.
      b. Surgery.
         i.   Angle surgery may be considered in selected cases but results are poor compared to PCG.
         ii. Filtering surgery: trabeculectomy with antiscarring agents for mild Peters anomaly or glaucoma drainage surgery for moderate to severe forms can be first line.
         iii. Transscleral cyclophotocoagulation: considered in cases of very advanced refractory glaucoma and/or poor visual potential.
5. Visual rehabilitation.
   A. Chronic pupil dilation or broad optical iridectomy is indicated for dense central opacities and when the lens is clear. Consider a scleral incision for the optical iridectomy so as to prevent further corneal scarring and place it at the site of maximum corneal clarity.

    B. Consider medically lowering IOP in the absence of glaucoma to improve corneal clarity. Successful glaucoma surgery can significantly reduce corneal opacification.

    C. Penetrating keratoplasty

       i. Is associated with disappointing results especially in infants.

      ii. Consider in cases of bilateral dense corneal opacities so as to clear the visual axis in at least one eye when a dedicated caregiver exists.

     iii. In cases of unilateral disease, the pros and cons of corneal transplant need to be carefully discussed with the parents.

     iv. IOP control is essential for subsequent corneal graft survival.

6. Ametropic correction and amblyopia therapy.

Aniridia

Definition

Aniridia is a bilateral ocular disorder characterized by the congenital, variable absence of a normal iris. Its incidence ranges from 1:64.000 to 1:100.000. The term aniridia is incorrect, as the iris is not completely absent. It is usually extremely hypoplastic with some rudimentary iris stump of variable width identified gonioscopically, or it is sometimes only partially absent. Aniridia is often associated with foveal and optic-nerve hypoplasia (present at birth), keratopathy, early-onset cataract and glaucoma. Additional associations include nystagmus, retinal detachment and ptosis.[23] Aniridia-associated keratopathy is due to limbal stem-cell deficiency. A large study in Sweden and Norway found that corneal involvement was present in 80% of aniridic individuals and that in 26%, the corneal abnormality caused visual disturbance. The general pattern was for peripheral thickening and pannus formation, which progressed centrally with eventual development of persistent corneal erosions and corneal opacity.[24] Central corneal thickness is known to be greater than normal in aniridic patients. [25]

Inheritance and associated conditions

In about two-thirds of cases the inheritance pattern is autosomal dominant with high penetrance and variable expression. Most of the remaining one third of cases result from sporadic mutations and are then passed on in an autosomal-dominant pattern with variable expressivity. Those individuals with sporadic mutations are at markedly increased risk of Wilms tumor (nephroblastoma) and WAGR syndrome (30%). This syndrome is a contiguous gene syndrome where the *PAX6* gene and *WT1* gene are both deleted along with other genes. The clinical features include: Wilms tumor (80% before the age of five), aniridia, genitourinary abnormalities and mental retardation. A very rare condition associated with aniridia is the autosomal recessive Gillespie syndrome, which includes aniridia, cerebellar ataxia, ptosis and mental retardation. The typical presentation is the discovery of fixed dilated pupils in a hypotonic infant.[26]

Most aniridic patients have mutations in the *PAX6* gene on 11p13. *PAX6* expression level appears to be critical for eye development and small variations in *PAX6* levels may result in subtly different phenotypes.[27] *PAX6* mutations have a high degree of phenotypic variability, with variable degrees of iris preservation and severity of macular and optic nerve maldevelopment. In addition, aniridia and Peters anomaly may be present in the same pedigree. The aniridia phenotype has been noted in several pedigrees of individuals without *PAX6* abnormality, but with *PITX2* and *FOXC1* mutations.[28,29] Recessive *CYP1B1* mutations can cause a distinct phenotype of partial aniridia, ectropion uveae, and central keratopathy[30] (*see* Section 3).

Incidence of glaucoma

Glaucoma occurs in 50% to 75% of patients. Early onset is unusual and in most cases, it usually appears in childhood or adolescence.

Mechanism of glaucoma

Both open-angle and angle-closure glaucoma occurs in aniridia. Open-angle glaucoma is more common and thought to be caused by poor development of the drainage system. Angle-closure glaucoma develops in a subset of patients when the iris gradually migrates over the trabecular meshwork resulting in progressive angle closure and elevated IOP.[31]

Management

Children with sporadic aniridia should be screened for Wilms tumor by renal ultrasound and urinalysis every three months until the age of six years[32] or until genetic test results become available. If the genetic test result for Wilms tumor is negative, that is, a sporadic aniridic patient does not have the *WT1* deletion, then monitoring for genitourinary complications may not be warranted.[32] The decision to discontinue tumor surveillance should be made by the pediatrician and the clinical geneticist.

Visual acuity can be poor in patients with aniridia due to foveal or optic nerve hypoplasia, cataract, ectopia lentis, glaucoma, keratopathy and photophobia. When media are clear, symptomatic relief of photophobia can be achieved with lubricants and tinted prescription glasses. Prescription cosmetic contact lenses may also be considered and their potential advantages/disadvantages discussed with the parents. Cataract surgery is demanding in aniridia because of frequently reduced visibility of intraocular structures due to keratopathy, lens subluxation and a thinner, more fragile lens capsule. Consider a posterior approach for cataract removal if ectopia lentis is present. If cataract surgery needs to be performed, the possibility of implanting segmental iris prosthetic devices (Morcher aniridia rings) or iris diaphragm lens (Morcher aniridia IOL) needs to be balanced against the significant risk of elevated IOP or worsening IOP control.[33-35] There are no reports of their use in children. Keratopathy increases with age and, irrespective of age, after intraocular surgery. Treatment of severe keratopathy is difficult. In one long-term study of patients with aniridic keratopathy, those undergoing surgery (23 eyes), either limbal transplant (10 eyes) or penetrating keratoplasty (13 eyes), and no surgery (25 eyes) were compared.[36] In terms of long-term visual prognosis, there was no significant difference between the limbal transplant and penetrating keratoplasty groups, but a slight improvement in the ocular surface of the limbal transplant group was noted in the first five years, after which there was worsening due to the recurrence of aniridic keratopathy. The median survival time for limbal transplant (48 months) was double that of penetrating keratoplasty (24 months) but this was not statistically significant. Furthermore, there was no significant difference in the long-term visual outcome between patients who had surgery and those patients who had no surgery for aniridic keratopathy.

Children with aniridia need to be monitored regularly for elevated IOP. If IOP begins to rise or glaucoma is present, medical therapy, including miotic drops,[31] should be initiated. Angle surgery, in particular goniotomy, has been reported both as therapy (with poor results)[31,37] and as prophylaxis against glaucoma in selected cases (modified goniotomy in children over a year old with greater than 180° angle closure and documented progression).[38] The latter is not widely practiced due to the potential risk of intraocular trauma. Trabeculectomy with antiscarring agents can be first line especially in the absence of a cataract. In theory, antimetabolites, especially 5FU, may aggravate existing keratopathy. Glaucoma drainage devices may be a better option especially in the presence of a cataract that will need extraction in the future, and can be associated with favorable results.[39] Care should be taken to place the tube far from the endothelium and away from the lens by oblique tube placement, over zonular fibers. Postoperative hypotony with any surgery should be avoided at all costs due to the danger of lens-corneal touch, which will cause both cataract and corneal decompensation. Transscleral cyclophotocoagulation is an option after a failed trabeculectomy or glaucoma drainage surgery.

Management summary (*see* Fig. 2)

1. Refer patients with sporadic aniridia for appropriate renal assessment and follow up.
2. Genetic screening if available.
3. Assess for presence of glaucoma.
   A. If glaucoma is absent: monitor for elevated IOP and treat medically if it develops.
   B. If glaucoma is present or develops:
      a. Medical therapy.
      b. Surgery.

   i. Angle surgery (goniotomy) has been reported both as therapy (with lack of a reported effect) and as prophylaxis in specific cases but the latter is not widely practiced due to the potential risk of intraocular trauma.

   ii. Trabeculectomy with antiscarring agents can be first-line, especially in the absence of a cataract but may aggravate existing keratopathy.

   iii. Glaucoma drainage surgery may be indicated if significant cataract is present or trabeculectomy fails and can be associated with favorable results. Aim for oblique tube placement in the AC, over zonule fibers rather than the lens.

   iv. Transscleral cyclophotocoagulation: consider after failed trabeculectomy or glaucoma drainage surgery.

   v. Avoid hypotony due to the increased risk of lens-corneal touch

4. Visual rehabilitation.

   A. Symptomatic relief of photophobia/glare can be achieved with lubricants and tinted glasses. Consider prescription cosmetic contact lenses following detailed discussion with parents.

   B. Cataract surgery.

     a. Anterior vs. posterior approach (ectopia lentis).

     b. Avoid Morcher aniridic IOL and iris rings because of risk to IOP control.

5. Ametropic correction and amblyopia therapy.

Congenital ectropion uveae

Definition and associations

Congenital ectropion uveae is rare and characterized by iris pigment epithelial hyperplasia from the pigment ruff which is present on the anterior iris stroma. It is typically non-progressive, but progression has been reported.[40] It can be associated with neurofibromatosis Type I (NF1), Axenfeld-Rieger anomaly or aniridia.[41,42]

Inheritance

Congenital ectropion uveae is usually sporadic (new case with no family history) and unilateral. The primary form of inheritance is autosomal dominant as part of NF-1. Additionally, *PAX6* mutations have been found in a father and son in whom the iris was present, though with ectropion uveae, and were so thought to have a variant of aniridia.[42]

Incidence of glaucoma

The incidence of glaucoma with congenital ectropion uvea is unknown but thought to be high with a variable age of onset. In one series of eight eyes with unilateral congenital ectropion uveae, seven had glaucoma, while the eighth was only a ten-week infant at the time of presentation, suggesting that future glaucoma was possible.[41] However, there is likely some selection bias in these cases.

Mechanism of glaucoma

Pathology has been reported from a series of five enucleated NF-1 eyes with congenital ectropion uvea by Edward and colleagues.[43] All patients had endothelial cells staining positive for vimentin in the anterior chamber angle. Uveal neurofibromas were also detected in all patients along with an absence of Schlemm canal. In patients without NF-1, glaucoma is thought to be due to maldevelopment of the angle.

Management

There is a strong association between congenital ectropion uveae and glaucoma, and therefore children presenting with this finding should be followed carefully and considered for systemic syndromes (particularly NF-1). Roughly half of children with congenital NF-1 associated with congenital glaucoma have ipsilateral plexiform neurofibromas, and examination should be directed towards this possible finding. A detailed family history should be obtained as well, with specific inquiry regarding NF-1. Consideration should be given for examining both parents for highly penetrant findings of NF-1 (eg. café-au-lait spots, Lisch nodules).

Children not presenting with glaucoma on initial detection of ectropion uveae should be followed regularly for glaucoma onset. Pathology findings in the anterior chamber (endothelialization of the anterior chamber angle, absence of Schlemm canal) of NF-1 eyes with congenital ectropion uveae suggest that angle surgery is unlikely to be successful. Medical therapy is first line. Trabeculectomy with antiscarring agents may be successful. [44,45]

Persistent fetal vasculature

Definition

Persistent fetal vasculature [PFV, also known as persistent hyperplastic primary vitreous (PHPV)], is a congenital anomaly in which the primary vitreous and hyaloid vasculature fail to regress. The primary vitreous is formed during the first month of gestation and is vascularized mesodermal tissue between the developing lens and the neuroectoderm of the optic cup, containing the hyaloid artery. PFV is usually unilateral (90%) and sporadic. It is classified into anterior and posterior types although usually both features exist in the same eye (60%).[46,47] It is often an isolated anomaly but can occur with other ocular conditions. Systemic association is uncommon, but more likely with bilateral involvement.[46,47] There is a variable clinical spectrum and features can include: a retrolental fibrovascular mass, microphthalmos, elongated ciliary processes, a shallow anterior chamber, varying degrees of lenticular opacification, elevated vitreous membrane or stalk from optic nerve, retinal fold, retinal traction or detachment and severe intraocular hemorrhage. It is usually associated with cataract, which may be present at birth, and cataract surgery is usually performed.[48] However, the lens may be clear due to posterior segment involvement only or it may become cataractous with time. Glaucoma is sometimes present at diagnosis or it may develop over time associated with cataract or develop after cataract surgery.

The exact etiology remains unknown, but PFV may have a genetic basis in light of familial cases and its association with ocular anomalies and congenital syndromes.[49]

Mechanism of glaucoma

Glaucoma usually develops from angle closure as a result of lens enlargement from cataract and from contraction of the retrolental fibrovascular membrane with secondary forward iris-lens diaphragm movement.[50] It may also develop after lensectomy with either an open, closed or mixed angle appearance. Occasionally, PFV is associated with neovascular glaucoma or glaucoma occurs after repeated hyphemas.

Management

Untreated, the natural history of PFV in a significant percentage of patients is that of recurrent intraocular hemorrhage and glaucoma, leading to enucleation or phthisis.[50] The heterogeneity of clinical presentation can make PFV challenging to manage surgically.[46] Clinical findings should, where possible, be supported by ultrasound. Surgical treatment is aimed towards obtaining useful vision and preventing or treating secondary complications such as glaucoma. So PFV management and expectations are based on the extent of anterior and posterior segment involvement. For example, in eyes with mild anterior involvement (clear visual axis, open angle and non progressive signs) or with severe posterior involvement, surgery is not usually indicated. However, patients with significant anterior involvement only, may have a chance of useful vision after surgery and amblyopia therapy. As the prognosis is guarded, avoiding early lensectomy (less than four weeks of age) is advisable unless indicated for glaucoma. In those with a combination of anterior and posterior PFV, the main aim may be to save the eye by avoiding or treating complications. Surgery is recommended before the development of deprivational amblyopia or secondary complications.

For patients with a non-visually significant cataract and normal IOP, regular monitoring is required to assess anterior chamber depth and the angle for the risk of angle-closure glaucoma. If there is progressive angle closure, even without elevated IOP, then lens aspiration is recommended to avoid an acute angle closure presentation. This surgery may be combined with removal of the anterior persistent fetal vascular membrane or left behind if significant posterior segment involvement has been identified. The peripheral retina may be attached to the membrane resulting in a retinal detachment intraoperatively. Following lensectomy, cases with a normal posterior segment require follow-up as per other aphakic/pseudophakic infants (*see* Section 10). Consider referral to a geneticist for evaluation of possible syndromic associations with bilateral PFV such as Norrie disease.

Often eyes with PFV are included in series regarding congenital cataracts, and it is a known risk factor for developing glaucoma after lensectomy. There is a paucity of literature specifically regarding the management of glaucoma associated with PFV following surgery. However, the approach to glaucoma management once medical therapy fails can be either by cyclodiode or glaucoma drainage surgery depending on the visual potential of the eye. In the largest cohort of patients with PFV in the literature (165 eyes), 81 eyes had surgery of which 70 eyes had at least six months of postoperative follow-up (median 47 months) and 84 eyes were considered poor surgical candidates and observed.[46] 'Glaucoma' was present at baseline in 13% of the non-surgical group and 29% of the surgical group. Of the 70 eyes that had surgery, one eye had an aqueous shunt at the time of lensectomy and another eight eyes developed 'worsening glaucoma' postoperatively, of which six eyes had a glaucoma drainage device and two eyes trabeculectomy. Of these nine eyes with glaucoma, four (44%) had either perception or no perception of light vision. The higher incidence of glaucoma noted in the surgical group was thought to reflect selection bias, angle synechiae, the development of secondary membranes and observation bias in the surgical group. The non-surgical group had a higher incidence of ciliary body and retinal detachments, which was thought to balance the increase in IOP from angle closure. Furthermore, they found microphthalmic eyes were associated with greater posterior involvement and significantly worse visual and anatomic outcomes. Along with microphthalmia, posterior disease, glaucoma and amblyopia also limited visual outcomes even after aggressive intervention.

In another retrospective series of 55 eyes with PFV followed over a ten-year period, eight eyes (14.5%) had glaucoma: three eyes had angle closure glaucoma prior to surgery, two eyes with shallow anterior chambers developed glaucoma after surgery, two eyes developed glaucoma after lensectomy and one eye conservatively managed developed glaucoma. Glaucoma was managed either medically, with photocycloablation or with trabeculectomy (57%).[47]

Microcornea

Definition

Microcornea is defined as a cornea less than ten mm in horizontal diameter at birth. As an isolated finding with the rest of the eye being normal, it is termed microcornea but if associated with a small anterior segment and eye then it is termed microphthalmos. It may occur as an isolated anomaly or be associated with other ocular conditions such as PFV, nanophthalmos, aniridia, congenital rubella, and Axenfeld Rieger syndrome. It may be associated with systemic conditions, such as fetal alcohol syndrome, myotonic dystrophy, achondroplasia. Microcornea is usually associated with hypermetropia.

Several rare, specific syndromes are associated with microcornea such as the microcornea-glaucoma-absent frontal sinus syndrome.[51] The mode of transmission appears to be autosomal dominant. The congenital cataract-microcornea syndrome is an association of congenital cataract and microcornea without any other systemic anomaly or dysmorphism. It is a genetically heterogeneous condition with inheritance being autosomal dominant. [52]

Inheritance

Most cases of microcornea are sporadic. A minority of patients demonstrate autosomal dominant or autosomal recessive inheritance.

Mechanism of glaucoma

Both open-angle and angle-closure mechanisms can cause glaucoma in individuals with microcornea. In extremely small eyes, including nanophthalmic eyes, angle closure is of particular concern. It can be difficult to visualize the drainage system by gonioscopy, and ultrasound biomicrosopy or other imaging techniques may be necessary. Microcornea is an significant risk factor for development of glaucoma following congenital cataract surgery especially if performed early (less than 12 weeks of age)[53] (*see* Section 10).

Management

If angle closure is present, then relief of pupillary block by iridectomy or iridotomy or removal of the lens may be indicated. Medical treatment is first line. In eyes with very small corneas, goniotomy may be impossible without an endoscope. Trabeculotomy may be possible.

Microcornea may be associated with high hyperopia and appropriate refractive correction should be prescribed.

Sclerocornea

Definition

Sclerocornea refers to a non-progressive scleralization of the cornea in which the peripheral cornea and sometimes the entire cornea is opacified by thick collagen bundles and vascularization without antecedent inflammation. Depending on the degree of scleralization, the vision may be minimally affected or profoundly compromised. The most common ocular association is cornea plana, found in 80% of cases. Keratometry reveals low values between 20 and 39 D. The limbus or corneal scleral sulcus is usually poorly defined, with superficial vessels extending from sclera, episclera, and conjunctiva to traverse into part or the entire cornea. Visual symptoms are dependent on the associated corneal flattening and of course whether the visual axis is affected by scleralization. Associated ocular abnormalities include aniridia, Axenfeld-Rieger anomaly, cataract, coloboma, esotropia, glaucoma, microphthalmos, posterior embryotoxon, and strabismus.[54] Sclerocornea has also been associated with facial anomalies, mental retardation, deafness, and cerebellar anomalies.

A number of syndromes feature sclerocornea and include Dandy-Walker, Hurler, Hallermann-Streiff and many others.

Inheritance

Approximately half of the cases of sclerocornea are familial; autosomal dominant and recessive patterns of inheritance have been described. The remaining cases are sporadic. Males and females are equally affected.

Management

The corneal abnormality will affect IOP measurements, and if possible more than one instrument should be used. Echographic measurement of the axial length can be of particular value when IOP measurements are uncertain. Plotting of axial length over time can assist in determining if the pressure is causing structural change (*see* Section 2). Ultrasound biomicroscopy, if available, should be performed when the anterior segment cannot be visualized, and standard B scan examination can provide some information regarding the degree of cupping if not visualized.

There are no data on which to base recommendations for treatment of glaucoma associated with sclerocornea. Goniotomy is not likely to be possible, unless an endoscope is used. However, trabeculotomy may be possible. Transillumination may be used to locate the scleral spur.

The visual prognosis depends on disease severity. If the process is confined to the periphery, vision may be minimally affected and the central cornea might clear further with age.

The degree of corneal involvement and, particularly in unilateral or asymmetric cases, the findings in the fellow eye will determine what, if any, surgical treatment is undertaken to create or improve the visual axis. Optical iridectomy may be indicated if the peripheral cornea is clear. Penetrating keratoplasty has been performed for central corneal involvement. If glaucoma is associated with sclerocornea, and if keratoplasty is being considered, it is essential that the glaucoma be controlled before cornea surgery is performed. With success defined as graft clarity, the rate of success of penetrating keratoplasty in sclerocornea has been reported to be 50% with repeated transplants after a mean follow-up of 40 months.[55]

Unclassified anterior segment anomaly

Some children present with congenital or developmental ocular anomalies that do not fit into any of the recognized categorized, such as the Axenfeld-Rieger spectrum or Peters anomaly. This may be because the findings are not consistent with defined conditions or the visualization of intraocular structures is poor. These cases of unclassified anterior segment abnormalities vary widely.

There are no published statistics regarding such conditions. They may results from perinatal injury (*e.g.*, toxins, infections), chromosomal rearrangements/deletions, or gene mutations. If such abnormalities result from autosomal recessive mutation(s), they may be more likely in consanguineous marriages. A risk for glaucoma is expected as visual developmental abnormality of the visible anterior segment structures is often accompanied by maldevelopment of the outflow system. Such children should be followed for life for the possibility of glaucoma whether or not they have glaucoma as children. If glaucoma occurs, treatment should be tailored according to the specific findings (*see* Fig. 2).

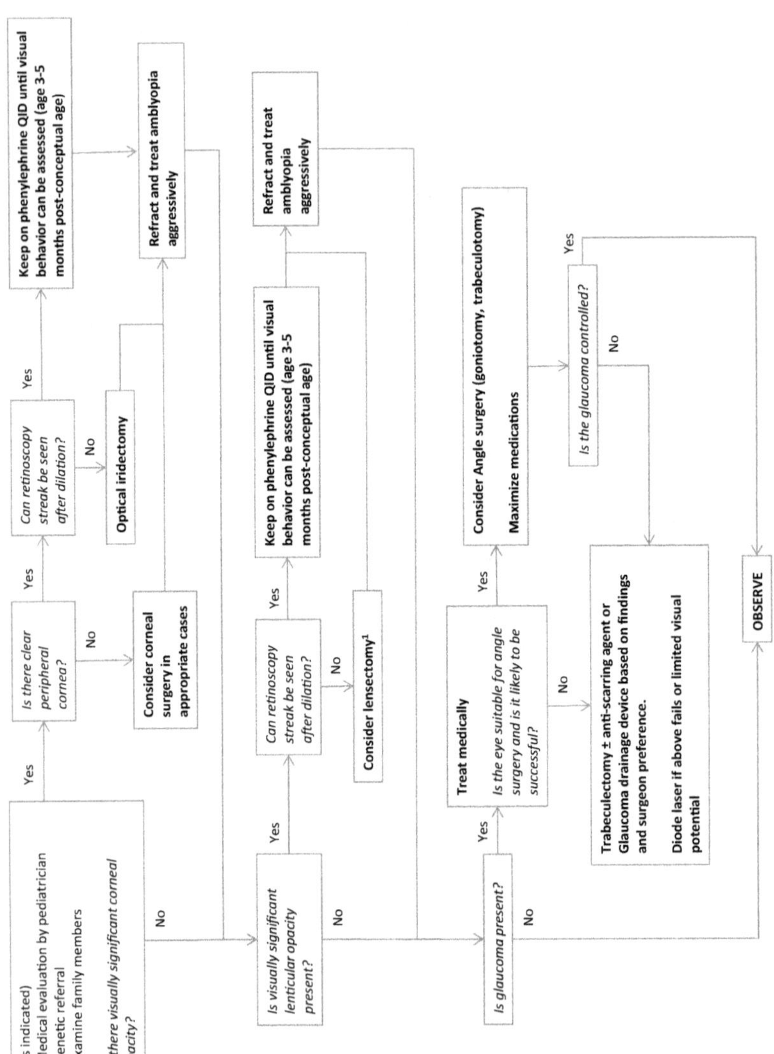

Fig. 2. A suggested approach to the management of glaucoma associated with a non acquired ocular anomaly. (It will be influenced by surgeon preference/experience and local facilities/equipment availability.)

References

1. Axenfeld T. Embryotoxon cornea posterius. Klin Monatsbl Augenheilkd 1920; 65: 381-382.
2. Rieger H. Verlagerung and Schlitzform der Pupille mit Hypoplasie des Irisvorderblattes. Z Augenheilkd 1934; 84: 98-103.
3. Reese AB, Ellsworth RM. The anterior chamber cleavage syndrome. Arch Ophthalmol 1966; 75: 307-318.
4. Rieger H. Dysgenesis mesodermalis corneae et iridis. Z Augenheilkd 1935; 86: 333.
5. Tripathi BJ, Tripathi RC. Neural crest origin of human trabecular meshwork and its implications for the pathogenesis of glaucoma. Am J Ophthalmol 1989; 107: 583-590.
6. www.ncbi.nlm.nih.gov/omim. OMIM, Online Mendelian Inheritance in Man.
7. Phillips JC, del Bono EA, Haines JL, et al. A second locus for Rieger syndrome maps to chromosome 13q14. Am J Hum Genet 1996; 59: 613-619.
8. Strungaru MH, Dinu I, Walter MA. Genotype-phenotype correlations in Axenfeld-Rieger malformation and glaucoma patients with FOXC1 and PITX2 mutations. Invest Ophthalmol Vis Sci 2007; 48: 228-237.
9. Idrees F, Vaideanu D, Fraser SG, et al. A review of anterior segment dysgeneses. Surv Ophthalmol 2006; 51: 213-231.
10. Rice NSC. The surgical management of congenital glaucoma. Aust J Ophthalmol. 1977; 5: 174-179.
11. Luntz MH. Congenital, infantile and juvenile glaucoma. Ophthalmology 1979; 86: 793-802.
12. Shields MB, Buckley E, Klintworth GK, Thresher R. Axenfeld-Rieger Syndrome. A spectrum of developmental disorders. Surv Ophthalmol 1985; 29: 387-409.
13. Ozeki H, Shirai S, Nozaki M, et al. Ocular and systemic features of Peters anomaly. Graefes Arch Clin Exp Ophthalmo 2000; 238: 833-839.
14. Heath DH, Shields MB. Glaucoma and Peters anomaly. A clinicopathologic case report. Graefes Arch Clin Exp Ophthalmol 1991; 229: 277-280.
15. Chang JW, Kim JH, Kim SJ, Yu YS. Long-term clinical course and outcome associated with Peters anomaly. Eye 2012; 26: 1237-1242.
16. Junemann A, Gusek GC, Naumann GO. Optical sector iridectomy: an alternative to perforating kerotoplasty in Peters anomaly. Klin Monbl Augenheilkd 1996; 209: 117-124.
17. Lowe MT, Keane MC, Coster DJ, Williams KA. The outcome of corneal transplantation in infants, children, and adolescents. Ophthalmology 2011; 118: 492-497.
18. Yang LL, Lambert SR, Lynn MJ, Stulting RD. Surgical management of glaucoma in infants and children with Peters anomaly: long-term structural and functional outcome. Ophthalmology 2004; 111: 112-117.
19. Rao KV, Fernandes M, Gangopadhyay N, et al. Outcome of penetrating keratoplasty for Peters anomaly. Cornea 2008; 27: 749-753.
20. Yang LL, Lambert SR, Lynn MJ, Stulting RD. Long term results of corneal graft survival in infants and children with Peters anomaly. Ophthalmology 1999; 106: 833-848.
21. Hashemi H, Ghaffari R, Mohebi M. Posterior lamellar keratoplasty (DSAEK) in Peters anomaly. Cornea 2012; 31: 1201-1205.
22. Quilendrino R, Yeh RY, Dapena I, et al. Large diameter Descemet membrane endothelial keratoplasty in buphthalmic eyes. Cornea 2013; 32: e74-8.
23. Lee H, Khan R, O'Keefe M. Aniridia:current pathology and management. Acta Ophthalmol 2008; 86: 708-715.
24. Eden U, Riise R, Tornqvist K. Corneal involvement in congenital aniridia. Cornea 2010; 29: 1096-1102.
25. Brandt JD, Casuso LA, Budenz DL. Markedly increased central corneal thickness: an unrecognized finding in congenital aniridia. Am J Ophthalmol 2004; 137: 348-350.
26. Nelson J, Flaherty M, Grattan-Smith P. Gillespie syndrome: a report of two further cases. Am J Med Genet 1997; 71: 134-138.

27. Kokotas H, Petersen MB. Clinical and molecular aspects of aniridia. Clin Genet 2010; 409-420.
28. Perveen R, Lloyd IC, Clayton -Smith J, et al. Phenotypic variability and asymmetry of Rieger syndrome associated with PITX2 mutations. Invest Ophthalmol Vis Sci 2000; 41: 2456-2460.
29. Ito YA, Footz TK, Berry FB, et al. Severe molecular defects of a novel FOXC1 W152G mutation result in aniridia. Invest Ophthalmol Vis Sci 2009; 50: 3573-3579.
30. Khan AO, Aldahmesh MA, Al-Abdi L, et al. Molecular characterization of newborn glaucoma including a distinct aniridic phenotype. Ophthalmic Genet 201; 32: 138-142.
31. Grant WM, Walton DS. Progressive changes in the angle in congenital aniridia, with development of glaucoma. Trans Am Ophthalmol Soc 1974; 72: 207-228.
32. Clericuzio C, Hingorani M, Crolla JA, et al. Clinical utility gene card for: WAGR syndrome. Eur J of Hum Genet 2011; 19. doi: 10.1038/ejhg.2010.220. Epub 2011 Jan 12.
33. Menezo JL, Martinez-Costa R, Cisneros A, Desco MC. Implantation of iris devices in congenital and traumatic aniridias: surgery solutions and complications. Eur J Ophthalmol 2005; 15: 451-457.
34. Reinhard T, Engelhardt S, Sundmacher R. Black diaphragm aniridia intraocular lens for congenital aniridia: long-term follow-up. J Cataract Refract Surg 2000; 26: 375-381.
35. Aslam SA, Wong SC, Ficker LA, MacLaren RE. Implantation of the black diaphragm intraocular lens in congenital and traumatic aniridia. Ophthalmology 2008; 115: 1705-1712.
36. de la Paz MF, Alvarez de Toledo J, Barraquer RI, Barraquer J. Long-term visual prognosis of corneal and ocular surface surgery in patients with congenital aniridia. Acta Ophthalmol 2008; 86: 735-740.
37. Walton DS. Aniridic glaucoma: the results of gonio-surgery to prevent and treat this problem. Trans Am Ophthalmol Soc 1986; 84: 59-70.
38. Chen TC, Walton DS. Goniosurgery for prevention of aniridic glaucoma. Arch Ophthalmol 1999; 117: 1144-1148.
39. Arroyave CP Scott IU, Gedde SJ, et al. Use of glaucoma drainage devices in the management of glaucoma associated with aniridia. Am J Ophthalmol 2003; 135: 155-159.
40. August PS, Niederberger H, Helbig H. Progression of congenital ectropion uveae. Arch Ophthalmol 2003; 121: 1511.
41. Ritch, R, Forbes M, Hetherington J Jr, et al. Congenital ectropion uveae with glaucoma. Ophthalmology 1984; 91: 326-331.
42. Willcock C, Grigg J, Wilson M, et al. Congenital iris ectropion as an indicator of variant aniridia. Br J Ophthalmol 2006; 90: 658-569.
43. Edward DP, Morales J, Bouhenni RA, et al. Congenital ectropion uvea and mechanisms of glaucoma in Neurofibromatosis Type 1: new insights. Ophthalmology 2012; 119: 1485-1494.
44. Seymenoğlu G, Başer E. Congenital iris ectropion associated with juvenile glaucoma. Int Ophthalmol 2011; 31: 33-38.
45. Liu XQ, Tang X. Congenital ectropion uvea and secondary glaucoma. Zhonghua Yan Ke Za Zhi 2009; 45: 888-891.
46. Sisk RA, Berrocal AM, Feuer WJ, Murray TG. Visual and anatomic outcomes with and without surgery in persistent fetal vasculature. Ophthalmology 2010; 117:2178-83.
47. Hunt A, Rowe N, Lam A, Martin F. Outcomes in persistent hyperplastic primary vitreous. Br J Ophthalmol 2005; 89: 859-863.
48. Amaya L, Taylor D, Russell-Egitt I, et al. The morphology and natural history of childhood cataracts. Surv Ophthalmol 2003: 48:125-144.
49. Shastry BS. Persistent hyperplastic vitreous: congenital malformation of the eye. Clin Experiment Ophthalmol. 2009; 37: 884-890.
50. Pollard ZF. Persistent hyperplastic primary vitreous: diagnosis, treatment and results. Trans Am Ophthalmol Soc 1997:95;487-549.
51. Chattopadhyay A, Kher AS, Bharucha BA, Nicholson AD. Microcornea, glaucoma, and absent frontal sinus. J Pediatr 1995: 127: 333.

52. Wang KJ, Wang S, Cao NQ, et al. A novel mutation in CRYBB1 associated with Congenital Cataract-Microcornea Syndrome: The p.Ser129Arg mutation destabilizes the βB1/βA3-crystallin heteromer but not the βB1-crystallin homomer. Hum Mutat 2011; 32:E2050-60.
53. Nishina S, Noda E, Azuma N. Outcome of early surgery for bilateral congenital cataracts in eyes with microcornea. Am J Ophthalmol 2007: 144: 276-280.
54. Ozeki H, Shirai S, Ikeda K, Ogura Y. Anomalies associated with Axenfeld-Rieger syndrome. Graefes Arch Clin Exp Ophthalmol 1999: 237: 730-734.
55. Michaeli A, Markovich A, Rootman DS. Corneal transplants for the treatment of congenital corneal opacities. J Pediatr Ophthalmol Strabismus 2005; 42: 34-44.

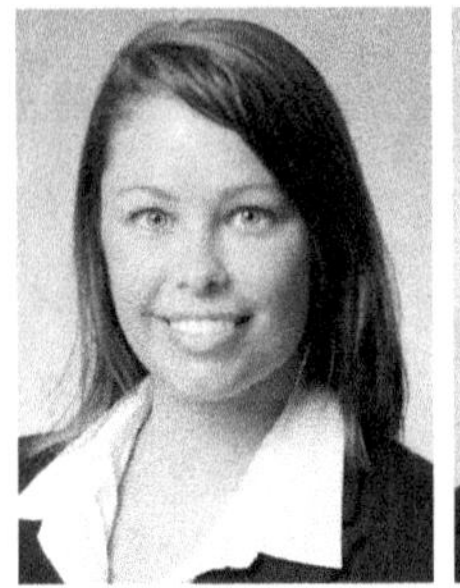

Caroline DeBenedictis

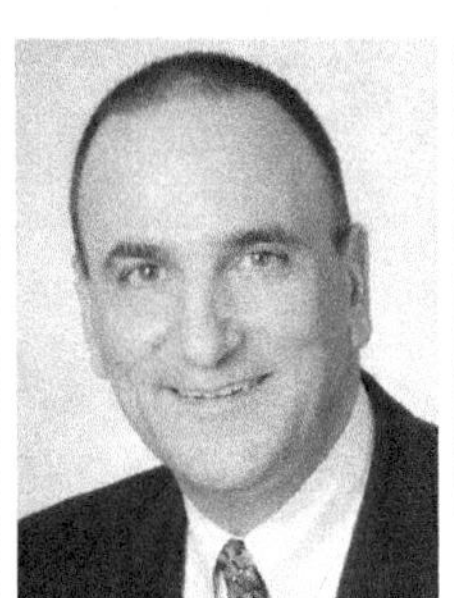

Alex Levin

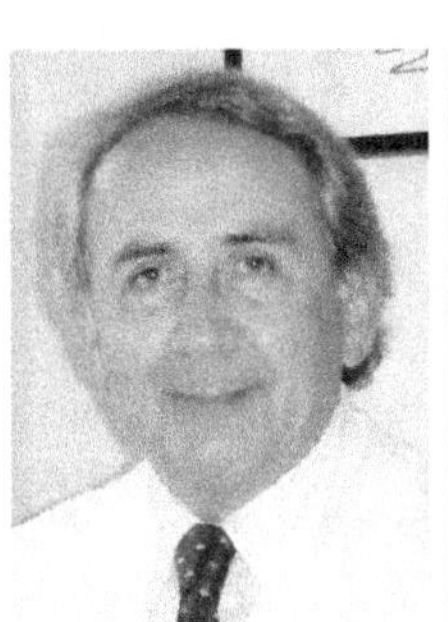

Eugenio J. Maul

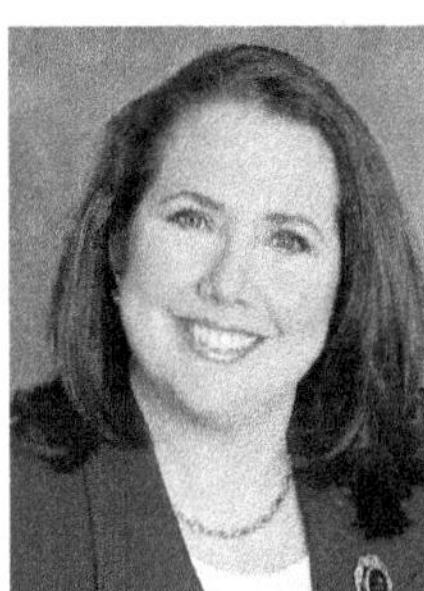

Alana L. Grajewski

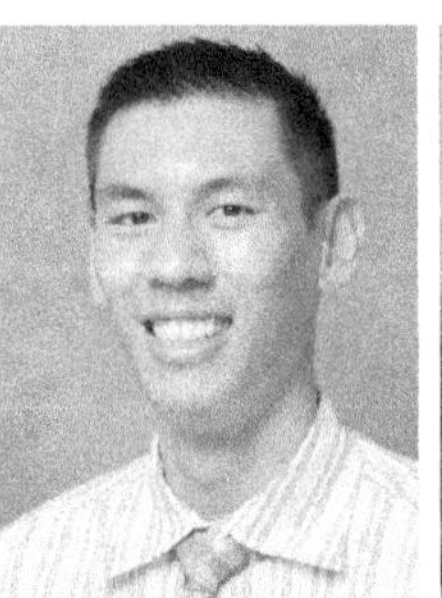

Ta Chen Peter Chang

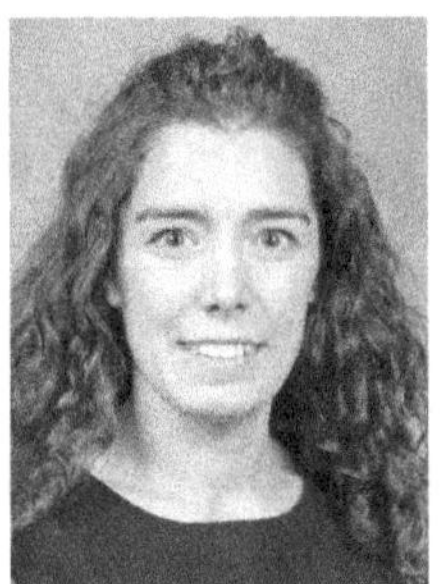

Elena Bitrian

8. GLAUCOMA ASSOCIATED WITH NON-ACQUIRED SYSTEMIC DISEASE OR SYNDROME

Alex Levin, Eugenio J. Maul, Ta Chen Peter Chang, Elena Bitrian, Caroline DeBenedictis, Alana L. Grajewski

Section Leaders: Alana L. Grajewski, Alex Levin, Eugenio J. Maul
Contributors: Allen Beck, Tam Dang, Teresa Chen, Vera Essuman, Arif Khan, Christiane Rolim de Moura, Jonathan Ruddle, Sirisha Senthil, Janet B. Serle, Luis Silva

Consensus statements

1. Syndromes with system anomalies or systemic diseases that are present at birth can be associated with ocular signs that include glaucoma.
   Comment: Patients should be regularly monitored for glaucoma throughout life and elevated intraocular pressure (IOP) treated, should it occur.
   Comment: Patients also should be assessed for systemic manifestations of their disease.
2. Sturge-Weber syndrome (SWS) is commonly associated with glaucoma.
   Comment: Periocular port-wine marks are associated with ipsilateral glaucoma. Lid involvement and/or episcleral capillary vascular malformation appear to further increase the risk of glaucoma.
   Comment: Choroidal hemangioma increases the risk of serous choroidal effusion and suprachoroidal hemorrhage with surgery, especially if the IOP drops precipitously or hypotony develops. Modifications to the surgical technique must be employed to minimize risk of hypotony.
   Comment: Patients should be assessed, perhaps including neuroimaging, for other manifestations of SWS.
3. Neurofibromatosis (NF1) is uncommonly associated with glaucoma.
   Comment: Optic pathway gliomas affect 12-15% of patients with neurofibromatosis and can present with decreased vision distinct from glaucoma.
4. Ectopia Lentis (EL) can present as an isolated ocular anomaly or be associated with other ocular or systemic findings.

Childhood Glaucoma, pp. 179-196
Edited by Robert N. Weinreb, Alana L. Grajewski, Maria Papadopoulos, John Grigg, and Sharon Freedman
2013 © Kugler Publications, Amsterdam, The Netherlands

Comment: Patients with EL are at risk of acute pupillary block.

Comment: All patients without a proven or obvious cause of EL should be tested for homocystinura by urine analysis and investigated for blood homocyteine levels prior to any anesthesia or sedation because of life-threatening vascular risks.

Comment: Patients with Marfan syndrome should have echocardiography and cardiology consultation prior to surgery.

5. Maintain close follow-up for infants with known or suspected congenital rubella, since glaucoma signs might be less evident at birth in some cases.

Comment: Rubella keratitis should be differentiated from corneal findings associated with IOP related corneal edema.

Introduction

The disorders discussed in this section are predominately syndromes, systemic anomalies or systemic diseases, which are present at birth and associated with ocular signs that may include glaucoma. The glaucoma may have an open or closed angle mechanism or may rarely resemble primary congenital glaucoma (PCG). Understanding the underlying relationship between the associated syndrome and the glaucoma is often helpful to determine the mechanism of the glaucoma. A thorough history, examination, and assessment of risk factors for surgical failure direct the management plan. Patients should be regularly monitored for glaucoma. Furthermore, ensure that patients are assessed for systemic manifestations of their disease.

Sturge-Weber syndrome

Caroline De Benedictis, Elena Bitrian, Alex Levin, Eugenio J. Maul, Alana L. Grajewski

Definition

Sturge-Weber syndrome (SWS), or encephalotrigeminal angiomatosis, is a congenital neurocutaneous vascular syndrome, which can potentially involve three organs: the skin, eye and brain. The most constant feature is a facial cutaneous vascular malformation [port-wine birthmark (PWM)] involving some portion of the trigeminal nerve distribution. There may or may not be ipsilateral leptomeningeal angiomatosis, brain atrophy, seizures or developmental delay. Ispilateral choroidal hemangioma (40%) and/or glaucoma (30%) also commonly occur. Other ocular features include prominent epibulbar blood vessels and conjunctival lesions, iris heterochromia, retinal vascular tortuosity, choroidal hemangiomas and visual field defects. Children with bilateral port-wine marks (10-30%) are more likely to have bilateral leptomeningeal lesions and greater risk of neurologic impairment, so should be referred for medical evaluation and ultimately for neuroimaging in consultation with the neurologist. Port-wine marks involving the ophthalmic division of V1 are more likely to have ipsilateral glaucoma, especially if the birthmark involves the upper eyelid. Choroidal hemangiomas are associated with an increased risk of ipsilateral glaucoma as well as choroidal effusions or suprachoroidal hemorrhages, especially during intraocular surgery or if there is postoperative hypotony.

The etiology of SWS remains unclear. No patterns of inheritance have been identified. The underlying pathogenesis has been most widely postulated to reflect primary venous dysplasia, with failure of regression of primordial embryonic venous plexus that are normally present at five to eight weeks of gestation. Other research highlights the ectatic capillaries and venules associated with a reduction in post-capillary venule neural density.[2] Localized primary venous dysplasia, with effects of venous hypertension transmitted to nearby venous passageways and compensatory collateral venous channels has been proposed as an alternative hypothesis.[3] The effect of these vascular abnormalities results in the defective structural differentiation of vessel walls, with functional abnormalities including increased capillary permeability, stasis and anoxia. Vessels undergo secondary fibrosis, hyaline deposition, dilation and calcification of vessel walls. This leads to venous stasis and obliteration of the lumen. Tissues supplied by these abnormal blood vessels manifest degenerative changes, especially in the cerebral cortex. The parietal and occipital lobes are most commonly affected. Venous stasis can lead to recurrent thrombotic episodes, transient ischemic episodes, and seizures.

Epidemiology

The incidence of SWS is estimated at one per 50,000. Men and women are affected equally. There is no recognized racial predilection or regional differences. Almost all patients have non-familial, sporadic disease, raising the hypothesis that the disorder is due to somatic post-zygotic mutation. The risk of glaucoma is highest in the first ten years of life, but patients need to be monitored throughout life as adult onset of glaucoma can also occur.

Mechanisms of glaucoma

There are two childhood peaks of glaucoma in SWS: congenital/infantile and juvenile onset. There are multiple mechanisms by which SWS glaucoma may occur. Patients with congenital/infantile onset glaucoma often have primary goniodysgenesis. Patients with SWS may have prominent iris processes that adhere to the trabecular meshwork, a gonioscopy pattern identical to that seen in primary congenital glaucoma (PCG). Schlemm canal can be attenuated and there can be a poorly developed scleral spur along with an anteriorly displaced iris root. After some years, usually towards the end of the first decade and into the second decade (especially around puberty), elevation of episcleral venous pressure can cause reduced outflow facility.[4,5] Less commonly, glaucoma may arise due to peripheral anterior synechiae (PAS) secondary to anterior rotation caused by choroidal hemangioma, low choroidal effusions, retinal detachment, or neovascular glaucoma. It is also possible that increased permeability of thin-walled blood vessels associated with a choroidal hemangioma cause an increase in aqueous production and therefore, intraocular pressure (IOP). There is an adult form of glaucoma associated with SWS that is similar to primary open-angle glaucoma and is associated with dilated conjunctival vessels, heterochromia iridis, choroidal hemangioma and abnormal retinal vessels.

Treatment

All patients should be assessed for other manifestations of SWS, in particular the involvement of the central nervous system by neuroimaging as indicated (*i.e.*, bilateral PWM or onset of seizures). Full systemic examination can help to differentiate overlap syndromes such as cutis marmorata telangiectasia, Klippel-Trenaunay-Weber, hereditary hemorrhagic telangiectasia and phakomatosis pigmentovascularis.

It is essential to preoperatively assess for the presence of choroidal hemangioma, which may be missed clinically, by indirect ophthalmoloscopy, ultrasound and/or enhanced-depth optical coherence tomography[6] or photography. The choroidal hemangioma may be localized to the posterior pole or extend to the whole fundus. Optic nerve cupping often looks larger in patients with choroidal hemangioma. This may be due to 'heaping' of the peripapillary hemangioma which bows the lamina cribosa backward. Therefore the optic nerve may look worse than expected. Additionally, it is more difficult to detect change by following the disc appearance alone. In patients where the choroidal hemangioma is causing angle closure or other posterior segment disease, such as submacular fluid, then treatment must be directed to reduce the hemangioma (*i.e.*, photodynamic or radiation therapy).[7]

Choroidal hemangioma is not a contraindication to surgery but does increase the risk of suprachoroidal hemorrhage, especially if the IOP drops precipitously or chronic hypotony develops. The risk of hemorrhage or choroidal effusion postoperatively is proportional to the size of the choroidal vascular malformation.

Glaucoma treatment options are usually determined by age of onset and mechanism of glaucoma. Congenital/infantile onset glaucoma is preferably treated with angle surgery[8,9] because of goniodysgenesis and the risks associated with more invasive surgery. Often medical treatment fails in these early onset cases but should be tried first before surgery. In older children with increased episcleral venous pressure as the main cause of glaucoma, often evident by the presence of blood in Schlemm canal on gonioscopy, medical management is recommended as the first approach. Alpha-agonists are relatively contraindicated if there is leptomeningeal angiomatosis, as the increased permeability of the blood-brain barrier can lead to significant central nervous system effects. Furthermore, medications which lower IOP significantly have been associated with serous non-rhematogenous retinal detachment and there are case reports of prostaglandin analogues causing serous retinal detachments in patients with choroidal hemangiomas.[10,11] As patients with SWS may have growth hormone deficiency, weight and growth should be monitored if oral acetazolamide is used. It should be noted that many of these patients are now on aspirin to reduce stroke-like episodes and this may need to be taken into consideration when surgery is planned.

When medical treatment fails in older children or after angle surgery, either trabeculectomy[9] or glaucoma drainage device (GDD) surgery[12-14] can be considered. Other surgical procedures reported in the literature include primary combined trabeculotomy-trabeculectomy[15] and non-penetrating deep sclerectomy.[16] Refractory glaucoma can be treated with ciliary body destruction, keeping in mind that inflammation may aggravate leakage from a choroidal hemangioma. Some surgeons advocate prophylactic measures, such as sclerotomies,[12] prior to intraocular surgery to help prevent suprachoroidal effusion and hemorrhage, but they are rarely necessary.[17] This is especially the case if measures are taken to prevent peri-operative hypotony which is paramount in these patients and can be achieved by tight scleral flap closure (*e.g.*, with trabeculectomy), an anterior chamber (AC) maintainer and other mechanisms for restricting postoperative GDD flow (*e.g.*, intraluminal stents with 3/0 supramid, ligatures with absorbable sutures around the tube and a tight tube tunnel into AC). The use of 'valved' (flow restricted) GDDs may not be effective in avoiding peri-operative hypotony, especially early in the postoperative period, but may be effective in avoiding late hypotony. Refer to Figure 1 for a suggested management algorithm.

Choroidal effusion is nonetheless common when the IOP is reduced in patients with choroidal hemangioma and so patients should be monitored closely. B-scan ultrasound is a useful tool to monitor these patients. Choroidal effusions can occur at higher than expected IOPs in the presence of a choroidal hemangioma. Conservative management and elimination of any aqueous suppressants usually results in resolution of the choroidal effusions.

Early skin laser treatment for children with PWM offers a better long-term prognosis for appearance. Ophthalmologists should ensure that patients get early dermatology consultation in infancy.[18] The Sturge-Weber Foundation is an excellent resource for families (http://www.sturge-weber.org/).

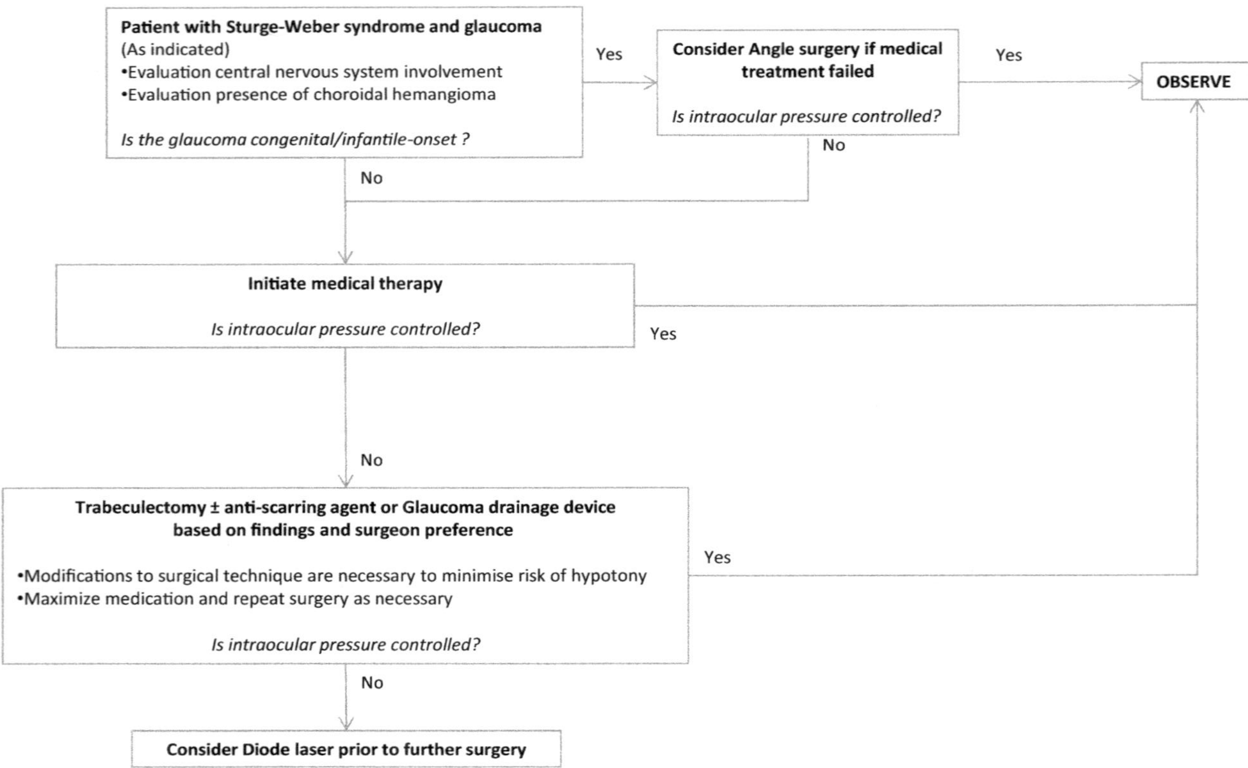

Fig. 1. A suggested approach to the management of glaucoma associated with Sturge-Weber syndrome. (It will be influenced by surgeon preference/experience and local facilities/equipment availability.)

References

1. Bodensteiner JB, Roach ES, eds. Sturge-Weber Syndrome. Mt. Freedom, NJ: The Sturge-Weber Foundation; 2010.
2. Breugem C, Hennekam R, van Gemert M, van der Horst C. Are Capillary Malformations Neurovenular or Purely Neural? Plast Reconstr Surg 2005; 115: 578-587.
3. Parsa C. Sturge-Weber Syndrome: A Unifified Pathophysiologic Mechanism. Curr Treat Options Neurol 2008; 10: 47-54.
4. Shiau T, Armogan N, Yan DB et al. The role of episcleral venous pressure in glaucoma associated with Sturge-Weber syndrome. JAAPOS 2012; 16: 61-64.
5. Phelps CD. The Pathogenesis of glaucoma in Sturge-Weber Syndrome. Ophthalmology 1978; 85: 276-286.
6. Arora KS, Quigley HA, Comi AM, et al. Increased Choroidal Thickness in Patients with Sturge-Weber Syndrome. JAMA Ophthalmol 2013; 4doi: 10. 1001/jamaophthalmol.2013.4044.
7. Tsipursky MS, Golchet PR, Jampol LM. Photodynamic therapy of choroidal hemangioma in Sturge-Weber syndrome, with a review of treatments for diffuse and circumscribed choroidal hemangiomas. Surv Ophthalmol 2011; 56: 68-85.
8. Olsen KE, Huang AS, Wright MM. The efficacy of goniotomy/trabeculotomy in early-onset glaucoma associated with Sturge-Weber Syndrome. JAAPOS 1998; 2: 365-368.
9. Iwach AG, Hoskins HD Jr, Hetherington J Jr, Shaffer RN. Analysis of surgical and medical management of glaucoma in Sturge-Weber syndrome. Ophthalmology 1990; 97: 904-909.
10. Addison PK, Papadopoulos M, Nischal KK, Hykin PG. Serous retinal detachment induced by topical bimatoprost in a patient with Sturge-Weber Syndrome. Eye (Lond) 2011; 25: 124-125.
11. Gambrelle J, Denis P, Kocaba V, Grange JD. Uveal effusion induced by topical travoprost in a patient with Sturge-Weber-Krabbe syndrome. J Fr Ophtalmol 2008; 31: e19.
12. Budenz DL, Sakamoto D, Eliezer R, Varma R, Heuer DK. Two-staged Baerveldt glaucoma implant for childhood glaucoma associated with Sturge-Weber syndrome. Ophthalmology 2000; 107: 2105-2110.
13. Hamush NF, Coleman AL, Wilson MR. Ahmed glaucoma valve implant for management of glaucoma in Sturge-Weber syndrome. Am J Ophthalmol 1999; 128: 758-760.
14. Amini H, Razeghinejad MR, Esfandiarpour B. Primary single-plate Molteno tube implantation for management of glaucoma in children with Sturge-Weber syndrome. Int Ophthalmol 2007; 27: 345-350.
15. Mandal AK. Primary combined Trabeculotomy-Trabeculectomy for early-onset glaucoma in Sturge-Weber Syndrome. Ophthalmology 1999; 106: 1621-1627.
16. Audren F, Abitbol O, Dureau P et al. Non-penetrating deep sclerectomy for glaucoma associated with Sturge-Weber syndrome. Acta Ophthalmol Scand 2006; 84: 656-660.
17. Eibschitz-Tsimhoni M, Lichter PR, Del Monte MA, et al. Assessing the need for posterior sclerotomy at the time of filtering surgery in patients with Sturge-Weber syndrome. Ophthalmology 2003; 110; 1361-1363.
18. Lam SM, Williams EF 3rd. Practical considerations in the treatment of capillary vascular malformations, or port wine stains. Facial Plast Surg 2004; 20: 71-76.

Neurofibromatosis

Ta Chen Peter Chang, Alex Levin, Eugenio J. Maul, Alana L. Grajewski

Definition

The diagnostic criteria for NF1 [MIM 162200] [1] require two of the following: six or more café-au-lait spots (> 0.5 cm in greatest diameter before puberty and > 1.5

cm thereafter), axillary/inguinal freckling, two or more Lisch nodules, optic pathway glioma, plexiform neurofibroma/subcutaneous neuromas, osseus lesions (*e.g.*, sphenoid wind dysplasia, tibial pseudoarthrosis) and a positive family history in a first degree relative.[2] This is an autosomal dominant disorder characterized by variable expression. The manifestations reflect loss-of-heterozygosity (*i.e.*, 'second hit' to the unaffected allele) of the tumor-suppressor gene *NF1* at 17q11.2, which encodes the protein neurofibromin 1.[3]

Epidemiology

NF1 has an estimated world-wide incidence of 1:2,500-3,000 and prevalence of 1:4,000.[4] Lisch nodules increase in frequency with age so that by adulthood, 98% of affected individuals have them. Optic pathway gliomas affect 12-15% of NF1 patients (5% of whom are symptomatic), with onset usually before seven years old, although gliomas may present up to the age of 30 years.[2] Optic nerve gliomas are usually indolent and benign. One-third of optic pathway gliomas present with proptosis or decreased vision, while two-thirds of patients are asymptomatic at the time of diagnosis.[5] Rarely, headache or precocious puberty have been the presenting symptoms.[5]

The incidence and prevalence of childhood glaucoma associated with NF1 is unknown, but it is likely to be quite uncommon. Grant and Walton examined a series of 300 childhood glaucoma cases over a period of six years and noted only one case that was associated with NF1.[6] Glaucoma is mainly a manifestation of those patients who have significant orbital involvement including sphenoid wing dysplasia and plexiform neurofibroma. These patients also frequently have ectropion uvea.

Mechanisms of glaucoma

The mechanisms of glaucoma include developmentally malformed trabecular meshwork, infiltration of the angle by neurofibroma and secondary angle closure from ciliary body infiltration by neurofibroma. Histopathologic examination of eyes enucleated secondary to end-stage glaucoma revealed complete angle closure in most eyes, grossly or histologically-apparent ectropion uveae and neurofibroma infiltrating the ciliary body in all specimens.[7] Immunostaining of enucleated specimens suggests that angle endothelialization and fibrous contracture may be a mechanism of peripheral anterior synechiae (PAS) formation.[7] One series of 56 clinically-diagnosed NF1 patients with lid plexiform neurofibroma referred to a major ophthalmology center, found 13 patients (23%) with glaucoma. The disease was ipsilateral to the orbito-facial involvement in all patients (one patient had bilateral lid plexiform neurofibromas and bilateral glaucoma).[3] All but two of these patients were diagnosed by three years old. The outcome of these glaucomatous eyes was uniformly poor, with only one of the 14 affected eyes retaining vision better than 20/400. Despite IOP control, both the affected eye and the non-glaucomatous eye exhibited abnormal continued increase in axial length.[3] It has been suggested that the presence of plexiform neurofibroma in the ocular adnexa may stimulate ocular growth via a paracrine mechanism.[8]

Treatment

Routine ophthalmologic examination should always include assessment of globe position, pupils, color vision and optic nerve appearance. Although routine neuro-imaging is not recommended for all children, any concerns of orbital involvement or abnormal optic nerve function should result in imaging.[5] A comparison of optical coherence tomography (OCT) measurement of circumpapillary retinal nerve fiber layer (RNFL) thickness of NF1 patients with known optic pathway gliomas, NF1 patients without gliomas and normal controls, showed significant RNFL thinning in NF1 patients with optic pathway gliomas. This suggests that serial OCT-RNFL analysis may be useful in monitoring the onset and progression of optic pathway gliomas.[9] This must be considered when using OCT to monitor glaucoma. Similarly, abnormalities in visual fields can be due to visual pathway glioma rather than the glaucoma.

There is no systematic survey of medical or surgical treatment for glaucoma in these patients. As there are often local factors that make surgery difficult such as proptosis, lid or orbital plexiform neurofibroma and orbital dystopia, a trial of medical therapy is recommended. If severe cognitive impairment is present, alpha-agonists may be relatively contraindicated even in older children because of the difficulty of recognizing neurologic side effects. Approximately 2% of individuals with NF1 have either renal artery stenosis or pheochromocytoma, so vasoactive ocular medications should be used with caution. It is also important to consider the feasibility of manipulating thickened lids in administering topical IOP-lowering medications. When maximal medical therapy fails, or in the rare case of glaucoma due to isolated goniodysgenesis in a patient with NF1, then goniotomy or trabeculotomy should be considered. Gonioscopy and/or anterior segment imaging are helpful in surgical planning to rule out significant PAS, which would make angle surgery difficult to perform. During goniotomy, it is not uncommon for the surgeon to feel a 'gritty' sensation while cutting into the angle. There is a high incidence of hyphema after angle surgery, which can also occur spontaneously in these patients. Failing angle surgery, a GDD can be considered, although the comorbidities of a space-occupying optic pathway glioma or altered orbital anatomy in a patient with sphenoid wing dysplasia and plexiform neurofibroma may make the surgery difficult and undesirable. Trabeculectomy may be less difficult if posterior dissection is made difficult by orbital involvement. If the orbital disease precludes GDD placement or trabeculectomy, cyclodestructive procedures may be the only option. The goal of therapy must be carefully defined and surgical expectation clearly communicated to the patients and their guardians, keeping in mind that the visual prognosis is often quite guarded due to the orbital and visual pathway involvement as well as amblyopia in these NF1 eyes with glaucoma.

References

1. Online Mendelian Inheritance in Men (OMIM), #162200 Neurofibromatosis, type 1; NF1. http://omim.org/entry/16220
2. Ferner RE, Huson SM, Thomas N, et al. Guidelines for the diagnosis and management of individuals with neurofibromatosis 1. J Med Genet 2007; 44: 81-88.
3. Morales J, Chaudhry IA, Bosley TM. Glaucoma and globe enlargement associated with neurofibromatosis type 1. Ophthalmology 2009; 116: 1725-1730.
4. Carey JC, Baty BJ, Johnson JP, Morrison T, Skolnick M, Kivlin J. The genetic aspects of neurofibromatosis. Ann N Y Acad Sci 1986; 486: 45-56.
5. Albers AC, Gutmann DH. Gliomas in patients with neurofibromatosis type 1. Expert Rev Neurother 2009; 9: 535-539.
6. Grant WM, Walton DS. Distinctive gonioscopic findings in glaucoma due to neurofibromatosis. Arch Ophthalmol 1968; 79: 127-134.
7. Edward DP, Morales J, Bouhenni RA, et al. Congenital ectropion uvea and mechanisms of glaucoma in neurofibromatosis type 1: new insights. Ophthalmology 2012; 119: 1485-1494.
8. Hoyt CS, Billson FA. Buphthalmos in neurofibromatosis: is it an expression of regional giantism? J Pediatr Ophthalmol 1977; 14: 228-234.
9. Chang L, El-Dairi MA, Frempong TA, et al. Optical coherence tomography in the evaluation of neurofibromatosis type-1 subjects with optic pathway gliomas. J AAPOS 2010; 14: 511-517.

Connective tissue disorders

Eugenio J. Maul, Claudio I. Perez, Alex Levin, Alana L. Grajewski

Definition

Ectopia lentis (EL) describes a displacement of the lens from its normal position due to distended or broken zonules. Microspherophakia is included in this category although it is not clear whether the primary defect is a developmentally small lens or stretched zonules.[1] If part of the zonules are affected or the zonules are asymmetrically affected, lens displacement (subluxation) may occur in the vertical, oblique or horizontal direction or in the anteroposterior axis. If all zonules are broken the lens can completely dislocate (luxate) into the posterior or anterior chamber.[2,3] Bilateral EL usually has a genetic origin.

Recent advances have provided a better understanding of molecular mechanisms involved in zonular disease.[4,5] Lens zonules are formed by 10 nm tubular microfibrils of fibrillin-1, a glycoprotein, with elastic properties. Fibrillin-1 is encoded by the gene *FBN1* at 15q21. Fibrillin-1 microfibrils are widely distributed in the body including both elastic and non-elastic tissues such as the skin, aorta, periosteum, cartilage, and ciliary zonules.[6] The elastic properties of zonular microfibrils are independent of the presence of elastin. Fibrillin-1 is rich in cysteine and extensively disulfide bonded. Similarities between zonular fibers and the microfibrils of the elastic tissue are striking. Zonules may be considered part of an elastic microfibrillar system.[7]

Ectopia lentis has been reported in 31 heritable disorders. Fibrillin-1 abnormality and diseases of sulfite metabolism such as sulfite oxidase deficiency, lead to poorly formed microfibrils which disrupts the integrity of the zonules causing a spectrum of lens displacements.[8,9] More than 500 different mutations have been identified in the *FBN1* gene.[10] The non-pigmented epithelium of the ciliary body is the main source of fibrillin-1 secreted into the zonules.[11] Disruption of cysteine metabolism, for example Homocystinuria type I, due to cystathione-ß-synthetase deficiency leads to brittle zonules that may easily break. Homocystinuria types II, III and IV are due to NN-Methylene tetrahydrofolate reductase deficiency, methionine synthatase deficiency and defective absorption of vitamin B12 respectively. These patients have high levels of homocysteine but low levels of methionine and less difficulty with ectopia lentis.[12]

Other causes of EL include: isolated autosomal recessive or autosomal dominant EL, ectopia lentis et pupillae, buphthalmos, coloboma, persistent fetal vasculature and systemic disorders such as lysyl oxidase deficiency, hyperlysinemia and syndromes such as EL with spontaneous filtering blebs, EL with craniosynostosis, or Kneist-like dysplasia. Acquired EL may also be caused by other ocular conditions such as pseudoexfoliation syndrome, trauma, intraocular tumors and uveitis among others.[2] Microspherophakia can be isolated or part of the autosomal recessive or autosomal dominant forms of Weill-Marchesani syndrome (WMS). Mutation in *LTBP2* causes primary megalocornea, zonular weakness and a secondary lens-related glaucoma.

Minimal absence or stretching of the zonules may be asymptomatic. Increasing compromise of the zonules leads to a proportional increase in sphericity of the lens, with progressive myopia and astigmatism. The main effect of ectopia lentis is a decrease in visual acuity.

Epidemiology

A national survey in Denmark revealed a prevalence of congenital ectopia lentis of 6.4/100,000. Estimated prevalence rate at birth was 0.83/10,000 live born.[13] In 274 of 396 cases a nosologic classification was possible. Marfan syndrome was found in 68.2% (187/274), ectopia lentis et pupillae in 21.2%, simple dominant ectopia lentis in 8%, homocystinuria in 1.1%, sulfite oxidase deficiency and Weill-Marchesani 0.7% each.[13]

Mechanism of glaucoma

Glaucoma is a common and often a serious complication of EL. The mechanism can be either angle closure from a displaced lens or an open-angle mechanism.[14,15]

Angle-closure glaucoma

The mechanism of secondary angle closure in ectopia lentis is multifactorial. Loose or broken zonules allow the lens to move forward, increasing both its area of contact with the pupil, and existing relative pupillary block (iris bombe). The increased pupillary block and/or repeated acute angle closure attacks can result in the development of peripheral anterior synechiae (PAS) and chronic angle closure.[2] PAS can also develop secondary to sustained axial anterior subluxation of the lens, 'pushing' the angle closed from behind.[17]

Acute angle closure can occur from secondary pupillary block caused by the subluxed lens in posterior chamber or by a disclocated lens within the pupil (lens-pupil capture) or into the anterior chamber (AC). It can also result from pupillary strangulation of the vitreous as it moves forward through the pupil into the AC with the lens. In children adhesion of the vitreous to the posterior lens surface is quite robust.[16] Dislocation into the AC may be spontaneous, after trauma, or with pupil dilatation. Pupillary block by a dislocated lens is common in late onset, simple ectopia lentis.[6] Secondary pupillary block is more common in microspherophakia and disorders with broken zonules such as homocystinuria or trauma.[16]

Open-angle glaucoma

A primary open-angle mechanism has been observed in Marfan syndrome. In a series of 573 patients 29 (5%) patients were diagnosed with glaucoma. Only two presented with acute angle closure. Open-angle mechanism was found in 44.8% of this series.[15]

When there is longstanding EL complicated by secondary cataract, phacolytic glaucoma may ensue[18] and the diagnosis may be easily missed if the lens is dislocated posteriorly. All children who have lens extraction are also at risk for aphakic glaucoma, independent of the underlying cause of their EL.

Treatment

Prophylaxis

In patients with EL without glaucoma and without the need to remove the lens, but in whom there is evidence of a shallow chamber, narrow angle, or impending forward luxation of the lens, a peripheral laser iridotomy is recommended to relieve pupillary block and minimize the risk of an acute attack of angle closure. Pilocarpine should not be used in these cases as it may precipitate acute angle closure by further loosening zonular support, especially in microspherophakia.[19] Early lensectomy, prior to chronic angle closure should be strongly considered, in particular with autosomal recessive WMS or EL with shallowing of the anterior chamber.[17]

Acute angle closure

Acute angle closure caused by secondary pupillary block from the lens trapped in the pupil or lens dislocation in the anterior chamber, must be treated with clear cornea or pars plana lensectomy.[20] Before resorting to immediate surgery, the lens may be repositioned by placing the patient in the supine position, dilating the pupil pharmacologically and allowing the lens to spontaneously (or with the assistance of manual massage) return to the posterior chamber, after which pilocarpine is applied to constrict the pupil and reduce the risk of recurrence. If the pressure remains elevated, anti-glaucoma medication may be of use as may topical anti-inflammatories such as prednisolone acetate. Mannitol may be particularly helpful as it shrinks the vitreous to aid in its retraction back into the posterior chamber. Peripheral laser iridotomy may also be useful to prevent recurrent acute secondary pupillary block. If lensectomy is then chosen, be particularly careful in recognizing the life-threatening risks in patients with homocystinuria who undergo anesthesia as this disorder has an associated platelet aggregation defect. All patients without a proven or obvious cause of their EL should be tested for homocystinuria by urine analysis and blood homocyteine levels prior to any surgery. Consideration should be given to bilateral simultaneous surgery in patients with increased risk for general anesthesia such as those with homocystinuria or significant aortic root dilation due to Marfan syndrome. Simultaneous glaucoma surgery is usually not recommended but in cases of increase anesthetic risk as above it should be considered. However, postoperative care could potentially be challenging.

Chronic glaucoma

Cases with glaucoma due to open-angle or chronic angle-closure mechanism may benefit from medical treatment before considering surgery. Lensectomy is not indicated in the treatment of open-angle glaucoma and is rarely of significant benefit once there is 360 degrees synechial angle closure. If medical management of the glaucoma fails, then glaucoma surgery is indicated and should be conducted in accordance with general principles discussed elsewhere. It is wise to avoid endoscopic diode cyclophotablation through an anterior approach if the ectopic lens is still present as this may precipitate acute luxation posteriorly. GDD implantation into a shallow anterior chamber (AC) or through extensive PAS may result in chronic low grade uveitis or corneal decompensation. Trabeculectomy may require a generous peripheral iridectomy to prevent iris from plugging the sclerostomy. Before performing sclerostomy, presence of vitreous in the anterior chamber should be determined by injecting an air bubble into the anterior chamber or via sponge traction techniques. If present, an anterior vitrectomy should precede sclero-corneal excision. Tight closure of the flap will minimize complications. Releasable sutures or laser suture lysis of the scleral flap may allow postoperative titration of IOP if needed while considering the risk of further vitreous prolapse.

Given the high risk of retinal detachment in these patients, especially those with Marfan syndrome, some have recommended inferior drainage placement in case silicone oil surgery becomes necessary in the future.[15]

Conditions associated with ectopia lentis (EL)

Simple ectopia lentis

EL may present as a congenital disorder or not until later adulthood with the former usually representing autosomal recessive disease and the latter autosomal dominant. Angle-closure glaucoma may be due to anterior axial lens subluxation. Early lensectomy may prevent development of chronic angle closure.[21]

Ectopia lentis et pupillae

Glaucoma is a rare manifestation.[22] Surgery may be complicated by the presence of extensive persistent pupillary membrane that may not be readily evident until after pharmacologic dilation.

Marfan syndrome

All patients should have echocardiography and cardiology consultation prior to surgery to ensure safety. Other systemic manifestations which might increase systemic risk should also be explored such as recurrent pneumothorax and dural ectasia. Some patients, especially those with neonatal Marfan, may have severe miosis. These patients are unlikely to have anterior lens subluxation (which is generally uncommon in Marfan syndrome). In any case, children with ectopia lentis from *FBN1* mutation need echocardiogram whether or not they meet diagnostic criteria for Marfan syndrome. The most common mechanism for late onset glaucoma is primary open angle.[14]

Homocystinuria

Mental retardation or learning disability occurs in 50% of patients with cystathione-ß-synthetase deficiency. In homocystinuria types II, III and IV there is no mental retardation due to a decrease in plasma levels of methionine. As discussed above one must remember that there is a thrombotic tendency, which creates a higher risk for general anesthesia.[23,24] This risk can be mitigated by admitting the child the day before surgery and hyper-hydrating with 1.5 times maintenance fluids intravenously. This should be continued throughout surgery and until the day after surgery. During surgery, wrap one limb with a tensor bandage to encourage venous return. Then unwrap the limb and move to another limb repeating this procedure. The wrapping-unwrapping should continue for all four limbs in succession throughout the procedure. The use of anti-thrombotic medication (*e.g.*, heparin) may also be considered. Consultation with a hematologist and/or metabolic specialist as well as the anesthesiologist is advised.

Despite popular preconceptions to the contrary, the lens may move in any direction including into the AC. Fifty percent of 45 cases dislocated their lens into the AC, with 11 complicated by secondary pupillary block glaucoma.[25]

Weill-Marchesani syndrome

Microspherophakia usually precedes EL and it is considered a prerequisite for the diagnosis of WMS.[16,26] Glaucoma is due to angle closure in 84.6% of the patients.[27] The AC shallowing over time can be impressively rapid and severe. Posterior synechiae may develop from chronic and repeated lens-iris touch. Early lensectomy should be encouraged when shallowing or posterior synechiae begin to develop. Often the AC will not deepen even after lensectomy if significant PAS have already formed. IOL implantation is not advised. Preoperative consultation to investigate for heart defects is advised. Blindness affects 20% of eyes with microspherophakia. Glaucoma is the cause of blindness in 77% of these eyes. In a series, 56 of 80 eyes with microspherophakia were isolated cases.[28]

References

1. Loeys BL, Dietz HC, Braverman AC, et al. The revised Ghent nosology for the Marfan syndrome. J Med Genet 2010; 47: 476-485.
2. Ritch R, Shields MB, Krupin T (Eds.), The Glaucomas. St. Louis: Mosby 1996.
3. Allingham RR, Damji KF, Freedman SF, Moroi SE, Rhee DJ, Shields MB (Eds.), Shield's Textbook of Glaucoma. Philadelphia: Lippincott Williams & Wilkins 2005.
4. Albert DM, Miller JW, Azar DT, Blodi BA (Eds.), Principles and Practice of Ophthalmology. New York: Elsevier 2008.
5. Dureau P. Pathophysiology of zonular disease. Curr Opin Ophthalmol 2008; 19: 27-30.
6. Deng T, Dong B, Zhang X, Dai H, Li Y. Late-onset bilateral dislocation and glaucoma associated with a novel mutation in FBN1. Mol Vis 2008; 14: 1229-1233.
7. Streeten BW. The nature of the ocular zonule. Trans Am Ophthalmol Soc 1982; 80: 823-854.
8. Wheatley HM, Traboulsi EI, Flowers BE, et al. Immunohistochemical localization of fibrillin in human ocular tissues. Arch Ophthalmol 1995; 113: 103-109.
9. Traboulsi EI (ed). Genetic Diseases of the Eye. New York: Oxford University 2012.
10. Boileau C, Jondeau G, Mizuguchi T, Matsumoto N. Molecular genetics of Marfan syndrome. Curr Opin Cardiol 2005; 20: 194-200.
11. Hansen E, Franc S, Garrone R. Synthesis and structural organization of zonular fibers during development and aging. Matrix Biol 2001; 20: 77-85.
12. Ramakrishnan S, Sulochana KN, Lakshmi S, Selvi R, Angayarkanni N. Biochemistry of homocisteine in health and disease. Ind J Biochem Biophys 2006; 43: 275-283.
13. Fuchs J, Rosenberg T. Congenital ectopia lentis. A Danish national survey. Acta Ophthalmol Scand 1998; 76: 20-26.
14. Izquierdo NJ, Traboulsi EI, Enger CH, Maumenee IH. Glaucoma in the Marfan syndrome. Transactions of the American Ophthalmological Society 1992; 90: 111-122.

15. Nemet AY, Assia EI, Apple DJ, Barequet IS. Current concepts of ocular manifestation in Marfan syndrome. Surv Ophthalmol 2006; 51: 561-575.
16. Nelson LB, Maumenee IH. Ectopia lentis. Surv Ophthalmol 1982; 27: 143-160.
17. Dagi LR, Walton DS. Anterior axial lens subluxation, progressive myopia, and angle closure glaucoma: recognition and treatment of atypical presentation of ectopia lentis. J AAPOS 2006; 10: 345-350.
18. Rossiter JD, Morris AH, Etchells D, Crick MP. Vitrectomy for phacolytic glaucoma in a patient with ectopia lentis et pupillae. Eye 2003; 17: 243-244.
19. Madill SA, Bain KE, Patton N, Bennett H, Singh J. Emergency use of pilocarpine and pupil block in ectopia lentis. Eye 2005; 19: 105-107.
20. Reese PD, Weingeist TA. Pars plana management of etopia lentis in children. Arch Ophthalmol 1987; 105: 1202-1204.
21. Konradsen T, Kugelberg M, Zetterström S. Visual outcomes and complications in surgery for ectopia lentis in children. J Cataract Refract Surg 2007; 33: 819-824.
22. Goldberg MF. Clinical manifestation of ectopia lentis et pupillae in 16 patients. Ophthalmology 1988; 95: 1080-1087.
23. Yamada T, Hamada H, Mochizuki S, et al. General anesthesia for patients with type III homocystinuria (tetrahydrofolate reductase deficiency). J Clin Anesth 2005; 17: 565-567.
24. Asghar A, Ali FM. Anaesthetic management of a young patient with homocystinura. J Coll Physicians Surg Pak 2012; 22: 720-2. doi: 11.2012/JCPSP.720722
25. Harrison DA, Mullaney PB, Mesfer SA, Awad AH, Dhindsa H. Management of ophthalmic complications of homocystinuria. Ophthalmology 1998; 105: 1886-1890.
26. Asaoda R, Kato M, Suami M, et al. Chronic angle closure glaucoma secondary to frail zonular fibres and spherophakia. Acta Ophthalmol Scand 2003; 81: 533-535.
27. Morales J, Al-Sharif L, Khalil DS, et al. Homozygous mutations in ADAMTS10 and AD-AMTS17 cause lenticular myopia,ectopia lentis,glaucoma spherophakia and short stature. Am J Hum Genet 2009; 85: 558-568.
28. Senthil S, Rao HL, Hoang NT, et al. Glaucoma in microspherophakia: presenting features and treatment outcome. J Glaucoma 2012 Oct 10. [Epub ahead of print].

Infection: Congenital rubella

Alana L. Grajewski, Elena Bitrian, Alex Levin, Eugenio J. Maul

Definition

Congenital rubella is seen in newborns of mothers infected with rubella during pregnancy. Congenital rubella is caused by a virus of the Togaviridae family that is transmitted through the placenta during the viremic phase in the mother, resulting in fetal viremia.[1]

Epidemiology

The use of rubella vaccine has had an enormous impact on the incidence of congenital rubella syndrome (CRS), with the last major United States outbreak occurring in 1964.[2] Infection in the third world, where vaccination is less common, continues to be a significant cause of ocular morbidity. It has been estimated that in 1996, approximately 22,000 children with CRS were born in Africa, 46,000 in South-East Asia, and 12,634 in the Western Pacific region.[3] Girls or females in the fertile age who test negative for rubella IgG antibodies should be vaccinated against rubella.

The transmission rate of congenital infection is dependent on the month of gestation during exposure. Ninety percent of fetuses will be affected if infection occurs in the first 11 weeks of gestation, 50% in weeks 11-20, 37% in weeks 20-35 and 100% during the last month of pregnancy.[2]

The rate of congenital defects and glaucoma is higher if the exposure is earlier gestation: 100% in the first 11 weeks, 30% in weeks 11-20, and none after week 20.[2] Cataracts and glaucoma appear when the exposure is in the first two months and retinopathy if the exposure is within the first five months. The earlier during gestation infection occurs, the more severe the ocular disease.[4]

The diagnosis is made by the presence of IgM antibodies to rubella in cord blood. Also, viral throat culture or serum sampling may be performed for serially rising IgG titers.[5]

Clinical findings

Systemic signs of congenital rubella present at birth include 'blueberry muffin' rash (dermal erythropoiesis), lymphadenopathy, hepatosplenomegaly, thrombocytopenia, interstitial pneumonitis and radiolucent bone lesions. The most common systemic finding is hearing loss (44%).[5] Intrauterine growth retardation, congenital heart defects, microcephaly and mental retardation are also often present.

Associated ocular abnormalities include pigmentary retinopathy (25%), strabismus (20%), cataracts (15%), microphthalmia (15%), optic atrophy (10%), corneal haze with or without glaucoma (10%), glaucoma (10%) and phthisis bulbi (2%).[6] Cataracts are caused by invasion of virus inside of the lens and are usually bilateral (80%).[7] The virus may persist for months to years after birth, so appropriate precautions should be taken by vulnerable contacts of the patient. The diagnosis of congenital rubella may be confirmed by lens culture or PCR for rubella virus. Cataracts are often accompanied by microphthalmia and/or microcornea. Corneal edema can be caused by endotheliopathy secondary to the virus or glaucoma. Rubella keratitis can be confused with corneal edema of primary congenital glaucoma. Less common ocular findings include iris hypoplasia, and chronic iridocyclitis. Gonioscopically and histopathologically the anterior chamber angle is similar to that seen in primary congenital glaucoma.[8]

Mechanism of glaucoma

The mechanism of glaucoma may be goniodysgenesis, uveitic, or phakomorphic. Glaucoma following congenital cataract surgery may also occur. Glaucoma seems to be more associated with more advanced cases of the disease.

Elevated IOP can be transient or permanent. An inflammatory reaction is the probable mechanism for the transient condition. The iritis, which may become chronic, is nongranulomatous with infiltration of the anterior uvea by lymphocytes, plasma cells and histocytes.[9]

Treatment

Systemic evaluation is critical to identify other findings secondary to congenital rubella, in particular cardiac and hematologic assessment. Developmental progress must also be followed, as delay is common. Early audiology assessment is also essential.

It is important to maintain close follow-up for infants with known or suspected congenital rubella, since glaucoma symptoms might be less evident at birth in some cases. Inflammation is managed medically with corticosteroids and associated elevated IOP with antiglaucoma therapy. If the IOP is unresponsive to medical therapy, angle surgery (goniotomy or trabeculotomy) should be considered for goniodysgenesis as it is often successful but multiple surgeries may be needed. Postoperative uveitis is common so a more intense postoperative steroid protocol may be indicated.[9] Phakomorphic glaucoma requires cataract extraction. Given the propensity to corneal disease, microphthalmia, and uveitis, leaving the child aphakic may be prudent. Children with CRS may be more prone to glaucoma after cataract removal, as they have a predisposition to glaucoma from their underlying systemic condition.

References

1. Arnold J. Ocular manifestations of congenital rubella. Curr Opin Ophthalmol 1995; 6: 45-50.
2. Mets MB, Chhabra MS. Eye manifestations of intrauterine infections and their impact on childhood blindness. Surv Ophthalmol 2008; 53: 95-111.
3. Taneja DK, Sharma P. Targeting rubella for elimination. Indian J Public Health 2012; 56: 269-272.
4. Khandekar R, Al Awaidy S, Ganesh A, Bawikar S. An epidemiological and clinical study of ocular manifestations of congenital rubella syndrome in Omani children. Arch Ophthalmol 2004; 122: 541-545.
5. Del Pizzo J. Focus on diagnosis: congenital infections (TORCH). Pediatr Rev 2011; 32: 537-542.
6. Givens KT, Lee DA, Jones T, Ilstrup DM. Congenital rubella syndrome: ophthalmic manifestations and associated systemic disorders. Br J Ophthalmol 1993; 77: 358-363.
7. Wolff SM. The ocular manifestations of congenital rubella. Trans Am Ophthalmol Soc 1972; 70: 577-614.
8. O'Neill JF. The ocular manifestations of congenital infection: a study of the early effect and long-term outcome of maternally transmitted rubella and toxoplasmosis. Trans Am Ophthalmol Soc 1998; 96: 813-879.
9. Ritch R, Shields B. The secondary glaucomas. St. Louis: Mosby 1982.

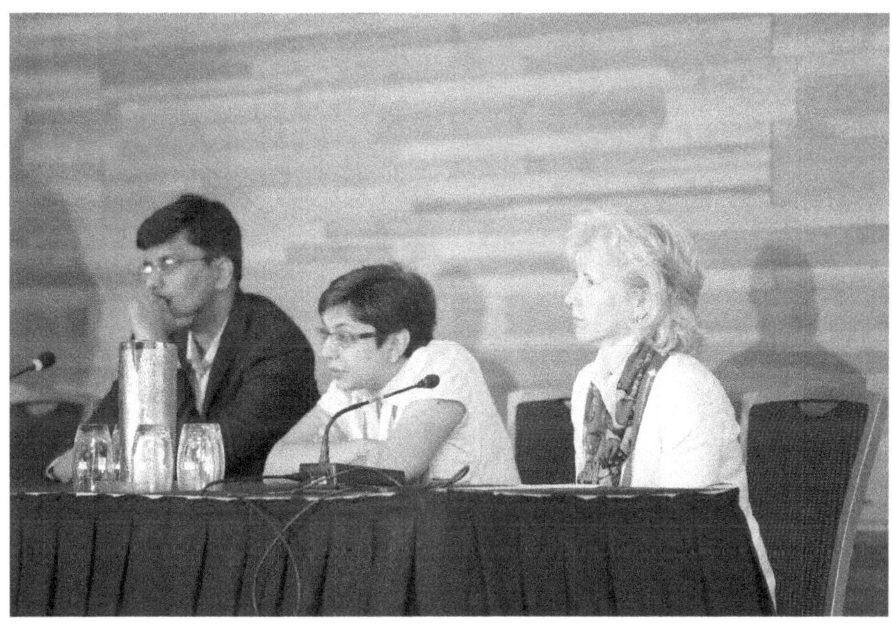

Viney Gupta, Sushmita Kaushik, Deborah Vanderveen (L-R)

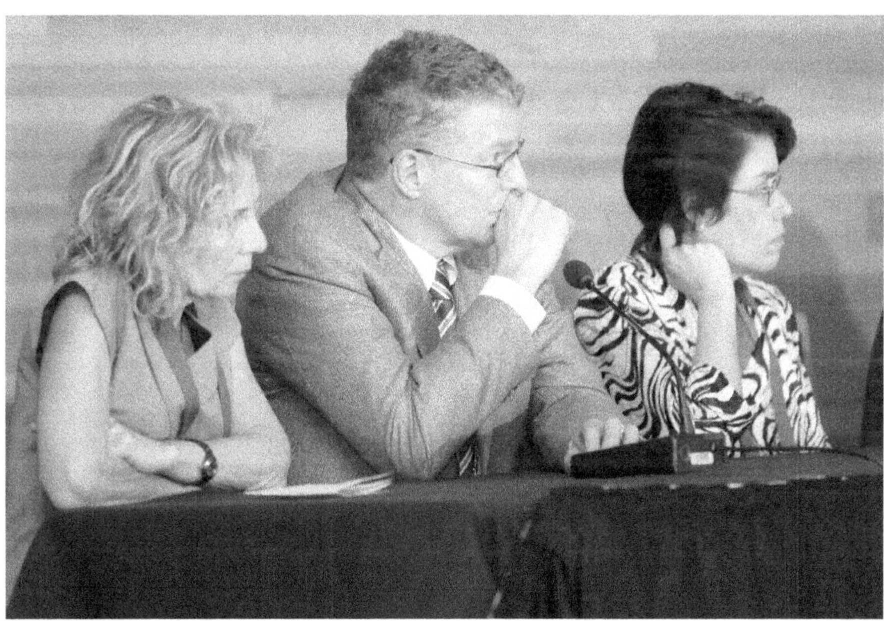

Orna Geyer, Allen Beck, Karen Joos (L-R)

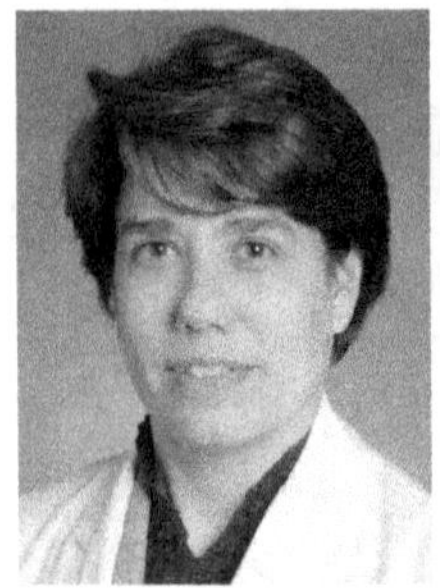

Karen Joos

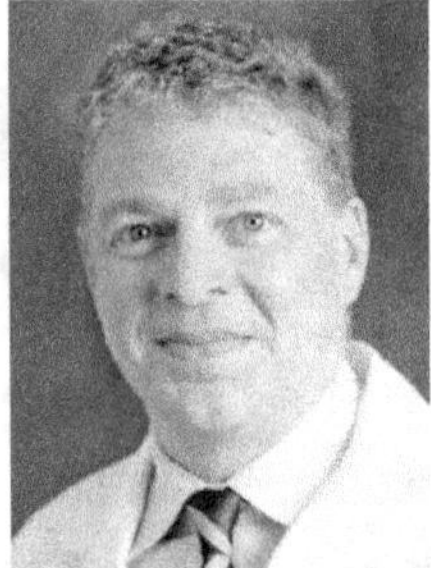

Allen Beck

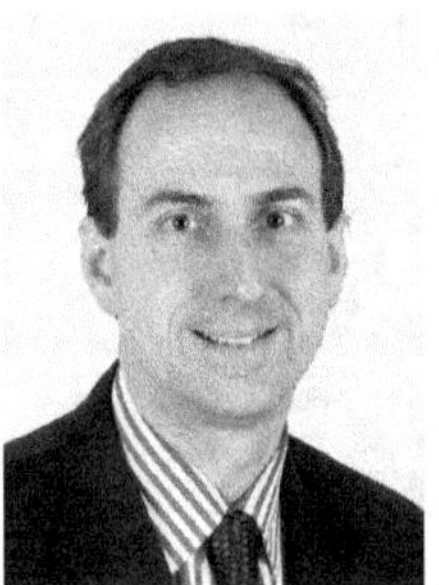

John Grigg

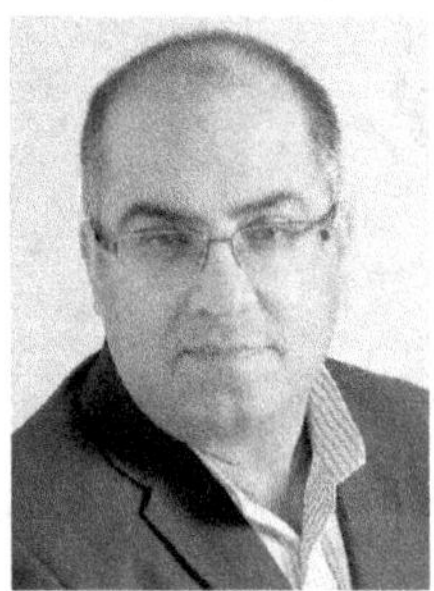

Ken Nishal

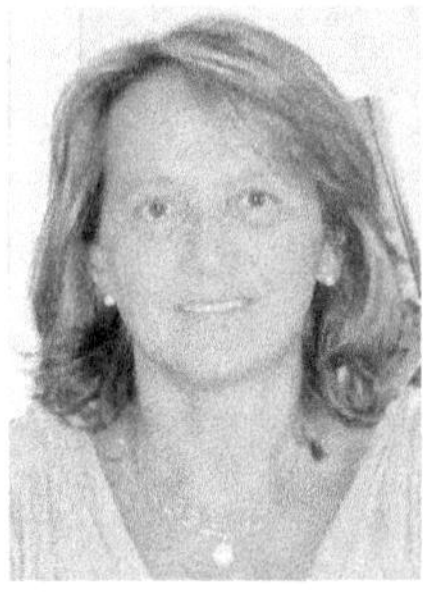

Alicia Serra-Castanera

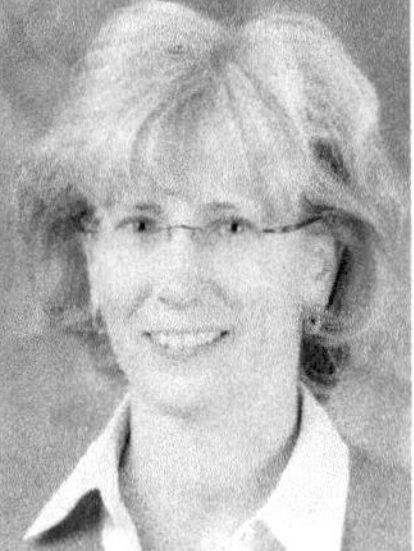

Deborah Vanderveen

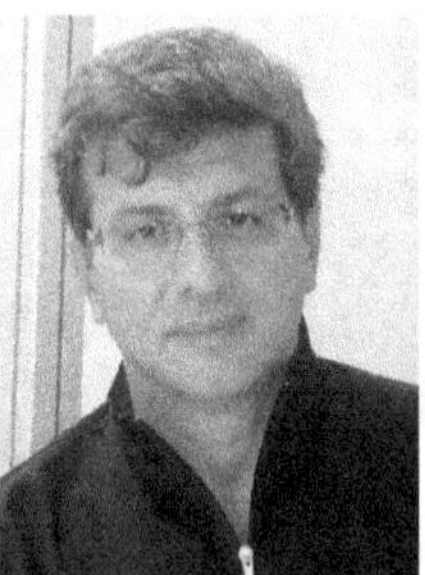

Paolo Nucci

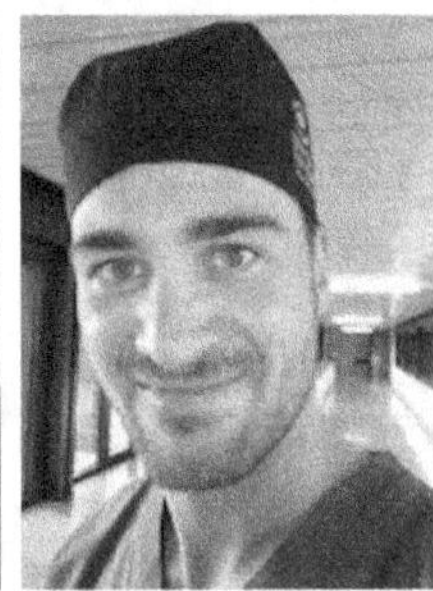

Matteo Sacchi

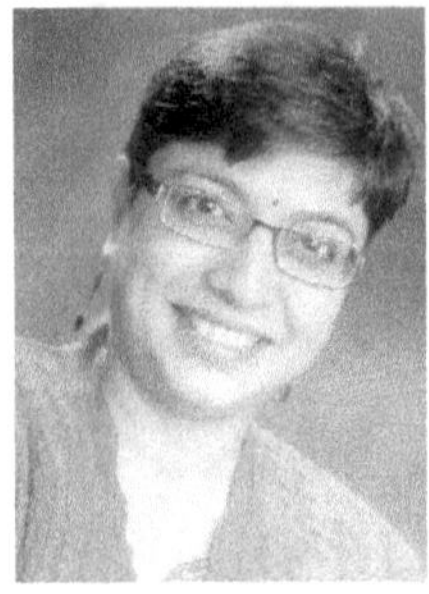

Sushmita Kaushik

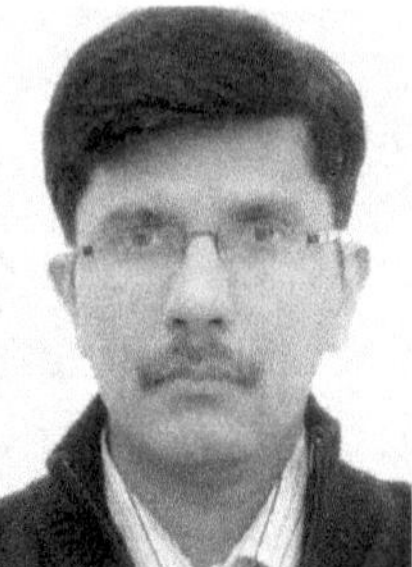

Viney Gupta

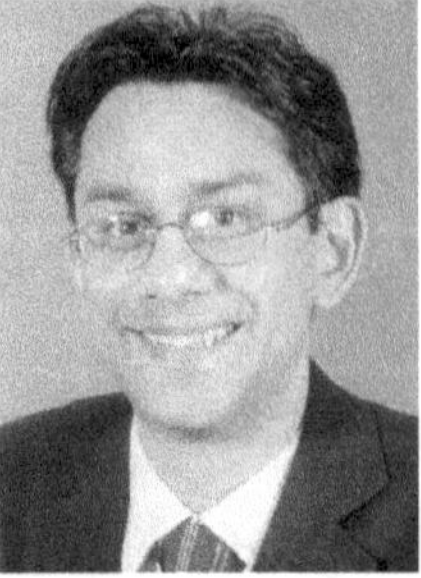

Susmito Biswas

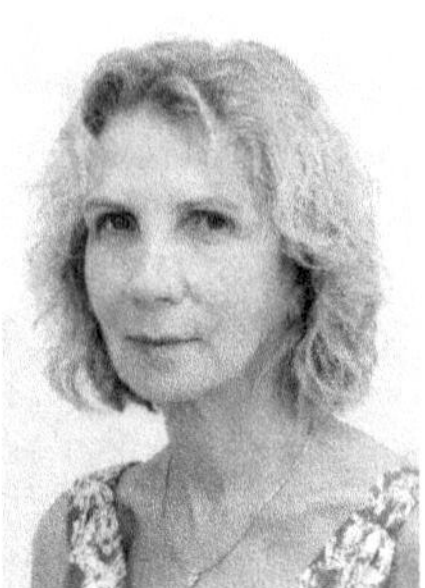

Orna Geyer

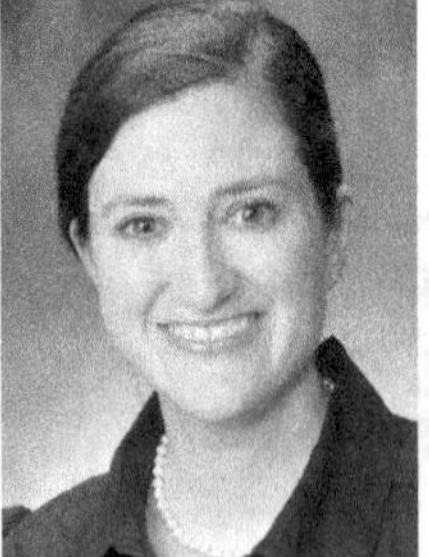

Kimberley Miller

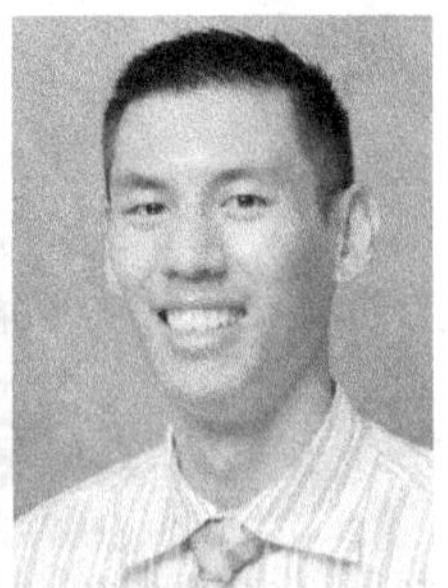

Ta Chen Peter Chang

9. GLAUCOMA ASSOCIATED WITH ACQUIRED CONDITIONS

Karen Joos, Allen Beck, John Grigg, Ken Nischal, Alicia Serra-Castanera, Deborah Vanderveen, Paolo Nucci, Matteo Sacchi, Sushmita Kaushik, Viney Gupta, Susmito Biswas, Orna Geyer, Kimberley Miller, Ta Chen Peter Chang

Section Leaders: John Grigg, Ken Nischal

Consensus statements

1. Managing uveitic glaucoma in children is challenging. The control of intraocular inflammation with adequate immunosuppression, topical and/or systemic agents, is a crucial part of management.
   Comment: Hypotony is a particular concern with surgery and modifications to the surgical technique must be employed to minimize its risk.
2. Traumatic glaucoma pathogenesis is multifactorial.
   Comment: Patients with sickle cell disease (not trait) are at higher risk for re-bleed and are likely to develop glaucomatous optic nerve damage, even with only moderately raised intraocular pressure (IOP).
   Comment: Management is aimed at controlling IOP and minimizing damage to the cornea and optic nerve. Consider surgical intervention with sustained elevated IOP > 30 mmHg unresponsive to maximum medical therapy or if corneal staining is present.
3. Steroid-induced elevated IOP is not uncommon and may be severe in children treated with ocular and systemic corticosteroids.
   Comment: Consider discontinuing the corticosteroid if possible or switching to a steroid sparing agent to ensure underlying disease control, which takes priority.
   Comment: IOP elevation may persist for months, years or even become permanent, requiring medical or surgical intervention.
4. Glaucoma secondary to intraocular tumors in children is a relatively rare event.
   Comment: Patients can be symptomatic with acute glaucoma due to the fast growth of the tumor, or symptom free in the case of a progressive, slow growing tumor.

Childhood Glaucoma, pp. 199-231
Edited by Robert N. Weinreb, Alana L. Grajewski, Maria Papadopoulos, John Grigg,
and Sharon Freedman
2013 © Kugler Publications, Amsterdam, The Netherlands

Comment: In cases of unexplained glaucoma, the possibility of an intraocular tumor should be considered, especially when a child presents with a severe chronic uveitis associated with high IOP.

Comment: Incisional surgical intervention to lower IOP is contra-indicated for glaucoma secondary to malignant ocular lesions.

5. The causes of retinopathy of prematurity (ROP) induced glaucoma are multi-factorial in nature but largely due to secondary angle closure.

Comment: Glaucoma may develop years or decades later in patients with treated or untreated Stage-4 or -5 ROP, so long-term surveillance is warranted.

Comment: IOP elevation may follow laser therapy for threshold ROP.

Introduction

This section deals with acquired conditions in which glaucoma or ocular hypertension are recognized associations. The acquired conditions are grouped into uveitis, trauma, steroid responsiveness, ocular tumors and retinopathy of prematurity.

For each of these groups it is important to recognize the association with glaucoma. When managing individual patients it is important to determine the mechanism underlying or predisposing to glaucoma. Once identified, any elevated IOP (*i.e.*, secondary ocular hypertension) should be treated before glaucoma develops and, if possible, the underlying risk factors managed.

Uveitis

Etiology of pediatric uveitis

Pediatric uveitis is rare.[1] Although the majority of cases of pediatric uveitis are idiopathic,[2] most published series report juvenile idiopathic arthritis (JIA) as the most common identifiable cause of uveitis in children with sarcoidosis being a remote second.[3-6] The etiology of the uveitis varies between studies depending on whether the cohort was from a pediatric referral center or a general pediatric ophthalmology clinic.[7,8] The etiology also varies with geographic location. Table 1 provides a guide to etiology for a uveitis referral center.

Table 1. Uveitis etiology

Juvenile idiopathic arthritis (JIA) associated uveitis (most frequent)	41-67%
Idiopathic uveitis (most frequent in general practice)	29%
Sarcoidosis	3-6%
Behçet disease	3%
Enthesis (ligament-bone junction)-related arthritis	2%

Mechanisms of glaucoma

- Open-angle glaucoma is the most common.[9,10] The mechanisms include:
  1. Trabecular meshwork (TM) damage/obstruction
     a. Inflammatory materials (*e.g.*, neutrophils, macrophages)
     b. Proteins
     c. Chemical mediators (cytokines, prostaglandins, nitric oxide)
  2. Trabecular cell dysfunction (trabeculitis)
  3. Altered vascular permeability
  4. Steroid response

- Angle closure
  1. Posterior synechiae (seclusio pupillae pupillary block)
  2. Peripheral anterior synechiae (PAS)
  3. Fibrin membrane over the pupil (occlusio pupillae pupillary block)
  4. Forward rotation of the ciliary body

Management

The management of pediatric patients with uveitis falls into two groups based on their clinical course and management challenges. These are JIA-associated uveitis and non-JIA-associated uveitis.

Juvenile idiopathic arthritis (JIA)-associated uveitis

Juvenile idiopathic arthritis is a heterogeneous group of diseases with seven subtypes including pauciarticular, polyarticular, and systemic forms with onset in a child younger than age 16 years.[11] (Table 2) The highest risk of uveitis is in pauciarticular ANA-positive JIA with onset < 6 years old and disease duration < 4 years. The inflammation is silent in greater than 50% of patients. Ophthalmic screening is recommended every 3 months. In older onset or longer disease duration, the screening is reduced to every 6 months and then to every 12 months.[12] (Table 3) Children with pauciarticular JIA have up to 20% risk of developing uveitis.[13] Anterior chamber (AC) cells have been used to determine the severity of the disease.[14] Other studies report that the amount of flare correlates with ocular complications and poor visual acuity.[15,16]

Table 2. International League of Associations for Rheumatology Classification of Juvenile Idiopathic Arthritis

Category	Definition	Frequency (% of all JIA)	Age of Onset	Sex Ratio
Systemic onset Juvenile idiopathic arthritis (JIA)	Arthritis in one or more joints with or preceded by fever of at least 2 weeks + one or more of the following: (1) rash; (2) lymphadenopathy; (3) hepatomegaly or splenomegaly; (4) serositis	4%-17%	Childhood	F=M
Oligo JIA	Arthritis affecting one to four joints during the first 6 months of disease	27%-56%	Early childhood: peak at 2-4 years	F>>>M
Polyarthritis (RF-negative)	Arthritis affects five or more joints in the first 6 months of disease. Tests for RF are negative	11%-28%	Biphasic: early 2-4 years and later 6-12 years	F>>M
Polyarthritis (RF-positive)	Arthritis affects five or more joints in the first 6 months of disease. Tests for RF are positive	2%-7%	Late childhood or adolescence	F>>M
Psoriatic arthritis	Arthritis and psoriasis	2%-11%	Biphasic : early 2-4 years and later 9-11 years	F>M
Enthesitis-related arthritis	Arthritis or enthesitis plus two of: (1) sacroiliac tenderness or lumbosacral pain; (2) HLA-B27 antigen; (3) arthritis in a male > 6 years old; (4) acute anterior uveitis; (5) family history HLA-B27-associated disease	3%-11%	Late childhood or adolescence	M>>F
Undifferentiated arthritis	Arthritis that fulfills criteria in no category or in two or more of the above categories	11%-21%		

(Adapted from Ravelli A, Martini A[17] and Petty R, Southwood T, Manners P, *et al.*[18])

Causes of vision loss in JIA-associated uveitis
These include: cataract, macular edema, glaucoma, band keratopathy, hypotony, optic nerve edema, and epiretinal membrane.

The incidence of vision loss in one study was 0.10/eye-year for vision 20/50 or worse, and was 0.08/eye-year for 20/200 or worse.[19]

Elevated intraocular pressure (IOP) is a common complication. Early detection and management of glaucoma is important with the prevalence of glaucoma up to

Table 3. American Academy of Pediatrics Guidelines for Screening Eye Examinations

Juvenile Idiopathic Arthritis (JIA)	Subtype Risk of Iritis	Examination Frequency
Oligoarticular or polyarticular, onset < 7 years of age and antinuclear factor (+)	High risk	Every 3–4 months
Oligoarticular or polyarticular and antinuclear antibody (–) regardless of age	Medium risk	Every 6 months
Onset > 7 years of age regardless of antinuclear antibody status	Medium risk	Every 6 months
Systemic onset JIA	Low risk	Every 12 months

(Adapted from Ravelli and Martini.[17])

20%.[9,20,21] The incidence of ocular hypertension in one study was reported to be 0.18/eye-year.[15]

Non-JIA uveitis

There are a number of systemic inflammatory disorders that have associated ocular involvement. The presentation of this group of inflammatory eye diseases is more likely to be associated with a red, painful, photophobic eye. The older the children the more likely are these symptoms.

Systemic inflammatory conditions associated with uveitis in children[5,22]

1. Sarcoidosis
2. Kerato-uveitis from herpes simplex
3. Juvenile Reiter syndrome
4. Lyme disease
5. Tubulointerstitial nephritis and uveitis syndrome in children
6. Trauma
7. Inflammatory bowel disease-associated anterior uveitis
8. Kawasaki disease

Principles of management

Manage inflammation with disease-modulating agents (DMAs)[23,24]

Non-steroidal anti-inflammatory drugs (NSAIDs) and corticosteroids (systemic or intra-articular) are only partially effective in treating the symptoms of JIA and its long-term complications. Treatment with systemic steroid-sparing drugs, also now referred to as disease-modifying antirheumatic drugs (DMARDs), are increasingly used because they appear to lead to better disease control. It is assumed that the more aggressive the control of inflammation early in the disease, the fewer or less severe the complications. DMARDs, which interfere directly with immune cells or their function to reduce inflammation, are typically classified as either biologic (*i.e.*, created by biologic processes) or non-biologic drugs, also referred to as synthetic DMARDs (*e.g.*, methotrexate, azathioprine).[23,25]

Disease-modulating agents (DMAs)

A. Corticosteroids (topical and systemic) and Non-steroidal anti-inflammatory drugs (NSAIDs)
  1. Mainstay of therapy for years.[26] Side effects of corticosteroids include steroid-responsive intraocular pressure elevation and cataract.
  2. Only partially effective in treating JIA symptoms.
  3. A topical cycloplegic agent may be added to treat uveitis.
  4. Intravitreal triamcinolone for chronic cystoid macular edema.[27]
B. Steroid-sparing therapy[23] [disease-modifying antirheumatic drugs (DMARDs)]
  1. Non-biological
     a. Methotrexate – FDA-approved – up to 25 mg weekly; there is some evidence that methotrexate is superior to NSAIDs.
     b. Sulfasalazine has its role in treating the arthritis.
  2. Biological
     a. Biologicals are being used for refractory JIA. These include etanercept (TNF-α blocker), infliximab (TNF-α antibody), anakinra (IL-1 receptor antagonist/off-label use), adalimumab (TNF-α antibody), abatacept (T-cell activation inhibitor), tocilizumab (IL-6 receptor antibody/approved April 2011 for systemic JIA), and rituximab (CD20 antibody).[28,29] Canakinumab and rilonacept (anti-IL-1 therapies) are in clinical trials in systemic JIA.[30] A_3 adenosine receptor agonists are being investigated as possible future therapies.[31]
     b. Commonly used agents in JIA associated uveitis are infliximab and adalimumab.

The management of the intraocular inflammation is crucial to reducing the vision-threatening complications of pediatric uveitis and in particular JIA-associated uveitis.[25] Immunosuppression follows a stepwise approach. If anterior segment inflammation is not controlled with topical steroid eye drops using a qid dosing schedule and local periorbital steroid injections,[26] then systemic immunosuppression is indicated. Another indication for systemic therapy is the child who is a steroid responder. This is best implemented in consultation with a pediatric rheumatologist or immunologist who is experienced in the management of these drugs in children.

If there is an acute flare up in inflammation then oral steroids are appropriate; however the use of a steroid sparing agent needs to be considered early in management. Methotrexate beginning with a low dose and gradually increasing is usually well tolerated in children. Nausea is a common problem at higher doses and may require discontinuation or change to subcutaneous administration. Subcutaneous methotrexate is often more potent at reducing intraocular inflammation than the same total weekly dosage given orally, and may diminish gastrointestinal side effects. Folic acid must be given as a daily supplement with methotrexate. Alternatives include mycophenolate which is well tolerated in children.[32]

If the anterior segment inflammation continues despite topical and systemic therapy, the addition of a biologic agent is indicated. Infliximab (monthly infusions) and adalimumab (fortnightly subcutaneous injections) are currently the most promising in pediatric uveitic patients. The long-term effectiveness of the newer biologic agents is dependent on the continuation of a non-biologic agent such as methotrexate to minimize the occurrence of an immune response to the biologic agent rendering it ineffective.

Manage elevated IOP

Managing uveitic glaucoma in children can be very challenging due to the multifactorial nature of the elevated IOP. Clinicians must be aware of the potential for the IOP to rise significantly and result in very rapid progression of the optic disc damage. Close monitoring and expedient intervention is required when this is the case.

Medications
Medications form the first line of therapy for elevated IOP related to uveitis in a child. Treatment must be commenced even if the optic discs are normal (secondary ocular hypertension). However, control of elevated IOP may not easily be achieved. Foster *et al.*[33] reported that only 17% of their cohort was controlled by topical medications alone; with the addition of oral carbonic anhydrase inhibitors this increased to 37%. The medication groups include: topical beta blockers, topical and oral carbonic anhydrase inhibitors, prostaglandin analogues and topical alpha-2 agonists.[34] There are theoretical and anecdotal risks of worsening uveitis or macular edema in patients taking prostaglandin analogues. Chang *et al.* suggest that in a tertiary uveitis clinical setting which included children, there was no increase in uveitis or macular edema in the group using prostaglandin analogues compared to the group using other glaucoma medications.[35] Caution is required in children using topical alpha-2 agonist due to somnolence in young children especially younger than six years.

Ensuring adequate immunosuppression is crucial in the management of these children. This means the early recognition of poor control with topical agents allowing the institution of systemic steroid sparing agents. Avoid the temptation to constantly change the steroid regime in an attempt to reduce IOP, unless clinically indicated for the inflammation, which takes priority. Beware of a lowered intraocular pressure in the setting of reduced steroid and increased uveitis, as the former may be a direct consequence of reduced aqueous production from the latter, rather than a reduced 'steroid response'. The only way to prove that elevated IOP in the setting of uveitis and steroid therapy is due to uveitis and not the steroid, is to eliminate the steroid with systemic steroid-sparing therapy.

Glaucoma surgery

Glaucoma surgery is often needed. One study reported an incidence of 0.05/eye-year.[15] The principles of treatment are to operate on 'a quiet eye' to reduce complications. Adequate immunosuppression, both topical and systemic, is crucial to managing the uveitis to minimize intraocular damage and risk for glaucoma as well as maximizing the success of any glaucoma surgical procedure in both the short and long term.

Surgical risks include: increased inflammation, ciliary body shutdown, cataract, corneal decompensation, retinal detachment, cystoid macular edema, choroidal effusion, flat AC, encapsulated bleb, extruded glaucoma drainage device (GDD), infection and amblyopia. Hypotony is a significant common complication in pediatric uveitic patients post glaucoma surgery[19] even in the absence of overdrainage. Adjustments need to be made to surgical techniques to minimize the occurrence of hypotony. If trabeculectomy is performed then tight scleral flap sutures are mandatory. The use of an intraluminal stent (*e.g.*, 3/0 supramid or 3/0 nylon) in addition to an extraluminal occlusive suture (*e.g.*, 6/0 vicryl) in non-flow restricted GDDs, assist in reducing the risk of postoperative hypotony. Refer to Figure 1 for a suggested management algorithm.

Surgical outcomes in pediatric uveitic glaucoma

The surgical options include angle surgery, trabeculectomy, GDDs and ciliary body destruction. Published studies are few in number, retrospective, usually combine multiple uveitic etiologies and have short follow-up.

Angle surgery

A significant advantage of angle surgery (goniotomy) is a lower complication rate although a transient postoperative hyphema is common. After one to three goniotomies, Ho *et al.* found qualified success rates (≤ 21 mmHg) of 72% overall in 40 eyes with 86% in phakic eyes and 36% in aphakic eyes over a mean 99-month follow-up. Significantly better outcomes were associated with being less than ten years old, phakic and having few PAS and no prior surgery. The ten-year Kaplan-Meier survival probability was 0.71.[36] Likewise, Bohnsack *et al.* found the ten-year Kaplan-Meier survival probability (≤ 21 mmHg) to be 0.69 in their study of 31 eyes following treatment with one or two goniotomies. [37]

Trabeculectomy

The literature is sparse regarding trabeculectomy surgery in children with uveitic glaucoma. Lam *et al.* found a postoperative IOP range of 9-22 mmHg in three patients following combined cataract and trabeculectomy procedures for unknown follow-up duration.[38] Heinz *et al.* found 88% success (< 21 mmHg, no medication) with trabeculectomy and Mitomycin C (MMC) (0.2mg/ml) and 50% success with modified deep sclerectomy and MMC (0.2 mg/ml) over a mean of 25 months.[39]

However, the trabeculectomy group needed further glaucoma surgery in 50%. The rate of shallow AC and choroidal detachment was 50% in the trabeculectomy group versus 20% modified deep sclerectomy group.

Glaucoma drainage devices

Bohnsack *et al.* found 4/5 eyes (80%) had successful IOP control after a mean follow up of 27 months.[37] Välimäki *et al.* found a success rate (≤ 21 mmHg) of 89% in 27 eyes with a mean 40-month follow-up in secondary glaucoma associated with JIA.[40] Kafkala *et al.* found a 7/7 patient success rate (≤ 21 mmHg with medication) with an Ahmed implant at a mean 37-month follow-up, with 2/6 developing limited suprachoroidal hemorrhage postoperatively which resorbed in a month without clinical sequelae.[41] Consider GDDs with smaller surface areas, *e.g.*, Baerveldt 250 mm^2, Ahmed 184 mm^2 and modify non-flow restricted GDD to minimize the risk of hypotony. A desirably low IOP often results after GDD surgery, due to limited aqueous production in many uveitic glaucoma cases.

Ciliary body destruction

Heinz *et al.* found a high failure rate after short-term follow-up in his study of 19 eyes which were treated 41 times with diode laser as primary treatment with a 32% qualified success (IOP ≤ 21 mmHg) on glaucoma medications at the end of 10 months mean follow-up.[42] They concluded that it was unsatisfactory treatment due to its poor success rate in controlling IOP in uveitic eyes with glaucoma. Furthermore, its use should be dissuaded as it aims to reduce the function of the ciliary body which is already compromised by inflammation, and may lead to problems with chronic hypotony with future more invasive surgery.

Management of cataract

Cataracts are among the most common ocular complication of JIA. Risk factors include posterior synechiae, long-standing ocular inflammation, and topical corticosteroids. Studies report up to 80% by adulthood with a JIA history.[38,43] Screening for uveitis and adequate immunosuppression are proposed as strategies to reduce cataract formation.[43] The uveitis is recommended to be quiescent for at least 3 months prior to cataract surgery and additional immunosuppression is given perioperatively with close postoperative monitoring for flare-ups.[43] New onset of ocular hypertension and secondary glaucoma may occur after cataract surgery, particularly when intravitreal triamcinolone is used as an adjunct to surgery.[44] The role of intraocular lenses in pediatric uveitis remains controversial. Recent studies found no difference in complications between aphakic and pseudophakic eyes in children with JIA uveitis.[45,46]

Pediatric cataract surgical tips to minimize inflammation and thus reduce glaucoma risk include: AC maintainer to avoid intra-operative hypotony and chamber

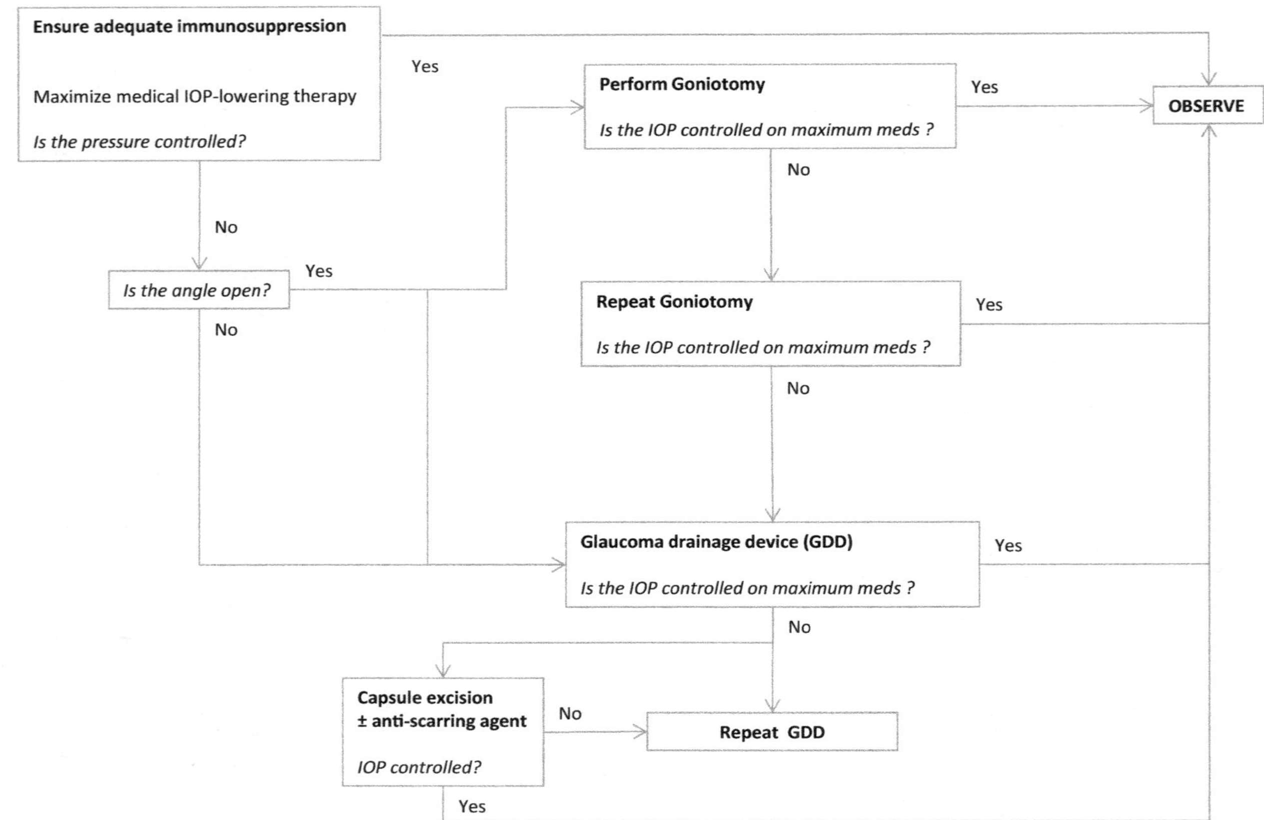

Fig. 1. A suggested approach to the management of uveitic glaucoma. (It will be influenced by surgeon preference/experience and local facilities/equipment availability.)

collapse, heparin in BSS infusion (1 unit/ml)[47-49] and the use of intravitreal triamcinolone.

Trauma

Definition

Raised intraocular pressure (> 21 mmHg) secondary to ocular trauma which may be acute or chronic in onset, and blunt or penetrating in nature.

Mechanisms of glaucoma

Blunt trauma

There are two peaks for glaucoma, within 1 year and after 10 years.[50]

Mechanism of raised IOP includes:

Uveitis
The initial IOP in cases of traumatic iritis is often low presumably due to transient ciliary body shutdown. This may be followed by a rise in IOP in the few days after injury secondary to obstruction of trabecular meshwork by inflammatory debris or even swelling of the trabecular meshwork contributing to the outflow obstruction.[51] The IOP elevation is usually mild and easily controlled. Steroids used to treat inflammation may cause elevated IOP.

Hyphema
The mean incidence of hyphema is 17/100,000 population (20/100,000 males and 4/100,000 females).[52,53] Blunt injury results in antero-posterior compression of the globe and equatorial globe expansion which induces stresses in the anterior chamber angle structures, which may lead to iris stromal and/or ciliary body vessel rupture with subsequent hemorrhage.[54] Re-bleeding may be due to clot lysis and/or retraction and is associated often with raised IOP.

Acutely, the intraocular pressure may be raised due to: occlusion of the trabecular meshwork by clot, inflammatory cells, or red blood cell debris; pupillary block secondary to a clot involving both the anterior and posterior chambers and large hyphemas. The larger the hyphema, the greater the chance of raised IOP. In patients with sickle cell disease, high IOP can be seen with a small hyphema.

Total vs. partial hyphema
Usually visual prognosis and complications are worse in the presence of total hyphema as opposed to subtotal hyphema.[55] Eyes with total hyphemas are more likely to require surgery than eyes with partial hyphemas. Persistence of the hyphema for more than one week can result in the formation of peripheral anterior synechiae (PAS). Posterior synechiae also can form.

Re-bleed vs. no re-bleed
Since a re-bleed can cause a substantial increase in hyphema size, re-bleeding may be associated with complications such as increased IOP, corneal blood staining, optic atrophy and PAS. The incidence of surgical intervention is higher in re-bleeds.[56] The use of medication that significantly reduces the incidence of re-bleeding should be considered regardless of hyphema size since risk of re-bleed is not related to size of hyphema.

Sickle cell disease
The term sickle cell disease (SCD) encompasses a group of disorders characterized by the presence of at least one hemoglobin S (Hb S) allele, and a second abnormal allele (frequently another HbS) allowing abnormal hemoglobin polymerization leading to a symptomatic disorder. Sickle cell trait patients are heterozygous for HbS and hemoglobin A (HbA).[57] Patients with sickle cell disease are at higher risk for a re-bleed and likely to develop glaucomatous nerve damage, even with only moderately raised IOP. [58] Optic nerve perfusion can be significantly compromised with only modest IOP elevations due to the vascular occlusive effects of sickle cell disease. In patients where the hyphema doesn't resolve in the expected time frame then an additional etiology should be considered. Sickle cell disease is one such condition. [59] Carbonic anhydrase inhibitors will potentiate the sickling process thus worsening the raised IOP; so should be avoided in patients with sickle cell disease.

Angle recession
The incidence of angle recession after eye trauma ranges from 20-94%. In patients with traumatic angle recession, 5-20% will go on to develop glaucoma.[60] The possibility of developing glaucoma in an eye with angle recession appears to be related to the extent of angle recession. The greater the circumferential extent of angle recession, the greater the chance of subsequently developing glaucoma; this is not a steadfast rule but is more reliable if greater than 180 degrees of the anterior chamber angle is involved. The glaucoma onset may be delayed many years after original injury.

Ghost cell glaucoma
After vitreous hemorrhage, erythrocytes degenerate from biconvex cells into spherical khaki colored ghost cells and if the anterior hyaloid face is ruptured, these ghost cells can migrate into the anterior chamber and obstruct the trabecular meshwork because ghost cells are more rigid than normal red blood cells. Red blood

cells take one to two weeks to degenerate into ghost cells so the onset of ghost cell glaucoma is usually around three weeks post-trauma.[61] It is rare in children and in one review of over 200 cases of traumatic and non-traumatic vitreous hemorrhage in children, no case of ghost cell glaucoma was reported.[62]

Dislocated lens

Rupture of the zonules can lead to anterior or posterior dislocation of the lens. Forward displacement of the lens or vitreous prolapse through the ruptured zonules can lead to pupillary block and angle-closure glaucoma. Total anterior dislocation can lead to acute angle-closure glaucoma secondary to pupillary block, or open-angle glaucoma due to direct angle obstruction by the whole lens or lens fragment. Posterior dislocation is less likely to cause glaucoma. However, if associated with vitreous prolapse, pupillary block glaucoma may ensue or if the dislocated lens becomes cataractous and lens proteins leak, phacolytic glaucoma may occur.

Penetrating trauma

Following repair of penetrating ocular trauma glaucoma may develop. Risk factors for developing glaucoma include: uveitis, hyphaema and epithelial/stromal down growth.

In one of the few prospective studies looking for early predictors of chronic post-traumatic glaucoma, Sihota *et al.*[63] reported them to be increased pigmentation of the angle on gonioscopic findings, a higher baseline IOP, the absence of a cyclodialysis cleft on UBM or gonioscopic findings, hyphema, angle recession > 180 degrees and lens injury.

Management

General measures

Management is aimed at controlling IOP and minimizing damage to the cornea and angle structures.[64] Hyphema patients need to be followed closely in the first week. Most children can be managed at home if appropriate support is available.[65] Clinic follow-up to monitor for re-bleeding and for IOP checks is suggested on the first day following trauma and then two to three times in the first ten days depending on progress. While there are no controlled studies, rest and avoidance of physical activity is advised. Many clinicians also prescribe cycloplegics (*e.g.*, atropine) and topical steroids for post-traumatic inflammation and hyphema.[66] Pressures over 25 mmHg should be treated.

Management of raised IOP

Medical treatment
Topical
- Unless there are contraindications, β-blockers are usually used first line. Adrenergic agonists such as apraclonidine or brimonidine may be used as second line. Brimonidine should be avoided in young children. Pilocarpine is avoided as this increases vascular permeability and makes the possibility of occlusio pupillae higher. Prostaglandin analogues theoretically should be avoided but there is no published evidence to suggest there is an increased inflammatory response in such circumstances.
- The use of cycloplegics is likely to reduce pain in cases of hyphema and also reduce the incidence of occlusio/seclusio pupillae.

Systemic
- Oral or intravenous acetazolamide. In cases of sickle cell disease the use of systemic acetazolamide can cause a sickle crisis and should be avoided. Local sickling of the blood in the AC may occur with the use of systemic CAIs prolonging clearance of the hyphaema. Its use in sickle cell trait is not contraindicated but the child should be well hydrated. IV mannitol can be used but needs hematological surveillance in the presence of sickle cell disease. The use of agents to prevent re-bleeds (*e.g.*, tranexamic acid) has no absolute evidence to advise its mandatory use.[67]

Surgical treatment
The decision to intervene surgically is determined by the risk of permanent blood staining of the cornea and the risk of optic nerve damage from raised IOP. In attempting to predict who may need surgical intervention, a number of risk factors have been identified.[68] These include hyphema, corneal injury, presence of optic atrophy, visual acuity < 20/200 and a history of penetrating ocular trauma. There is general agreement on the timing for intervention in the acute situation. These include cases of total hyphema or partial hyphema with sustained IOP greater than 30 mmHg on maximum medical therapy including oral CAIs, or any evidence of corneal staining.

There is no universal agreement on the method of intervention in hypertensive hyphaema. Surgical washout of the anterior chamber is recommended. The role and outcome of trabeculectomy at the time of washout has been reported by some.[69] Other authors have reported the use of gonioaspiration (AC/angle washout under the guidance of a Koeppe lens) in cases of small hyphemas with high IOP (> 30 mmHg)[70] without trabeculectomy.

Corticosteroid-induced ocular hypertension and glaucoma

Definition

Corticosteroid-induced ocular hypertension: An increase in IOP only, as a result of oral, intravenous, inhaled, topical, periocular, and intravitreal corticosteroid therapy.[71]

Corticosteroid-induced glaucoma: Glaucoma resulting from corticosteroid-induced ocular hypertension (*see* Section 1).

Background

The first associations between the use of steroids and IOP were reported by McLean who identified an increase in IOP after systemic administration of ACTH in 1950.[72] Treatment of adult patients with topical corticosteroids for four to six weeks leads to an increase in IOP greater than 16 mmHg in 5% of the population, and 6 to 15 mmHg in 30% of the population.[73-75]

Potency and mode of administration of corticosteroids plays a major role in the degree of corticosteroid response. Higher potency corticosteroids administered to the eye are most likely to exhibit elevated IOP.[71]

Children have been noted to have a higher frequency and worse severity of corticosteroid response. Lam *et al.* noted 71% of children treated with dexamethasone 0.1% qid had an IOP of greater than 21 mmHg, and 36% had an IOP greater than 30 mmHg. In children less than six years of age, the net increase was greater and the time to peak IOP was shorter.[76]

Pathophysiology: proposed mechanisms

1. Increased aqueous outflow resistance.[71]
2. Changes in TM microstructure.
3. Increase in the deposition of extracellular matrix material in the TM.
4. Reduced degradation of substances in the TM.

Corticosteroid preparations and method of administration

The topical route is the most common of all modes of administration of steroids in the pediatric population,[76-81] and therefore more likely to be the one to induce IOP elevation in children.[76,82] The severity of the IOP increase resulting from topical corticosteroid correlates with the anti-inflammatory potency of the preparations. Lam *et al.*[76] reported an IOP greater than 30 mmHg in 36% of children treated with dexamethasone 0.1% qid, [76] compared to Fan *et al.*[82] who reported this in only 6.5% of children treated with the less potent corticosteroid fluorometholone 0.1% instilled six times daily. The IOP response to topical steroids is dose- and age-dependent. A higher frequency of corticosteroid application is associated with greater ocular hypertension, and younger-aged children have a higher peak of IOP and attain peak IOP earlier.[76] Infants may have a more rapid and severe increase in IOP. Buphthalmos and glaucoma were reported in a three-week-old infant following one week of topical steroids[83] and in a six-month-old infant after four months treatment with topical steroids.[84]

Increased IOP after sub-tenon injection of triamcinolone has been reported in adults.[85] Pediatric patients with uveitis experienced an IOP rise more frequently when treated with periocular steroid injections shortly after the onset of the disease. The number of peri-ocular injections had no influence on the development of elevated IOP.[77] There is one case report in the literature which describes a child who developed glaucoma following topical corticosteroids and sub-tenon injection of triamcinolone.[86]

Intravitreal sustained-release steroid implants frequently cause increased IOP in adults.[87] Patel *et al.* [78] reported IOP spikes in the range of 30-45 mmHg following implantation of a fluocinolone acetonide implant in four of six eyes of children aged 6 to 13 years. The IOP of two of those eyes was controlled successfully with medical therapy, while the other two required GDD placement. The two remaining eyes had GDDs placed for poor IOP control before the implantation of the steroid implant and did not develop IOP elevation.

Prolonged systemic corticosteroid therapy may also induce IOP elevation in children. Hayasaka *et al.*[79] reported that 20% of pediatric patients developed IOP in the range of 22-30 mmHg after long-term use (mean 4 years) of oral prednisolone. One of their patients developed glaucoma and required glaucoma surgery. Age, dosage or duration of treatment did not correlate with the high IOP in that study. Yamashita *et al.*[88] observed an IOP rise higher than 21 mmHg, with a mean maximum increase to 39 mmHg in all five children receiving high-dose oral or intravenous dexamethasone intermittently for 2.5 to 3 years. One patient developed glaucomatous optic neuropathy. Although rare, a rapid (7-8 days after initiating treatment) and severe rise in IOP in the range of 38-56 mmHg has been described following high-dose oral prednisolone (60 mg/day).[89,90]

Chronic intermittent (over two years) use of inhaled or nasal corticosteroids did not cause ocular hypertension in children,[80,81] however, there is one anecdotal report describing IOP elevation following administration of nasal and inhalation steroids in an eight-year-old girl.[91]

Treatment

Initial treatment consists of discontinuing the corticosteroid if possible. However, IOP elevation may persist for months, years or even become permanent, requiring medical or surgical intervention.

Medical treatment

The underlying disease that necessitated steroid treatment should be treated as needed with other agents systemically (immunosuppressive and biologics), avoiding corticosteroids by any route of administration.

If corticosteroid treatment is necessary, sometimes the route can be changed and the dosage minimized if it does not compromise disease control.[89,92] Rates of corticosteroid-induced IOP elevation are dependent on dose and route of administration.[82,93-96] The patient will need close supervision during corticosteroid treatment in case any side effects occur.

Persistent elevated IOP or pathology causing elevated IOP may require IOP-lowering therapy. Typically, medical therapy is initiated with aqueous suppression.[90,97] Prostaglandins may be used[83] depending on the underlying pathology which resulted in initial corticosteroid use.

Surgical treatment

When medical therapy is inadequate, surgical intervention is required. Angle surgery is the initial choice if there are no PAS from underlying inflammatory ocular disease. Angle surgery makes sense since the pathology is changes in the TM and there is no reason to believe there is pathology further down the outflow pathway.

Glaucoma filtering surgery (glaucoma drainage device or trabeculectomy) may be effective if angle surgery is inadequate. A trabeculectomy can often be done without antiscarring agents if there is systemic immune suppression. Smaller sized GDDs are typically adequate, especially if corticosteroids were initially used to treat uveitis or the patient is systemically immunosuppressed.

Following trabeculectomy there is some evidence that the steroid response can continue to affect the IOP in the presence of a patent ostium and diffuse filtration bleb.[98] Identifying the steroid responder prior to filtration surgery will assist in the post-op management.

Tumors

Introduction

Given the relative infrequency of intraocular tumors, secondary glaucoma as a result of intraocular tumors is a relatively rare event. Patients with acquired glaucoma secondary to tumors can be symptomatic with acute glaucoma due to the fast growth of the tumor, or symptom-free in case of progressive, low growing tumor. Retinoblastoma, medulloepithelioma and intraocular melanoma are the most common tumors leading to secondary glaucoma. Development of secondary acquired glaucoma can result from: direct trabecular meshwork infiltration by the tumor;

tumor cells seeding into the angle; pigment/inflammatory cell dispersion into the anterior chamber and angle or angle closure due to anterior displacement of lens-iris diaphragm. Other mechanisms are: melanophagic, ghost cells, suprachoroidal hemorrhage, iris neovascularization and choroidal detachment.

In cases of unexplained glaucoma, the possibility of an intraocular lesion should be considered and the differential diagnosis of an intraocular neoplasm should be taken into account when a child presents with a severe chronic uveitis associated with high IOP.

Types of tumors

Benign tumors

Iris and ciliary body cysts

Iris cysts are uncommon in childhood.[99,100] The usual age of onset of primary cysts is infancy to adolescence but may present much later. The iris cysts can be classified as primary cysts, which occur in eyes without prior trauma or surgery, and secondary cysts. Primary cysts are further divided into congenital and acquired cysts (depending on age of onset) and pigment epithelial or stromal cysts (depending on location and histopathology).[101,102]

Primary cysts of the iris pigment epithelium (60-70%) occur at characteristic locations: peripheral (iridociliary), midzonal (Fig. 2), central (pupillary), or dislodged (fixed or free-floating). Additionally, because they are lined by pigment epithelium, they usually present as colored masses that do not transmit light.[103] Most of these cysts have been reported to remain stable over time and do not require treatment.[99,101]

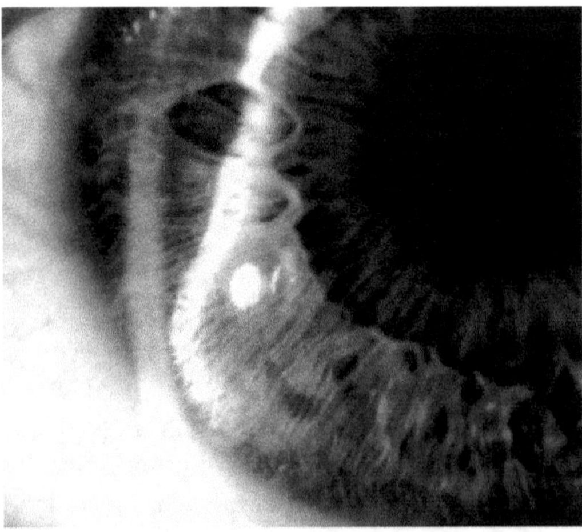

Fig. 2. Midzonal iris cyst.

In contrast, primary iris stromal cysts (20-30%) arise anterior to the pigment epithelium, usually present as translucent masses, and often progress in size and thus require intervention.[100]

Although iris cysts arising from the iris pigment epithelium are considered common in adults, and iris stromal cysts are considered typical of childhood, in a series of 57 iris cysts in children, Shields *et al.* found pigment epithelial cysts to be more common than iris stromal cysts.[100]

Secondary iris cysts can occur in children after trauma, surgery, malignancy, or parasitic infection.[100]

Diagnosis

The majority of the primary iris cysts are asymptomatic and may be detected on routine examination.[99,103] Most cysts of the iris pigment epithelium come to the clinician's attention during routine eye examination, when they may represent a diagnostic challenge considering they must be differentiated from malignant intraocular tumors, especially uveal melanoma or medulloepithelioma.[103]

The symptoms depend on the size of the lesion and extent of involvement and may range from none to marked decreased vision. The primary cysts may rarely increase in size with time resulting in symptoms in adolescence or adulthood.

When assessing an iris cyst it is important to remember intraocular tumors as a differential diagnosis (Table 4). Investigations, in particular ultrasound biomicroscopy (UBM), are very helpful in this regard.[104]

Treatment

The choice of treatment of iris cyst largely depends on the cause and extent of the cyst. Various modalities of treatment have been used, ranging from conservative

Table 4. Distinguishing features between iris cysts and malignancy. (Adapted from Rao *et al.*[99])

	Iris cyst	Malignancy
Consistency	Cystic	Solid (rarely cavitation)
Borders	Regular	Irregular
Surface	Smooth	Rough and irregular
Vascularization	No	Surface vessels
Contents	Variable	Solid lesion
Iris	displacement	Arising from the iris stroma
Associated findings	Variable	Ectropion uvea, cataract, neovascular glaucoma
Documented growth	Occasionally	Usually positive
UBM		
Walls	Thin	Thick
Contents	Clear	Suspended particles
Contour	Regular	Irregular with extension over cornea lens iris
Posterior extension	Rare	Common
Angle	No/Minimal invasion	Angle distortion common

to extensive surgical approaches. Although a conservative approach is usually recommended for asymptomatic lesions, intervention is necessary when elevated IOP, amblyopia or corneal decompensation occurs.

The decision to intervene should be considered in the following circumstances: large cysts involving more than half of the anterior chamber, a documented increase in size that is symptomatic, evidence of recurrent iridocyclitis, corneal decompensation due to endothelial touch by the cyst, or in cases with secondary glaucoma.[105-107]

Iridociliary cysts may lead to secondary glaucoma by pushing the iris root anteriorly, and causing a pseudo-plateau iris configuration with angle closure. In a large series of young patients with angle-closure glaucoma, iridociliary cysts were found to be the second most common cause of angle closure glaucoma.[108] Iridociliary cysts causing angle closure are usually multiple, extending around the angle circumference.[108]

Lasers play a major role in management of iris cysts. Both the Argon laser and Nd:Yag laser have roles in the management of iris cysts.[109,110] Argon laser is used to photocoagulate, devitalize the epithelium, and shrink the size of cyst.[111,112] Nd:YAG laser is used to perforate the cyst.

In the presence of angle closure glaucoma, laser is the mainstay of treatment including cyst puncture and argon laser peripheral iridoplasty in patients with persistent appositional angle closure.[108]

Surgical excision of iris cysts offers a more definitive management option. Surgical excision can be used in all types of cysts. The surgical excision may involve one or more of the following procedures: sector iridectomy, iridectomy with corneal curettage, excision plus posterior corneal lamellar resection, iridectomy plus cryotherapy, iridocyclectomy, and penetrating keratoplasty plus iridocyclectomy.[104,113]

The management of iris cysts is challenging as they may recur following more conservative treatments or surgical excision of the cyst alone. Significant intraocular inflammation can follow the release of cyst contents with conservative or surgical treatment. Surgical options have the potential to compromise the integrity of the globe. This risk increases with size of the lesion.

Juvenile xanthogranuloma (JXG)
This is a benign skin disorder that affects infants in 80-90% of the cases.[114] Ocular involvement appears in 10% of cases, sometimes before the skin lesions, and includes iris infiltrates, uveitis, hyphema, heterochromia and rarely posterior segment involvement (Fig. 3).[115]

Glaucoma is a common complication and the postulated mechanisms are: TM obstruction by histiocytic cells and red blood cells from the AC hemorrhage; PAS due to recurrent TM inflammation and neovascular glaucoma.

Prompt diagnosis of this condition is of great importance, as JXG may lead to severe eye complications, with secondary glaucoma being the most sight threatening. Glaucoma associated with iris lesions or spontaneous hyphema is strongly

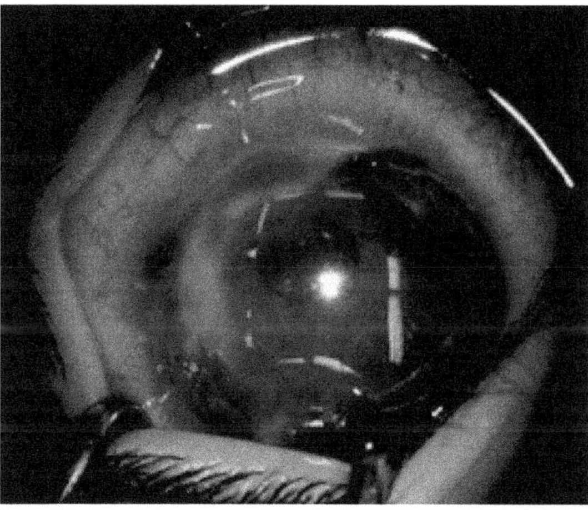

Fig. 3. Anterior segment juvenile xanthogranuloma with hyphema and buphthalmos.

suspicious of JXG.[115] To confirm the diagnosis, a thorough skin examination is important, searching for cutaneous lesions to biopsy, especially in the region of the head and neck. The absence of skin involvement at the time of eye involvement does not, however, rule out the disease,[116] since the skin lesions can regress spontaneously or appear later in the evolution of the disease process. In those cases an aqueous aspiration or iris biopsy can help to establish the diagnosis.[115,117]

Treatment
  Medical
  - Topical and/or oral hypotensive medication;
  - Steroids: topical, subconjunctival (with both short-acting steroid such as dexamethasone and a long-acting steroid such as betamethasone);[118]
  - Systemic administration.
In refractory cases, stronger medication (*i.e.*, vinblastine or methotrexate) or irradiation may be required.

  Surgery
In refractory cases, glaucoma surgery may be needed. Glaucoma drainage devices can be effective, although trabeculectomy without anti-scarring agents may be considered as a temporizing measure. The decision as to whether to proceed with a trabeculectomy or a primary glaucoma drainage device depends on the anatomy of the anterior segment. In particular how distorted the anatomy is following the recurrent hyphemas and associated inflammation.

Malignant lesions

Systemic neoplasia

The eye can be involved secondarily in some systemic neoplasia in children. One fourth of children with acute leukemia, were found to have cells or flare in anterior chamber.[119,120]

The development of the glaucoma may be due to the presence of tumor cells in the anterior segment leading to an hypopyon or due to hyphema. In rare cases choroidal infiltration produces hemorrhagic retinal detachment and acute angle closure glaucoma.[119] Glaucoma should be treated conservatively to prevent extraocular seeding.

Retinoblastoma

Glaucoma is the presenting sign of retinoblastoma (RB) in 5-7% of cases. Glaucoma has been reported as the most common clinical finding at presentation for retinoblastoma patients apart from leukocoria.[121] Ocular hypertension is documented in 17-23% of eyes,[122] and histologic signs of glaucoma in the optic nerve are found in half of cases enucleated.[123]

Mechanisms of glaucoma[122,123]
- Neovascularization of the iris (NVI), a frequent finding
- Angle closure due to a large tumor or associated retinal detachment
- Obstruction of the angle by tumor cells

A shallow AC in a child presenting with buphthalmos[124] must lead to the suspicion of a posterior segment occupying lesion, and ultrasound examination is mandatory (especially if corneal edema prevents ophthalmoscopy). Also, examination of the fundus of the fellow eye may show other tumors.

The appropriate management for RB takes priority over that for glaucoma. Generally, glaucoma is managed medically with aqueous suppressants, but once neovascular glaucoma develops, medical management usually fails and enucleation is often required. Glaucoma filtration or drainage device operations are absolutely contraindicated because of the risk of extraocular spread of viable tumor cells.

A significant association between elevated IOP and high risk histopathology has been reported.[125] In addition, the presence of raised IOP and NVI is predictive of choroidal invasion,[126] therefore enucleation is indicated in most cases.[127]

Medulloepithelioma

Medulloepithelioma is the commonest ciliary body neoplasm in childhood.[128,129] It can be benign or malignant. It occurs sporadically during the first decade as unilateral solid lobulated lesion arising from the ciliary body. Diagnosis of medulloepithelioma is usually unequivocal when a ciliary body mass presents in childhood. Masquerade signs include sectorial cataracts in children, which should raise suspicion in the absence of trauma history. Excision or local radiation with iodine plaques is the preferred treatment for small tumors and the prognosis is excellent. Enucleation is the treatment for larger tumors, a painful eye with poor visual potential, and for strong clinical suspicion of malignancy due to fast tumor growth.

Patients with medulloepithelioma often show high IOP and AC reaction, with no evidence of lesion, resulting in misdiagnosis as uveitic glaucoma or endophthalmitis.[130] Neovascular glaucoma can also be the presenting sign of this condition.

Because of the rarity of the tumor, there is lack of large series of patients with this condition and it is difficult to draw strong evidence about the best treatment for these patients. However, glaucoma drainage device and filtering surgery should be avoided in patients with malignant tumors such as medulloepithelioma, as they increase the risk of tumor seeding.

Uveal melanoma

Uveal melanoma can develop within the iris, ciliary body, choroid or in a combination of these. It occurs rarely in the pediatric age group.[131] Although anterior uveal melanoma affecting the iris or ciliary body is less common than choroidal melanoma, (5-8%)[132] due to the close anatomical relationship with the TM, it is more commonly associated with elevated intraocular pressure (IOP).[133]

Iris melanoma represents approximately 4% of all uveal melanomas both in children and in adults.[134] Acquired secondary glaucoma has been found in 14 to 30% of eyes with iris melanoma.[122,133-137]

Treatment of iris melanoma depends on tumor size, tumor seeding, intraocular pressure and age of patients. Local resection can be used in young patients with small sized tumors and no sign of tumor seeding. Plaque radiotherapy is preferred in older patients with large tumor size and increased tumor seeding, whereas primary enucleation is advised for patients showing larger size, extensive tumor seeding and advanced secondary glaucoma.[138]

The prevalence of secondary glaucoma increases with patient age. Secondary glaucoma was found in 17% of patients younger than 20 years, in 25% of patients aged 21 to 60 years and in 38% of patients older than 60 years.[134] Iris melanoma causes glaucoma by a number of means including TM infiltration with neoplastic cells leading to outflow obstruction. In a recent published case series of 144 patients with iris melanoma Shields found that 40% of patients at diagnosis were affected by glaucoma secondary to the tumor. Mechanisms of glaucoma development were: angle infiltration by the tumor (86%), angle neovascularization (7%) and glaucoma secondary to hyphema (7%).[138]

Patients treated with radiotherapy may experience ocular hypertension in the immediate follow-up period due to a direct effect of the radiotherapy on the iridocorneal angle, resulting in trabecular meshwork inflammation and scarring. Irradiation therapy results in very low tumor recurrence rate.[139] Treatment approaches for secondary glaucoma associated with iris melanoma include IOP lowering medications, surgery and ciliary body ablation.[140] The role of surgery has been restricted in these patients as glaucoma surgery has traditionally been considered high risk for tumor seeding. Recently Sharkawi *et al.* showed that Baerveldt implants were able to control IOP in 86% of patients with anterior uveal melanoma and uncontrolled IOP following anterior segment proton beam irradiation.[141] Tumor recurrence and metastases were not observed during the short 12-month study follow-up period. Although studies (largely in adults) exist to suggest no or minimal risk of tumor seeding with incisional glaucoma surgery, the risk cannot be ruled out and should be considered significant in the child's lifetime. Until we have studies with longer follow-up and larger sample size showing that systemic metastatic rates of shunted eyes is comparable with non-shunted eyes, drainage glaucoma surgery for malignant ocular lesions should be avoided in children.

Retinopathy of prematurity (ROP)

Definition

ROP-induced glaucoma occurs in an eye with a history of retinopathy of prematurity and anatomic changes due to the ROP or treatment for ROP. Visual field defects in ROP may be difficult to assess or detect due to: structural changes resulting from ROP (*e.g.*, optic nerve distortion due to tractional changes, corneal opacities); low vision, or neurologic sequelae of prematurity confounding visual field interpretation.

Background

ROP is a disease of the retinal vasculature found in infants born prematurely, which in severe cases results in retinal detachment, sometimes despite treatment with cryotherapy or laser photocoagulation. Use of intravitreal anti-vascular endothelial growth factor medications for severe ROP also shows promise.[142] While current management of prematurity and ROP has significantly reduced the rate of unfavorable outcomes in developed countries, individuals born in emerging countries and adult patients with history of premature birth may experience significant ocular complications, including glaucoma.

The Cryotherapy for Retinopathy of Prematurity randomized trial, in which eyes of infants < 1251 g at birth with threshold ROP were randomized to cryotherapy or observation, 5% of treated eyes and 10% of untreated eyes were diagnosed with glaucoma by ten years of age.[143] In the Early Treatment for Retinopathy of Prematurity randomized trial, in which eyes of infants < 1251 g at birth with high-risk pre-threshold ROP were randomized to treatment or observation until threshold ROP developed, six-year outcomes showed that nearly 2% of eyes had developed glaucoma. Of these, about half had shallow anterior chambers and only one eye had measurable vision.[144]

Diagnosis of angle closure glaucoma in neonate with ROP

Angle-closure glaucoma in ROP can occur due to a number or reasons and the diagnosis should be suspected with the occurrence of the following clinical findings: corneal edema, enlarged corneal diameter, severe shallowing of the anterior chamber and abnormally elevated IOP.

Mechanisms and pathophysiology of glaucoma

There are three stages or time points when glaucoma or ocular hypertension is likely to occur. Each is associated with its own underlying mechanisms. The time points include:

1. Associated with laser retinal photocoagulation;
2. Associated with treatment for stage 4 and 5 ROP;
3. Associated with untreated stage 4 or 5.

Early related to laser treatment for threshold ROP

Shallow anterior chambers in ROP patients are known to be caused by various factors for example, choroidal detachment after excessive photocoagulation, development of retrolental mass, or relative increment in lens thickness. But the cause of a shallow anterior chamber may not be determined.[145] In ROP patients, the lens and its ligaments are elastic, and therefore secondary angle-closure glaucoma from lens displacement may occur.

It is important that ophthalmologists be aware of the possible development of angle closure glaucoma following retinal photocoagulation for ROP. Several explanations may account for the development of angle-closure following laser photocoagulation treatment for ROP.

- Thermal injury to the choroidal vasculature may possibly result in vascular occlusion with choroidal congestion and subsequent anterior displacement of the lens-iris diaphragm.[146]
- Ciliary body edema may contribute to anterior displacement of the lens-iris diaphragm.
- Hyphema (more common in cases with prominent tunica vasculosa lentis), with blockage of trabecular meshwork and transient disruption in aqueous outflow or formation of synechiae and pupillary block.[145]
- Potentially, lenticular changes resulting in increased size of the lens could cause or exacerbate angle closure (phacomorphic glaucoma).
- Leakage of lens material may induce intraocular inflammation and phacolytic glaucoma.

These mechanisms can all result in narrowing of the angle with the potential for secondary angle closure and peripheral anterior synechiae formation. Additionally, intraocular inflammation may promote the formation of both anterior and posterior synechiae and exacerbate acute angle-closure glaucoma following laser treatment for ROP.[147] Ultrasound biomicroscopy may be useful to help determine the cause of the elevation in IOP/glaucoma.[145,148]

Associated with treatments for stage 4 and 5 ROP
This group relates to those individuals in whom there is progressive posterior-type ROP that is refractory to laser treatment and rapidly progresses to tractional retinal detachment with extensive fibrovascular proliferation.[146,149]

Glaucoma is a common complication following surgery for stage 4/5 ROP, which may be delayed in onset. IOP elevation after vitrectomy for may occur in up to 22%, and is associated with the findings of a poor visual outcome,[150] a young gestational age and aphakic status.[151] Additionally, glaucoma may occur after scleral buckling procedures for ROP.[152]

Late effects of ROP
Secondary angle-closure glaucoma with or without pupillary block has previously been recognized as a late complication of ROP.[147,148,153,154] In addition to an angle-closure mechanism, it has been suggested that abnormal angle structures or an arrest in angle development in this population may result in decreased outflow facility and glaucoma.[155]

Other mechanisms of glaucoma in ROP
Another described mechanism of angle closure in ROP is: relative anterior microphthalmos in the presence of myopia (relative anterior microphthalmos occurs secondary to structural consequences of ROP and its treatment).[156] Myopia in ROP is often associated with increased lens thickness and power with lesser contributions from corneal steepness, axial length and anterior displacement of the lens center.[157,158]

Glaucoma may develop years or decades later, so that long-term surveillance for patients with history of ROP and prematurity is warranted.[159] Neovascular glaucoma may also complicate ROP in the setting of traction retinal detachment that has been incompletely resolved, as can glaucoma in aphakia after retinal surgery that has removed the lens in infancy for ROP-related retinal detachment repair.

Management

Medical therapy and surgery in the form of peripheral iridectomy for pupillary block form the mainstay of treatment. Angle surgery may have a role following lens-sparing vitrectomy-related open angle glaucoma. The role of lensectomy in glaucoma management depends on the suspected etiology. Glaucoma drainage devices or ciliary body ablation may be considered for cases of chronic angle closure that have failed medical or primary procedures.

References

1. Chebil A, Chaabani L, Kort F, et al. [Epidemiologic study of pediatric uveitis: a series of 49 cases]. J Fr Ophtalmol 2012; 35: 30-34.
2. Edelsten C, Reddy M, Stanford M, et al. Visual loss associated with pediatric uveitis in English primary and referral centers. Am J Ophthalmol 2003; 135: 676-680.
3. Kim SJ. Diagnosis and management of noninfectious pediatric uveitis. Int Ophthalmol Clin 2011; 51: 129-145.
4. BenEzra D, Cohen E, Maftzir G. Patterns of intraocular inflammation in children. Bull Soc Belge Ophthalmol 2001; 279: 35-38.
5. Kanski J, Shun-Shin G. Systemic uveitis syndromes in childhood: an analysis of 340 cases. Ophthalmology 1984; 91: 1247-1252.
6. Azar D, Martin F. Paediatric uveitis: a Sydney clinic experience. Clin Experiment Ophthalmol 2004; 32: 468-471.
7. Holland GN, Stiehm ER. Special considerations in the evaluation and management of uveitis in children. Am J Ophthalmol 2003; 135: 867-878.
8. Tugal-Tutkun I, Havrlikova K, Power WJ, Foster CS. Changing patterns in uveitis of childhood. Ophthalmology 1996; 103: 375-383.
9. Heinz C, Mingels A, Goebel C, et al. Chronic uveitis in children with and without juvenile idiopathic arthritis: differences in patient characteristics and clinical course. J Rheumatol 2008; 35: 1403-1407.
10. Krupin T, Feitl M, Karalekas D. Glaucoma associated uveitis. In: Ritch R, Shields M, Krupin T (Eds.), The Glaucomas. Second ed. St Louis: Mosby 1996, pp. 1225-1258.
11. Espinosa M, Gottlieb BS. Juvenile idiopathic arthritis. Pediatrics in Review 2012; 33: 303-313.
12. American Academy of Pediatrics Section on Rheumatology and Section on Ophthalmology: Guidelines for ophthalmologic examinations in children with juvenile rheumatoid arthritis. Pediatrics in Review 1993; 92: 295-296.
13. Kotaniemi K, Savolainen A, Aho K. Severe childhood uveitis without overt arthritis. Clin Exp Rheumatol 2003; 21: 395-398.
14. Jabs D, Nussenblatt R, Rosenbaum J. Standardization of Uveitis Nomenclature (SUN) Working Group. Standardization of uveitis nomenclature for reporting clinical data. Results of the First International Workshop. Am J Ophthalmol 2005; 140: 509-516.
15. Thorne J, Woreta F, Kedhar S, et al. Juvenile idiopathic arthritis-associated uveitis: incidence of ocular complications and visual acuity loss. Am J Ophthalmol 2007; 143: 840-846.
16. Tappeiner C, Heinz C, Roesel M, Heiligenhaus A. Elevated laser flare values correlate with complicated course of anterior uveitis in patients with juvenile idiopathic arthritis. Acta Ophthalmol (Oxf) 2011; 89: e521-527.
17. Ravelli A, Martini A. Juvenile idiopathic arthritis. Lancet 2007; 369: 767-778.
18. Petty R, Southwood T, Manners P, et al. International League of Associations for Rheumatology classification of juvenile idiopathic arthritis: second revision, Edmonton, 2001. J Rheumatol 2004; 31: 390-392.
19. Daniel E, Pistilli M, Pujari SS, et al. Risk of hypotony in noninfectious uveitis. Ophthalmology 2012; 119: 2377-2385.
20. Key Sr, Kimura S. Iridocyclitis associated with juvenile rheumatoid arthritis. Am J Ophthalmol 1975; 80: 425-429.
21. Lovell D. Update on treatment of arthritis in children: new treatments, new goals. Bull NYU Hosp Jt Dis 2006; 64: 72-76.

22. van der Horst-Bruinsma I, Nurmohamed M. Management and evaluation of extra-articular manifestations in spondyloarthritis. Ther Adv Musculoskelet Dis 2012; 4: 413-422.

23. Kemper A, Van Mater H, Coeytaux R, et al. Systematic review of disease-modifying anti-rheumatic drugs for juvenile idiopathic arthritis. BMC Pediatr 2012; 12: 29.

24. Kemper A, Coeytaux R, Sanders G, et al. Disease-Modifying Antirheumatic Drugs (DMARDs) in Children With Juvenile Idiopathic Arthritis (JIA). [Internet]2011 September Contract No.: 11-EHC039-EF.

25. Cantarini L, Simonini G, Frediani B, et al. Treatment strategies for childhood noninfectious chronic uveitis: an update. Expert Opin Investig Drugs 2012; 21: 1-6.

26. Habot-Wilner Z, Sallam A, Roufas A, et al. Periocular corticosteroid injection in the management of uveitis in children. Acta Ophthalmol (Oxf) 2010; 88: e299-304.

27. Sallam A, Comer RM, Chang JH, et al. Short-term safety and efficacy of intravitreal triamcinolone acetonide for uveitic macular edema in children. Arch Ophthalmol 2008; 126: 200-205.

28. Ungar W, Costa V, Burnett H, et al. The use of biologic response modifiers in polyarticular-course juvenile idiopathic arthritis: A systematic review. Semin Arthritis Rheum 2013; 42: 597-618.

29. Horneff G. Update on biologicals for treatment of juvenile idiopathic arthritis. Expert Opin Biol Ther 2013; 13: 361-376.

30. DeWitt E, Kimura Y, Beukelman T, et al. Consensus treatment plans for new-onset systemic juvenile idiopathic arthritis. Arthritis Care Res (Hoboken) 2012; 64: 1001-1010.

31. Fishman P, Bar-Yehuda S, Liang B, Jacobson K. Pharmacological and therapeutic effects of A3 adenosine receptor agonists. Drug Discov Today 2012; 17: 359-366.

32. Klisovic DD. Mycophenolate mofetil use in the treatment of noninfectious uveitis. Dev Ophthalmol 2012; 51: 57-62.

33. Foster CS, Havrlikova K, Baltatzis S, et al. Secondary glaucoma in patients with juvenile rheumatoid arthritis-associated iridocyclitis. Acta Ophthalmol Scand 2000; 78: 576-579.

34. Heinz C, Pleyer U, Ruokonnen P, Heiligenhaus A. Secondary glaucoma in childhood uveitis. Ophthalmologe 2008; 105: 438-444.

35. Chang J, McCluskey P, Missotten T, et al. Use of ocular hypotensive prostaglandin analogues in patients with uveitis: does their use increase anterior uveitis and cystoid macular oedema? Br J Ophthalmol 2008; 92: 916-912.

36. Ho CL, Walton DS. Goniosurgery for glaucoma secondary to chronic anterior uveitis: prognostic factors and surgical technique. J Glaucoma 2004; 13: 445-449.

37. Bohnsack BL, Freedman SF. Surgical outcomes in childhood uveitic glaucoma. Am J Ophthalmol 2013; 155: 134-142.

38. Lam LA, Lowder CY, Baerveldt G, et al. Surgical management of cataracts in children with juvenile rheumatoid arthritis-associated uveitis. Am J Ophthalmol 2003; 135: 772-778.

39. Heinz C, Koch J, Heiligenhaus A. Trabeculectomy or modified deep sclerectomy in juvenile uveitic glaucoma. J Ophthalmic Inflamm Infect 2011; 1: 165-170.

40. Välimäki J, Airaksinen P, Tuulonen A. Molteno implantation for secondary glaucoma in juvenile rheumatoid arthritis. Arch Ophthalmol 1997; 115: 1253-1256.

41. Kafkala C, Hynes A, Choi J, et al. Ahmed valve implantation for uncontrolled pediatric uveitic glaucoma. J AAPOS [Comparative Study] 2005; 9: 336-340.

42. Heinz C, Koch J, Heiligenhaus A. Transscleral diode laser cyclophotocoagulation as primary surgical treatment for secondary glaucoma in juvenile idiopathic arthritis: high failure rate after short term follow up. Br J Ophthalmol 2006; 90: 737-740.

43. Angeles-Han S, Yeh S. Prevention and management of cataracts in children with juvenile idiopathic arthritis-associated uveitis. Curr Rheumatol Rep 2012; 14: 142-149.

44. Cleary CA, Lanigan B, O'Keeffe M. Intracameral triamcinolone acetonide after pediatric cataract surgery. J Cataract Refract Surg 2010; 36: 1676-1681.

45. Sijssens KM, Los LI, Rothova A, et al. Long-term ocular complications in aphakic versus pseudophakic eyes of children with juvenile idiopathic arthritis-associated uveitis. Br J Ophthalmol 2010; 94: 1145-1149.

46. Terrada C, Julian K, Cassoux N, et al. Cataract surgery with primary intraocular lens implantation in children with uveitis: long-term outcomes. J Cataract Refract Surg 2011; 37: 1977-1983.
47. Sukhija J, Ram J. Anti-inflammatory effect of low-molecular-weight heparin in pediatric cataract surgery. Am J Ophthalmol 2012; 154: 1003-1004.
48. Rumelt S, Stolovich C, Segal ZI, Rehany U. Intraoperative enoxaparin minimizes inflammatory reaction after pediatric cataract surgery. Am J Ophthalmol 2006; 141: 433-437.
49. Wilson ME, Jr., Trivedi RH. Low molecular-weight heparin in the intraocular irrigating solution in pediatric cataract and intraocular lens surgery. Am J Ophthalmol 2006; 141: 537-538.
50. Blanton F. Anterior angle recession and secondary glaucoma: a study of the aftereffects of traumatic hyphemas. Arch Ophthalmol 1964; 72: 39-44.
51. De Leon-Ortega JE, Girkin CA. Ocular trauma-related glaucoma. Ophthalmol Clin North Am 2002; 15: 215-223.
52. Agapitos P, Noel L, Clarke W. Traumatic hyphema in children. Ophthalmology 1987; 94: 1238-1241.
53. Kennedy R, Brubaker R. Traumatic hyphema in a defined population. Am J Ophthalmol 1988; 106: 123-130.
54. Wilson F. Traumatic hyphema. Pathogenesis and management. Ophthalmology 1980; 87: 910-919.
55. Read J, Goldberg M. Comparison of medical treatment for traumatic hyphema. Trans Am Acad Ophthalmol Otolaryngol 1974; 78: 799-815.
56. Kutner B, Fourman S, Brein K, et al. Aminocaproic acid reduces the risk of secondary hemorrhage in patients with traumatic hyphema. Arch Ophthalmol 1987; 105: 206-208.
57. Bender M, Hobbs W. Sickle Cell Disease. Seattle (WA): University of Washington, Seattle 2013 [28th July 2013]; Available from: http://www.ncbi.nlm.nih.gov/books/NBK1377/.
58. Goldberg M. Sickled erythrocytes, hyphema, and secondary glaucoma: I. The diagnosis and treatment of sickled erythrocytes in human hyphemas. Ophthalmic Surg Lasers 1979; 10: 17-31.
59. Hooper CY, Fraser-Bell S, Farinelli A, Grigg JR. Complicated hyphaema: think sickle. Clin Experiment Ophthalmol 2006; 34: 377-378.
60. Salmon J, Mermoud A, Ivey A, et al. The detection of post-traumatic angle recession by gonioscopy in a population-based glaucoma survey. Ophthalmology 1994; 101: 1844-1850.
61. Montenegro M, Simmons R. Ghost cell glaucoma. Int Ophthalmol Clin 1995; 35: 111-115.
62. Spirn M, Lynn M, Hubbard Gr. Vitreous hemorrhage in children. Ophthalmology 2006; 113: 848-852.
63. Sihota R, Kumar S, Gupta V, et al. Early predictors of traumatic glaucoma after closed globe injury: trabecular pigmentation, widened angle recess, and higher baseline intraocular pressure. Arch Ophthalmol 2008; 126: 921-926.
64. Ashaye A. Traumatic hyphaema: a report of 472 consecutive cases. BMC Ophthalmol 2008; 8: 24.
65. Rocha K, Martins E, Melo LJ, Moraes N. Outpatient management of traumatic hyphema in children: prospective evalution. J AAPOS 2004; 8: 357-361.
66. Walton W, Von Hagen S, Grigorian R, Zarbin M. Management of traumatic hyphema. Surv Ophthalmol 2002; 47: 297-334.
67. Albiani D, Hodge W, Pan Y, et al. Tranexamic acid in the treatment of pediatric traumatic hyphema. Can J Ophthalmol 2008; 43: 428-431.
68. Ozer PA, Yalvac IS, Satana B, et al. Incidence and risk factors in secondary glaucomas after blunt and penetrating ocular trauma. J Glaucoma 2007; 16: 685-690.
69. Baig M, Ahmed J, Ali M. Role of trabeculectomy in the management of hypertensive traumatic total hyphaema. J Coll Physicians Surg Pak 2009; 19: 496-499.
70. Pandey P, Sung VCT. Gonioaspiration for refractory glaucoma secondary to traumatic hyphema in patients with sickle cell trait. Ophthalmic Surg Lasers Imaging 2010; 41: 386-389.

71. Jones RI, Rhee D. Corticosteroid-induced ocular hypertension and glaucoma: A brief review and update of the literature. Curr Op Ophthalmol 2006; 17: 163-167.
72. McLean J. Use of ACTH and cortisone. Trans Am Ophthalmol Soc 1950; 48: 293-296.
73. Armaly M. Statistical attributes of the steroid hypertensive response in the clinically normal eye. Invest Ophthalmol Vis Sci 1965; 4: 187-197.
74. Becker B. Intraocular pressure response to topical corticosteroids. Invest Ophthalmol Vis Sci 1965; 4: 198-205.
75. Schwartz B. The response of ocular pressure to corticosteroids. Int Ophthalmol Clin 1966; 6: 929-989.
76. Lam D, Fan D, Ng J, et al. Ocular hypertensive and anti-inflammatory responses to different dosages of topical dexamethasone in children: a randomized trial. Clin Exper Ophthalmol 2005; 33: 252-258.
77. Sijssens KM, Rothova A, Berendschot TT, de Boer JH. Ocular hypertension and secondary glaucoma in children with uveitis. Ophthalmology 2006; 113: 853-859.e2.
78. Patel CC, Mandava N, Oliver SCN, et al. Treatment of intractable posterior uveitis in pediatric patients with the fluocinolone acetonide intravitreal implant (Retisert). Retina 2012; 32: 537-542.
79. Hayasaka Y, Hayasaka S, Matsukura H. Ocular findings in Japanese children with nephrotic syndrome receiving prolonged corticosteroid therapy. Ophthalmologica 2006; 220: 181-185.
80. Behbehani AH, Owayed AF, Hijazi ZM, et al. Cataract and ocular hypertension in children on inhaled corticosteroid therapy. J Pediatr Ophthalmol Strabismus 2005; 42: 23-27.
81. Ozkaya E, Ozsutcu M, Mete F. Lack of ocular side effects after 2 years of topical steroids for allergic rhinitis. J Pediatr Ophthalmol Strabismus 2011; 48: 311-317.
82. Fan D, Ng J, Lam D. A prospective study on ocular hypertensive and anti-inflammatory response to different dosages of fluorometholone in children. Ophthalmology 2001; 108: 1973-1977.
83. Hutcheson KA. Steroid-induced glaucoma in an infant. J AAPOS 2007; 11: 522-523.
84. Salim S. What's your diagnosis? Steroid-induced glaucoma. J Pediatr Ophthalmol Strabismus 2006; 43: 270-284.
85. Kawamura R, Inoue M, Shinoda H, Shinoda K, et al. Incidence of increased intraocular pressure after subtenon injection of triamcinolone acetonide. J Ocul Pharmacol Ther 2011; 27: 299-304.
86. Romano P. Fluorinated ocular/periocular corticosteroids have caused death as well as glaucoma in children. Clin Exp Ophthalmol 2003; 31: 279-280.
87. Bollinger KE, Smith SD. Prevalence and management of elevated intraocular pressure after placement of an intravitreal sustained-release steroid implant. Curr Opin Ophthalmol 2009; 20: 99-103.
88. Yamashita T, Kodama Y, Tanaka M, et al. Steroid-induced glaucoma in children with acute lymphoblastic leukemia: a possible complication. J Glaucoma 2010; 19: 188-190.
89. Brito P, Silva S, Cotta J, Falcão-Reis F. Severe ocular hypertension secondary to systemic corticosteroid treatment in a child with nephrotic syndrome. Clinical Ophthalmology 2012; 6: 1675-1679.
90. Tham C, Ng J, Li R, et al. Intraocular pressure profile of a child on a systemic corticosteroid. Am J Ophthalmol 2004; 137: 198-201.
91. Desnoeck M, Casteels I, Casteels K. Intraocular pressure elevation in a child due to the use of inhalation steroids--a case report. Bull Soc Belge Ophtalmol 2001; 280: 97-100.
92. Mataftsi A, Narang A, Moore W, Nischal KK. Do reducing regimens of fluorometholone for paediatric ocular surface disease cause glaucoma? Br J Ophthalmol 2011; 95: 1531-1533.
93. Ng J, Fan D, Young A, et al. Ocular hypertensive response to topical dexamethasone in children: a dose-dependent phenomenon. Ophthalmology 2000; 107: 2097-2100.
94. Lee Y, Park C, Woo K. Ocular hypertensive response to topical dexamethasone ointment in children. Korean J Ophthalmol 2006; 20: 166-170.

95. Tripathi R, Kirschner B, Kipp M, et al. Corticosteroid treatment for inflammatory bowel disease in pediatric patients increases intraocular pressure. Gastroenterology 1992; 102: 1957-1961.

96. Tripathi RC, Kipp MA, Tripathi BJ et al. Ocular toxicity of prednisone in pediatric patients with inflammatory bowel disease. Lens Eye Toxic Res 1992; 9: 469-482.

97. Park J, Gole G. Corticosteroid-induced glaucoma in a child after a scleral reinforcement procedure. Clin Experiment Ophthalmol 2002; 30: 372-374.

98. Thomas R, Jay JL. Raised intraocular pressure with topical steroids after trabeculectomy. Graefes Arch Clin Exp Ophthalmol 1988; 226: 337-340.

99. Rao A, Gupta V, Bhadange Y, et al. Iris cysts: a review. Semin 2011; 26: 11-22.

100. Shields J, Shields C, Lois N, Mercado G. Iris cysts in children: classification, incidence, and management. The 1998 Torrence A Makley Jr Lecture. Br J Ophthalmol 1999; 83: 334-338.

101. Shields JA, Kline MW, Augsburger JJ. Primary iris cysts: a review of the literature and report of 62 cases. Br J Ophthalmol 1984; 68: 152-166.

102. Wong RK, Salchow DJ. Iris cyst after iris-sutured intraocular lens implantation in a child. J AAPOS 2012; 16: 199-200.

103. Lois N, Shields CL, Shields JA, Mercado G. Primary cysts of the iris pigment epithelium. Clinical features and natural course in 234 patients. Ophthalmology 1998; 105: 1879-1885.

104. Conway R, Chew T, Golchet P, et al. Ultrasound biomicroscopy: role in diagnosis and management in 130 consecutive patients evaluated for anterior segment tumours. Br J Ophthalmol 2005; 89: 950-955.

105. Shen CC, Netland PA, Wilson MW, Morris WR. Management of congenital nonpigmented iris cyst. Ophthalmology 2006; 113: 1639.e1-7.

106. Bruner W, Michels R, Stark W, Maumenee A. Management of epithelial cysts of the anterior chamber. Ophthalmic Surg 1981; 12: 279-285.

107. Badlani VK, Quinones R, Wilensky JT, et al. Angle-closure glaucoma in teenagers. J Glaucoma 2003; 12: 198-203.

108. Ritch R, Chang BM, Liebmann JM. Angle closure in younger patients. Ophthalmology 2003; 110: 1880-18889.

109. Cleasby G. Photocoagulation of iris-ciliary body epithelial cysts. Trans Am Acad Ophthalmol Otolaryngol 1971; 75: 638-642.

110. Honrubia F, Brito C, Grijalbo M. Photocoagulation of iris cyst. Trans Ophthalmol Soc U K 1982; 102: 184-186.

111. Xiao Y, Wang Y, Niu G, Li K. Transpupillary argon laser photocoagulation and Nd:YAG laser cystotomy for peripheral iris pigment epithelium cyst. Am J Ophthalmol 2006; 142: 691-693.

112. Kuchenbecker J, Motschmann M, Schmitz K, Behrens-Baumann W. Laser iridocystotomy for bilateral acute angle-closure glaucoma secondary to iris cysts. Am J Ophthalmol 2000; 129: 391-393.

113. Naumann G, Rummelt V. Block excision of cystic and diffuse epithelial ingrowth of the anterior chamber. Report on 32 consecutive patients. Arch Ophthalmol 1992; 110: 223-227.

114. Chang MW, Frieden IJ, Good W. The risk intraocular juvenile xanthogranuloma: survey of current practices and assessment of risk. J Am Acad Dermatol 1996; 34: 445-449.

115. Vendal Z, Walton D, Chen T. Glaucoma in juvenile xanthogranuloma. Semin 2006; 21: 191-194.

116. Liang S, Liu Y-H, Fang K. Juvenile xanthogranuloma with ocular involvement. Pediatr Dermatol 2009; 26: 232-234.

117. Zimmerman L. Juvenile Xanthogranuloma. Trans Am Acad Ophthalmol Otolaryngol 1965; 69: 412.

118. Casteels I, Olver J, Malone M, Taylor D. Early treatment of juvenile xanthogranuloma of the iris with subconjunctival steroids. Br J Ophthalmol [Case Reports] 1993; 77: 57-60.

119. Abramson A. Anterior chamber activity in children with acute leukemia. Ann Ophthalmol 1980; 12: 553.

120. Santoni G, Fiore C, Lupidi G, Bibbiani U. Recurring bilateral hypopyon in chronic myeloid leukemia in blastic transformation. Graefe's Arch Clin Exp Ophthalmol 1985; 223: 211-213.
121. Kashyap S, Meel R, Pushker N, et al. Clinical predictors of high risk histopathology in retinoblastoma. Pediatr Blood Cancer 2012; 58: 356-361.
122. Shields CL, Shields JA, Shields MB, Augsburger JJ. Prevalence and mechanisms of secondary intraocular pressure elevation in eyes with intraocular tumors. Ophthalmology 1987; 94: 839-846.
123. Yoshizumi MO, Thomas JV, Smith TR. Glaucoma-inducing mechanisms in eyes with retinoblastoma. Arch Ophthalmol 1978; 96: 105-110.
124. de Leon JMS, Walton DS, Latina MA, Mercado GV. Glaucoma in retinoblastoma. Semin 2005; 20: 217-222.
125. Chantada G, Gonzalez A, Fandino A, et al. Some clinical findings at presentation can predict highrisk pathology features in unilateral retinoblastoma. J Pediatr Hematol Oncol 2009; 31: 325-329.
126. Shields C, Shields J, Baez K, et al. Choroidal invasion of retinoblastoma: Metastatic potential andclinical risk factors. Br J Ophthalmol 1993; 77: 544-548.
127. Ellsworth R. The practical management of Retinoblastoma. Trans Am Ophthalmol 1969; 67: 462.
128. Shields JA, Eagle RC, Jr., Shields CL, Potter PD. Congenital neoplasms of the nonpigmented ciliary epithelium (medulloepithelioma). Ophthalmology 1996; 103: 1998-2006.
129. Broughton L, Zimmerman L. A clinicopathologic study of intraocular medulloepitheliomas. Am J Ophthalmol 1978; 85: 407-418.
130. Chua J, Muen W, Reddy A, Brookes J. The Masquerades of a Childhood Ciliary Body Medulloepithelioma: A Case of Chronic Uveitis, Cataract, and Secondary Glaucoma. Case Rep Ophthalmol Med 2012; Article ID 493493.
131. Kanthan GL, Grigg J, Billson F, et al. Paediatric uveal melanoma. Clin Experiment Ophthalmol 2008; 36: 374-376.
132. Wanner J, Pasquale L. Glaucomas secondary to intraocular melanomas. Semin Ophthalmol 2006; 21: 181-189.
133. Shields C, Materin M, Shields J, et al. Factors associated with elevated intraocular pressure in eyes with iris melanoma. Br J Ophthalmol 2001; 85: 666 -669.
134. Shields C, Kaliki S, Furuta M, et al. Iris melanoma features and prognosis in children and adults in 317 patients. J Am Assoc Pediatr Ophthalmol Strabismus 2012; 16: 10-16.
135. Shields C, Shields J, Materin M, et al. Iris melanoma: risk factors for metastasis in 169 consecutive patients. Ophthalmology 2001; 108: 172-178.
136. Khan S, Finger P, Yu B, et al. Clinical and pathologic characteristics of biopsy-proven iris melanoma. Arch Ophthalmol 2012; 130: 57-64.
137. Fernandes B, Krema H, Fulda E, et al. Management of iris melanomas with 125 Iodine plaque radiotherapy. Am J Ophthalmol 2010; 149: 70-76.
138. Shields C, Shah S, Bianciotto C, et al. Iris Melanoma Management with Iodine-125 Plaque Radiotherapy in 144 Patients: Impact of Melanoma-Related Glaucoma on Outcomes. Ophthalmology 2013; 120: 55-61.
139. Egger E, Zografos L, Schalenbourg A, et al. Eye retention after proton beam radiotherapy for uveal melanoma. Int J Radiat Oncol Biol Phys 2003; 55: 867-880.
140. Zhao H-S, Wei W-B. Dilemma in management of ocular medulloepithelioma in a child. Chin Med J 2012; 125: 392-395.
141. Sharkawi E, Oleszczuk J, Bergin C, Zografos L. Baerveldt shunts in the treatment of glaucoma secondary to anterior uveal melanoma and proton beam radiotherapy. Br J Ophthalmol 2012; 96: 1104-1107.
142. Mintz-Hittner H, Kennedy KA, Chuang A, for the BEAT-ROP Cooperative Group. Efficacy of Intravitreal Bevacizumab for Stage 3+ Retinopathy of Prematurity. N Engl J Med 2011; 364: 603-615.

143. Cryotherapy for Retinopathy of Prematurity Cooperative Group. Multicenter Trial of Cryotherapy for Retinopathy of Prematurity: ophthalmological outcomes at 10 years. Arch Ophthalmol 2001; 119: 1110-1118.

144. Bremer D, Rogers D, Good W, et al. Glaucoma in the Early Treatment for Retinopathy of Prematurity (ETROP) study. J AAPOS 2012; 16: 449-452.

145. Uehara A, Kurokawa T, Gotoh N, et al. Angle closure glaucoma after laser photocoagulation for retinopathy of prematurity. Br J Ophthalmol 2004; 88: 1099-1100.

146. Mensher J. Anterior chamber depth alteration after retinal photocoagulation. Arch Ophthalmol 1977; 95: 113-116.

147. Trigler L, Weaver RG, Jr., O'Neil JW, et al. Case series of angle-closure glaucoma after laser treatment for retinopathy of prematurity. J AAPOS 2005; 9: 17-21.

148. Pollard ZF. Secondary angle-closure glaucoma in cicatricial retrolental fibroplasia. Am J Ophthalmol 1980; 89: 651-653.

149. Choi J, Kim JH, Kim S-J, Yu YS. Long-term results of lens-sparing vitrectomy for progressive posterior-type stage 4A retinopathy of prematurity. Korean J Ophthalmol 2012; 26: 277-284.

150. Knight-Nanan DM, Algawi K, Bowell R, O'Keefe M. Advanced cicatricial retinopathy of prematurity – outcome and complications. Br J Ophthalmol 1996; 80: 343-345.

151. Iwahashi-Shima C, Miki A, Hamasaki T, et al. Intraocular pressure elevation is a delayed-onset complication after successful vitrectomy for stages 4 and 5 retinopathy of prematurity. Retina 2012; 32: 1636-1642.

152. Halperin LS, Schoch LH. Angle closure glaucoma after scleral buckling for retinopathy of prematurity. Case report. Arch Ophthalmol 1988; 106: 453.

153. Michael AJ, Pesin SR, Katz LJ, Tasman WS. Management of late-onset angle-closure glaucoma associated with retinopathy of prematurity. Ophthalmology 1991; 98: 1093-1098.

154. Faure C, Caputo G, Sahel JA, Paques M. [Retinopathy of prematurity complicated by late glaucoma: a case report]. J Fr Ophtalmol 2008; 31: 535.e1-3.

155. Hartnett ME, Gilbert MM, Richardson TM, et al. Anterior segment evaluation of infants with retinopathy of prematurity. Ophthalmology 1990; 97: 122-130.

156. Ziemssen F, Adam H, Bartz-Schmidt K, Schlote T. Angle closure glaucoma in association with relative anterior microphthalmos (RAM) after premature birth retinopathy (ROP). Klin Monatsbl Augenheilkd 2004; 221: 503-508.

157. Garcia-Valenzuela E, Kaufman L. High myopia associated with retinopathy of prematurity is primarily lenticular. J AAPOS 2005; 9: 121-128.

158. Jayaprakasam A, Martin KR, White AJR. Phacomorphic intermittent angle closure in a patient with retinopathy of prematurity and lenticular high myopia. Clin Experiment Ophthalmol 2012; 40: 646-647.

159. Smith J, Shivitz I. Angle-closure glaucoma in adults with cicatricial retinopathy of prematurity. Arch Ophthalmol 1984; 102: 371-372.

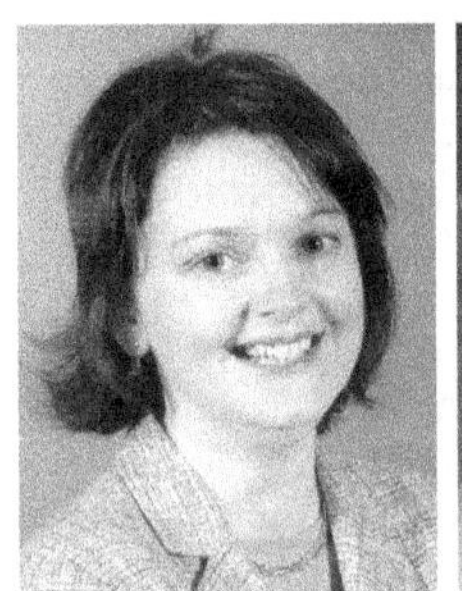

Cecelia Fenerty

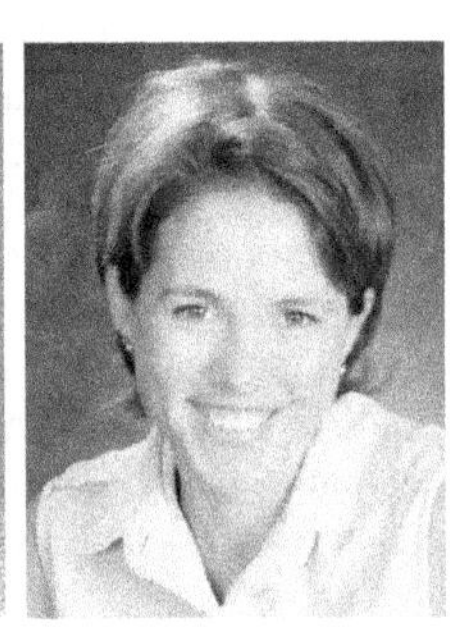

Nicola Freeman

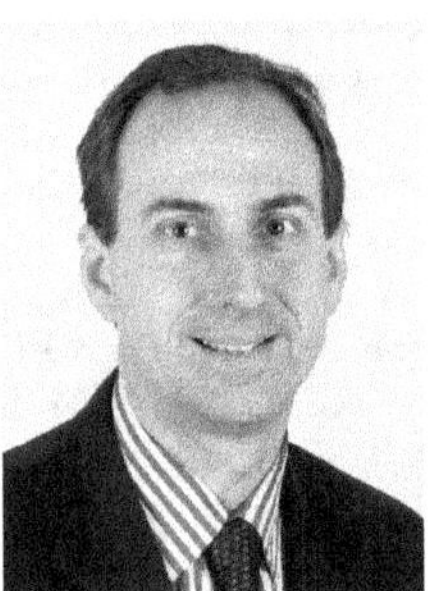

John Grigg

10. GLAUCOMA FOLLOWING CATARACT SURGERY

Cecilia Fenerty, Nicola Freeman, John Grigg

Section Leaders: John Grigg, Cecilia Fenerty, Nicola Freeman
Contributors: Allen Beck, Ta Chen Peter Chang, Teresa Chen, Tam Dang, Vera Essuman, Hernán Iturriaga-Valenzuela, Karen Joos, Ramesh Kekunnaya, Chan Yun Kim, Chris Lyons, Alicia Serra-Castanera, Ed Wilson

Consensus statements

1. Glaucoma following cataract surgery is that which occurs after pediatric cataract removal of either congenital idiopathic cataract, cataract associated with ocular or systemic syndromes and acquired cataract.
2. Glaucoma can occur in aphakic and pseudophakic eyes.
3. Young age at the time of cataract surgery and microcornea increase the risk of glaucoma.
4. Glaucoma usually occurs in eyes with open angles but angle closure can occur, and it is important to elucidate the underlying mechanism when possible (*e.g.*, by gonioscopy).
5. The risk of glaucoma following cataract surgery in children is lifelong, so regular monitoring is necessary.
6. Medical intraocular pressure (IOP) lowering therapy is usually first line treatment for glaucoma following cataract surgery. When medical therapy fails, surgical therapy is indicated but there is no consensus on the preferred approach.

Definition

This section addresses glaucoma after pediatric cataract removal and includes only those conditions in which there is no glaucoma prior to the cataract surgery. If glaucoma exists prior to cataract surgery then the condition is classified in a different category depending on the etiology. The effect of removing the lens therefore has a direct role in the development of glaucoma. This is one of the commonest

Childhood Glaucoma, pp. 233-247
Edited by Robert N. Weinreb, Alana L. Grajewski, Maria Papadopoulos, John Grigg, and Sharon Freedman
2013 © Kugler Publications, Amsterdam, The Netherlands

causes of secondary childhood glaucoma and hence the reason for its own category. Both aphakic and pseudophakic eyes may be affected. The different cataract etiologies include:

- Congenital idiopathic cataract;
- Congenital cataract in the setting of an ocular anomaly or systemic syndrome with a known glaucoma relationship [such as Lowe syndrome, congenital rubella syndrome, aniridia, or persistent fetal vasculature (PFV)];
- Acquired cataract.

This section will mainly review glaucoma following congenital cataract surgery.

Incidence of glaucoma following congenital cataract surgery

Glaucoma following pediatric cataract surgery is a frequent and lifelong risk.[1-4] During the past decade, the occurrence of glaucoma after cataract surgery was reported to be higher in patients who underwent cataract surgery at a younger age.[5-12] Trivedi *et al.* noted in their retrospective review that all patients who developed glaucoma had cataract surgery performed at 4.5 months of age or younger. The development of glaucoma was 24.4% in pseudophakic eyes and 19% in aphakic eyes.[13] The annual incidence of postoperative glaucoma was 5.25 per 100 surgeries in a review of 165 children with congenital cataract in the United Kingdom.[14] A younger age was associated with glaucoma. Glaucoma developed even 6.73 years following cataract surgery prompting continued vigilance in these patients.[14] The incidence of glaucoma was 3.9 cases per 100 person years in a retrospective Australian study of 147 eyes.[15] Risk was higher in children with bilateral cataract and surgery at a younger age.[15] Cataract surgery was performed in 113 patients in another retrospective review. Glaucoma developed in 9.7% of these eyes between six months and ten years postoperatively.[16] The glaucoma risk may also be related to surgeon factors.

Standards for congenital cataract surgery

Cataract removal is most commonly combined with primary posterior capsulotomy and anterior vitrectomy with or without a lens implant. Prevention of hypotony is crucial. Surgical factors to minimize this complication include the use of an anterior chamber (AC) maintainer or separate infusion line and securely suturing all wounds including paracentesis ports. Minimizing inflammation is also essential with the use of adequate topical steroids in the postoperative period. The use of heparin in the anterior chamber infusion line may assist with this process.[17,18]

Peripheral iridectomy may be used for prophylaxis against angle-closure glaucoma. When iridectomy is not routine practice, it should be considered for the following circumstances: sulcus lens inserted, poor pupil dilatation, shallow AC and when anterior vitrectomy is not possible.

Microcornea and congenital cataract

Cataracts in the presence of microcornea may require additional considerations. In the preoperative assessment, measurement of intraocular pressure (IOP), central corneal thickness (CCT), gonioscopy, axial length measurement and possibly ultrasound biomicroscopy (UBM) assist in determining the best surgical approach. Modification of the surgical technique may be required such as:

- Pupilloplasty if the pupil is not dilating adequately;
- Iris hooks or similar devices can be used as an alternative to pupilloplasty;
- Adequate care to avoid any damage to corneal endothelial cells;
- Intraocular lens implantation (IOL) is best avoided;
- Large capsulorhexis and postoperative use of atropine;
- Measurement and monitoring of IOP, CCT, axial length and refraction postoperatively.

Glaucoma has been recognized as a serious complication following surgery in the presence of microcornea. Wallace *et al.* in their series of forty-eight eyes identified 29 patients with aphakic glaucoma.[19] Forty-five of the 48 (94%) eyes were found to have microcornea when compared with the normal corneal diameter for their age. They recommended all children undergoing cataract surgery should have their corneal diameters recorded.[19] Patients with corneal diameters smaller than normal should be followed closely for the development of glaucoma throughout childhood and beyond.

Many studies report the association of microcornea and the development of glaucoma. It has been suggested that eyes with microcornea are predisposed to iridocorneal apposition and angle closure; conversely, the angle is often open in eyes with microcornea-associated aphakic glaucoma. Therefore the exact mechanism is still unknown. Microcornea can be associated with other risk factors for glaucoma such as poor pupillary dilation, retained lens cortex and coexisting ocular anomalies.

Mechanisms of glaucoma

The mechanism for glaucoma development following pediatric cataract surgery falls into two groups; open angle and angle closure often secondary to pupillary block.

Open angle presentations are the commonest, peripheral anterior synechiae (PAS) may be present, but the majority of the angle is open. The presentation may be any time after surgery.[3-5]

Angle-closure secondary pupillary block is a rare occurrence with modern pediatric cataract surgery. In general, presentation will be earlier. Risk factors for the development include: microcornea, poor pupil dilatation, retained lens matter, sulcus IOL and uveitis with pupillary membrane formation. Localized shallowing of the AC is most often due to secondary lens fiber proliferation, but may occur with forward movement of the vitreous face. If detected early, removal of the lens fibers combined with a surgical peripheral iridectomy will minimize the risk of angle-closure glaucoma. Post operative inflammation can also lead to progressive angle closure.

Pathogenesis of open angle glaucoma following pediatric cataract surgery

The removal of the pediatric cataract is the event that places the eye at risk from developing glaucoma.[20] There are no consistent preoperative angle findings on gonioscopy in older more co-operative children or at examination under anesthesia (EUA) to suggest a role in pathogenesis.[4] In the presence of an open angle the mechanism is poorly understood but may include the following:

- Trabecular meshwork (TM) dysfunction from inflammation and cellular obstruction;
- Corticosteroid-induced mechanism;
- Insult to developing angle structures from interaction with lens epithelial cells or vitreous leading to reduced outflow facility and/or developmental arrest;[21]
- TM collapse from lack of ciliary body traction.

Risk factors for open angle following pediatric cataract surgery glaucoma

Age at surgery and microcornea are the two risk factors most commonly associated with glaucoma (*see* Table 1).[22] In the Infant Aphakia Treatment Study (IATS) one-year results, corneal diameter was noted to be moderately correlated, and age at surgery and PFV were the only statistically significant risk factors in multivariate analysis.

The literature supports a younger age at surgery as having a greater risk for the development of glaucoma. A number of studies report an increased risk at different ages for surgery in the first 12 months of life. Surgery within four weeks of term is the first time point.[11,23] Only one study has not found a relationship between age at cataract surgery (prior to twelve weeks of age) and the development of glaucoma.[24] Others found that cataract surgery prior to nine months of age had a greater risk than surgery after this age.[1,3,25] Further studies report an increased incidence for those undergoing the cataract surgery prior to 12 months of age.[13,25-27]

Some initial small or non-randomized studies reported that the presence of an IOL was protective for the development of glaucoma.[28-30] Intraocular lens implantation in infants less than 12 months occurs only in selected cases. The criteria that many surgeons use in making the decision to implant an IOL means that many of the risk factors associated with the development of post-pediatric cataract surgery glaucoma are absent. The selection bias contributes to explaining the lower rate of glaucoma in pseudophakic infants reported in these studies. Three studies have reported that an IOL is not protective for the development of glaucoma.[12,13,31] Modern surgical techniques do not eliminate the early development of glaucoma following congenital cataract surgery with or without an IOL implant.[31] These studies highlight the need for lifelong surveillance for glaucoma.

PFV is a non-acquired ocular anomaly that has been associated with the development of glaucoma without cataract surgery.[32] Following lens removal these PFV cases have a significant risk for developing glaucoma.

Table 1. Risk factors for open angle glaucoma following pediatric cataract surgery

Age at cataract surgery (early surgery carries a higher risk of glaucoma)
Microcornea
Secondary membrane/iridectomy surgery
Chronic uveitis
Type of cataract (nuclear and persistent fetal vasculature)
Family history of secondary glaucoma after congenital cataract surgery

Presentation and monitoring

Symptomatic cases of significantly elevated IOP as occur in acute angle closure secondary to pupillary block or even with an open angle, are easier to detect. To detect elevated IOP early before glaucoma develops, the majority of open-angle cases depend on regular postoperative monitoring, so clinicians must be alert to the risk of glaucoma.

Recommendation for postoperative monitoring

- Although review intervals have not been studied, some experts suggest the following review intervals: week 1, month 1, and thereafter 2-4 monthly review.
- Subsequent monitoring intervals depend on clinical assessment of risk of glaucoma: high risk 2-4 monthly and low risk 6-12 monthly.
- Risk is determined by number of associations (Table 1).

Methods of assessment/monitoring

The majority of monitoring takes place in an outpatient setting. Measuring IOP is challenging for a number of reasons (*i.e.*, nystagmus). Monitoring with iCare rebound tonometry is increasingly common to facilitate outpatient assessment. Optic nerve assessment may be challenging due to the presence of miosis, nystagmus, lens/capsule remnants so an EUA may be necessary to obtain an adequate glaucoma assessment. It is important to differentiate the various mechanisms of raised IOP. In the postoperative period following pediatric cataract surgery, one of the most important differential causes of elevated IOP is steroid responsiveness. A persistently elevated IOP occurring post-surgery in a patient who has been off topical steroids for at least six weeks and has had documented normal IOP in the interval since stopping topical steroids, would tend to exclude steroids as an etiological factor.

The key features to monitor

1. IOP: measurement challenging.
   a. Monitoring with rebound tonometry is increasingly common enabling outpatient assessment.
2. Optic disc changes.
3. Corneal features.
   a. Corneal edema (common with raised IOP and often causes contact lens intolerance);
   b. Splits in Descemet membrane (Haab Striae);
   c. Corneal diameter;
   d. CCT measurement.
4. Refraction (myopic shift coupled with an increase in ocular dimensions out of keeping with normal growth).
5. Axial length.
6. Visual fields: in older more co-operative children but difficult because of poor visual acuity (VA), nystagmus, spectacle artifact.
7. Anterior segment UBM used by some for angle assessment when cornea cloudy.

Central corneal thickness (CCT)

In eyes with unoperated congenital cataracts, the CCT is in the normal range or similar to fellow eyes in unilateral cases. Thicker corneas have been measured in children following cataract surgery. Simon *et al.* found 42 eyes with either aphakia or pseudophakia to have a CCT average of 660 microns compared to 576 microns in the fellow phakic eye (P < 0.0001).[33] Likewise, Simsek *et al.* found thicker mean CCT post-cataract surgery, but noted a difference between aphakic and pseudophakic eyes with primary IOL implantation (P = 0.011).[34] Their report found an inverse correlation between the age of the patient at time of cataract surgery and CCT.[34] A multi-center study of CCT in 184 eyes with childhood glaucoma found significant differences in mean CCT of 651 microns in aphakic glaucoma when compared to 563 microns in primary congenital glaucoma (P < 0.0001) or to 529 microns in Axenfeld-Rieger glaucoma (P < 0.0001).[35]

Lim *et al.* found mean CCT was 552 microns in eyes with cataract versus 551 microns in fellow eyes. Following cataract surgery, affected eyes showed a mean increase of 29.7 microns while fellow eyes were unchanged (P = 0.03).[36] In addition, pseudophakic/aphakic eyes with glaucoma were found to have an average 56 micron thicker CCT than pseudophakic/aphakic eyes without glaucoma (P = 0.043).[36] Resende *et al.* prospectively also found increased mean CCT following cataract surgery in 37 eyes.[37] They measured a mean CCT change of 56 microns in aphakic eyes and 13 microns in pseudophakic eyes. Younger children were left aphakic. In addition, they found CCT increased more if cataract surgery was performed at less than one year of age than at older ages.[37] Ventura *et al.* found that intracameral triamcinolone injected in 53 eyes following cataract removal did not change CCT postoperatively.[38] Filous *et al.* reported that mean CCT in microphthalmic eyes after cataract surgery (635 microns) was similar to mean CCT in microphthalmic eyes without eye surgery (642 microns).[39] Following surgery with time the CCT increases and this effect is greater in aphakic than in pseudophakic eyes.[40] This gradual increase in CCT is despite other parameters including endothelial cell count and morphological features being similar to controls.[41]

Despite the theoretical overestimation of IOP that occurs in eyes with thick corneas, children with aphakia do develop glaucoma and visual field defects.[22] It appears this acquired increase in CCT does not necessarily cause an over-estimation of IOP in children and it may relate to the corneal properties of a pediatric eye. The definitive role for pachymetry in the evaluation of childhood glaucoma is currently uncertain. While CCT should be measured in all children with glaucoma or suspected glaucoma, it should not be used to 'adjust' an IOP measurement. Regardless of the CCT, the appearance of the optic disc remains the most important feature of the assessment.[22]

Treatment of glaucoma following congenital cataract surgery

The management of glaucoma or ocular hypertension following pediatric cataract surgery is one of the most challenging clinical problems.[3,42] Medical therapy remains the initial therapy for children with open-angle glaucoma, whereas surgery is required for definitive treatment of pupillary block glaucoma.

Pupil block glaucoma

Surgery is the primary approach for patients with pupillary block glaucoma. The surgery involves removing any secondary lens fiber proliferation that may be contributing to the pupil block and performing an adequate anterior vitrectomy which includes removal of vitreous from the AC. Goniosynechialysis may be useful to open the angle. The addition of sodium heparin to the balanced salt irrigating solution does reduce the inflammation and adhesiveness of the vitreous to the surgical incisions.

Open-angle glaucoma

The decision tree for medication, laser or surgery depends on social, family and economic factors in addition to glaucoma severity and ocular characteristics.

Medications

Medications are first line for treating a child with ocular hypertension or glaucoma following cataract surgery. A confounding factor may be the use of steroids both topical and systemic. Alternatives should be sought without compromising inflammatory control. Then choice of medication varies from clinician to clinician and is dependent on efficacy, potential side effects, cost and availability across different healthcare systems (*see* Section 4).

- Beta-blockers: First-line choice for some. Respiratory side effects may be a concern for young children even without a pre-existing diagnosis of asthma.
- Carbonic anhydrase inhibitors: Topical is first-line medication choice for some. Oral may be used in the short term pending surgery when maximally tolerated topical medication is not controlling IOP adequately.
- Miotics: Not first-line choice but may be effective particularly in aphakic cases as opposed to pseudophakic cases.
- Prostaglandin analogues: First-line choice for some. May have poor efficacy in some children. There is a theoretical risk of cystoid macular edema which is rare. If the vision is different from expected then consider this as a possibility. Cost is prohibitive in some healthcare systems.
- Adrenergic agonists: These are not first-line agents. They must be used with caution in children under six years of age or less than 20 kg because of the risks of somnolence and coma in very young patients.

Surgery

Published results of laser and surgical treatments for glaucoma following cataract surgery are limited by: (1) small numbers in most series; (2) varying surgical techniques or devices; and (3) varying criteria for success. Some data are reported within papers describing results for surgery for more than one type of childhood glaucoma where glaucoma following congenital cataract surgery is a subgroup. In the main, surgery and cyclodestructive laser are used when medications are insufficient to adequately control glaucoma. Glaucoma surgery in these children, especially in buphthalmic eyes is prone to higher rate of complications if hypotony occurs. Refer to Figure 1 for a suggested management algorithm.

Angle surgery

Although angle surgery (goniotomy and trabeculotomy) have been used to treat aphakic glaucoma following congenital cataract surgery, data documenting these treatment modalities in this setting are limited.[43] Angle surgery for pediatric cataract induced glaucoma has a reported qualified success rate of 42.9% (n = 11) after a single treatment increasing to a qualified success rate of success of 57% with up to two treatments after a median follow-up of 4.2 years.[43] However, success as low as 15 and 16% has been reported by Walton (n = 16)[4] and Chen (n = 24),[22] respectively.

Trabeculectomy

Trabeculectomy may be suitable for older and more co-operative children who have no need to wear contact lenses but results are poor with aphakia being a significant risk factor for failure. This was highlighted by Azuara-Blanco *et al.*,[44] who had a 0% success in aphakic eyes (n = 8) treated with trabeculectomy. Beck *et al.*[45] showed a significantly increased risk for failure with aphakic eyes treated with Mitomycin C (MMC) enhanced trabeculectomy. Cumulative probability of qualified success at 24 months for aphakia/pseudophakia was 46% over one year of age (17 eyes) and 0% for less than one year of age (three eyes) as compared to phakic eyes with 88% success over one year of age (24 eyes) and 20% for less than one year of age (five eyes). Similarly, Mandal *et al.*[46] reported a poor rate of success for trabeculectomy with or without MMC in aphakic Asian eyes. They found a complete success rate of 36.8% at the end of three years.

The most commonly reported complications after trabeculectomy with MMC include shallow anterior chambers and serous choroidal detachments, both signs of hypotony. Suprachoroidal hemorrhage is a particular risk in large (buphthalmic) eyes. Furthermore, if contact lens refractive correction is required, trabeculectomy is undesirable because of the risk of bleb related complications (especially blebitis and endophthalmitis).[31, 43, 46, 47]

Glaucoma drainage devices

Glaucoma drainage devices GDD have become the preferred primary surgical intervention for many patients with aphakic glaucoma.[48] They are especially indicated for aphakic eyes where contact lens wear is the preferred method of optical correction, younger patients not considered suitable for trabeculectomy and where other surgical options have failed or are not an appropriate option (*e.g.*, PAS preventing angle surgery). Placement of the tube may be in the AC or pars plana depending on clinical circumstance and anatomy of the AC.

A success rate of 68% for Ahmed glaucoma implant (AGI) with or without medications has been reported,[27] and another series reported a qualified success rate in 18/19 cases (IOP below 15 mmHg including topical medication).[49]

In one series where a mixture of GDDs were used, a 90% success rate was reported at one year falling to 55% success at ten years. A success rate of 85% with follow- up of over 11 years has been reported for Molteno tube implant in a series where 44% of cases were aphakic.[50]

Pakravan *et al.*[51] examined the success rate of trabeculectomy with MMC and AGI with MMC for glaucoma in aphakic eyes. At 14 months, the complete and qualified success for trabeculectomy with MMC was 33.3% and 40% respectively, with a complication rate of 40% whereas for the AGI with MMC group, they were 20% and 66.7% with a complications rate of 27% after a similar follow-up. Although the results were not statistically significant the lower complication rates do support the potential for better outcomes with GDDs.

Ciliary body destruction

Cyclophotocoagulation with the diode laser (transcleral, endoscopic) is an important modality for uncontrolled IOP in aphakic/pseudophakic eyes. The diode laser has replaced other cyclodestructive procedures such as cyclocryotherapy in most settings. Diode laser photoablation may also be considered as a temporizing measure in the pediatric age group.

Kirwan *et al.*[52] in one of the largest series reported a qualified success rate of 54% (plus medications) at two years in 77 eyes, and a re-treatment rate of 66%. Aphakic eyes showed a more sustained fall in IOP compared to other secondary glaucomas.

Retinal detachment is a recognized complication of cyclodiode procedures particularly in aphakic eyes. Kirwan *et al.*[52] reported 9% (3/34) of aphakic eyes developed a retinal detachment.

Endocyclophotocoagulation may have similar results to transscleral diode laser regarding success rate (43%) and complications, *e.g.*, retinal detachment rate 6% (2/36 eyes)[53] but with a lower re-treatment rate (25-38%).[53,54]

Summary of laser and surgical treatments

Prospective and randomized studies of surgical techniques for the treatment of glaucoma following congenital cataract surgery are not available to guide clinicians. For all laser and surgical interventions, supplementation with topical glaucoma medications may be required to achieve success. Current data suggest angle surgery may be suitable for some cases depending on gonioscopic appearance but success is variable. Filtration surgery with or without anti-scarring augmentation has limited success and is not appropriate where contact lens refractive correction is anticipated. GDD implantation carries the highest success rate and long-term benefits over trabeculectomy. Laser ablative procedures have limited success and carry significant risk of retinal detachment in aphakic cases.

Visual outcome and amblyopia

Amblyopia is a major cause of visual impairment in cases of glaucoma following cataract surgery and therapy should be instigated as early as possible in conjunction with treatment for glaucoma.[55] The visual outcome is also affected by the type of cataract,[56] corneal changes complicating glaucoma, refractive changes and the surgical procedures. Early detection of glaucoma and frequent vision monitoring is essential to maximize visual potential.

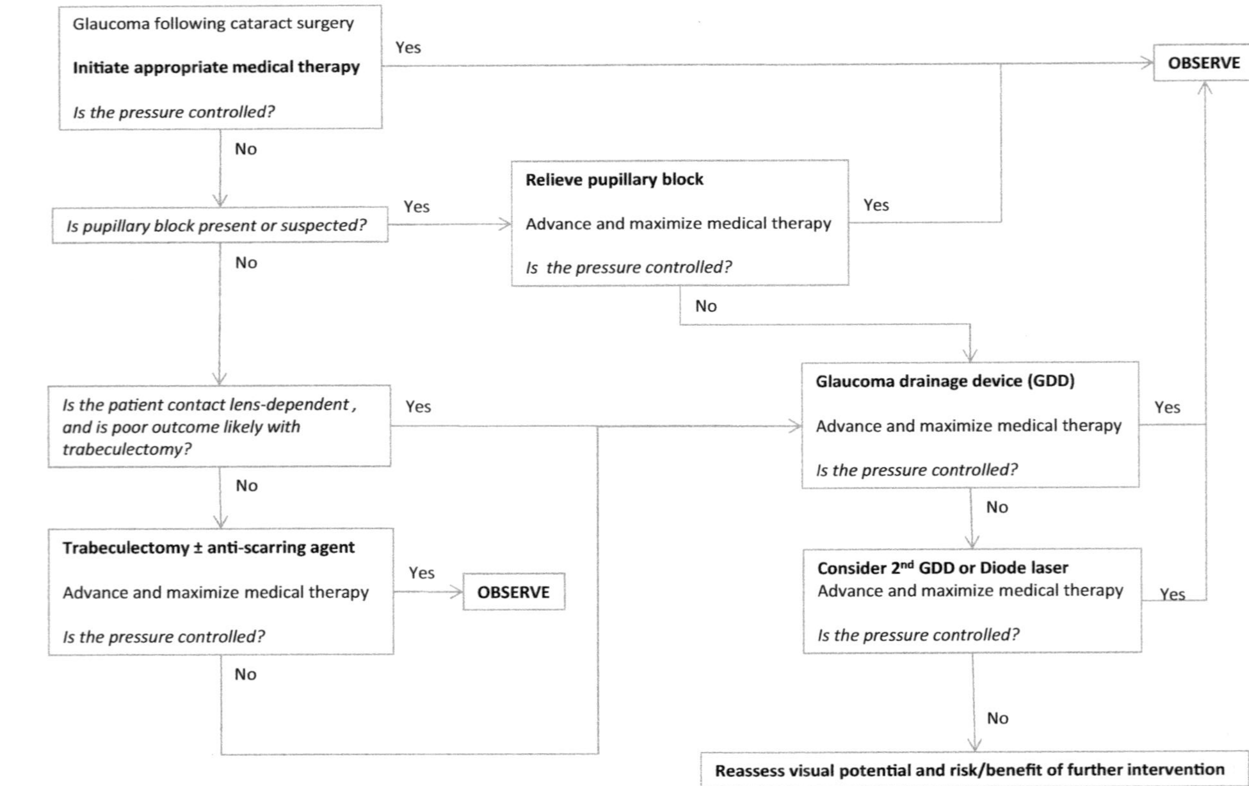

Fig. 1. A suggested approach to the management of glaucoma following cataract surgery. (It will be influenced by surgeon preference/experience and local facilities/equipment availability.)

References

1. Rabiah PK. Frequency and predictors of glaucoma after pediatric cataract surgery. Amer J Ophthalmol 2004; 137: 30-37.
2. Simon J, Mehta N, Simmons S, et al. Glaucoma after pediatric lensectomy/vitrectomy. Ophthalmology 1991; 98: 670-674.
3. Swamy BN, Billson F, Martin F, et al. Secondary glaucoma after paediatric cataract surgery. Br J Ophthalmol 2007; 91: 1627-1630.
4. Walton D. Pediatric aphakic glaucoma: a study of 65 patients. Trans Am Ophthalmol Soc 1995; 93: 403-413.
5. Comer RM, Kim P, Cline R, Lyons CJ. Cataract surgery in the first year of life: aphakic glaucoma and visual outcomes. Can J Ophthalmol 2011; 46: 148-152.
6. Egbert J, Wright M, Dahlhauser K, et al. A prospective study of ocular hypertension and glaucoma after pediatric cataract surgery. Ophthalmology 1995; 102: 1098-1101.
7. Kuhli-Hattenbach C, Luchtenberg M, Kohnen T, Hattenbach L-O. Risk factors for complications after congenital cataract surgery without intraocular lens implantation in the first 18 months of life. Am J Ophthalmol 2008; 146: 1-7.
8. Magnusson G, Abrahamsson M, Sjostrand J. Glaucoma following congenital cataract surgery: an 18-year longitudinal follow-up. Acta Ophthalmol Scand 2000; 78: 65-70.
9. Mills M, Robb R. Glaucoma following childhood cataract surgery. J Pediatr Ophthalmol Strabismus. 1994; 31: 355-360.
10. Miyahara S, Amino K, Tanihara H. Glaucoma secondary to pars plana lensectomy for congenital cataract. Graefes Arch Clin Exp Ophthalmol 2002; 240: 176-179.
11. Vishwanath M, Cheong-Leen R, Taylor D, et al. Is early surgery for congenital cataract a risk factor for glaucoma? Br J Ophthalmol 2004; 88: 905-910.
12. Wong IBY, Sukthankar VD, Cortina-Borja M, Nischal KK. Incidence of early-onset glaucoma after infant cataract extraction with and without intraocular lens implantation. Br J Ophthalmol 2009; 93: 1200-1203.
13. Trivedi RH, Wilson ME Jr., Golub RL. Incidence and risk factors for glaucoma after pediatric cataract surgery with and without intraocular lens implantation. J AAPOS 2006; 10: 117-123.
14. Chak M, Rahi JS, British Congenital Cataract Interest G. Incidence of and factors associated with glaucoma after surgery for congenital cataract: findings from the British Congenital Cataract Study. Ophthalmology 2008; 115: 1013-8.e2.
15. Ruddle J, Staffieri S, Crowston J, et al. Incidence and predictors of glaucoma following surgery for congenital cataract in the first year of life in Victoria, Australia. Clin Experiment Ophthalmol 2013.
16. Urban B, Bakunowicz-Lazarczyk A. Aphakic glaucoma after congenital cataract surgery with and without intraocular lens implantation. Klin Oczna 2010; 112: 105-107.
17. Vasavada V, Praveen M, Shah S, et al. Anti-inflammatory Effect of Low-Molecular-Weight Heparin in Pediatric Cataract Surgery: A Randomized Clinical Trial. Am J Ophthalmol 2012; 154: 252-258.
18. Dada T, Dada V, Sharma N, et al. Primary posterior capsulorhexis with optic capture and intracameral heparin in pediatric cataract surgery. Clin Exp Ophthalmol 2000; 28: 361-363.
19. Wallace DK, Plager DA. Corneal diameter in childhood aphakic glaucoma. J Pediatric Ophthalmol Strabismus 1996; 33: 230-234.
20. Levin AV. Aphakic glaucoma: a never-ending story? Br J Ophthalmol 2007; 91: 1574-1575.
21. Michael I, Shmoish M, Walton DS, Levenberg S. Interactions between trabecular meshwork cells and lens epithelial cells: a possible mechanism in infantile aphakic glaucoma. Invest Ophthalmol Vis Sci 2008; 49: 3981-3987.
22. Chen TC, Walton DS, Bhatia LS. Aphakic glaucoma after congenital cataract surgery. Arch Ophthalmol 2004; 122: 1819-1825.

23. Lambert S, Lynn M, Drews-Botsch C, et al. A comparison of grating visual acuity, strabismus, and reoperation outcomes among children with aphakia and pseudophakia after unilateral cataract surgery during the first six months of life. J AAPOS 2001; 5: 70-75.
24. Watts P, Abdolell M, Levin AV. Complications in infants undergoing surgery for congenital cataract in the first 12 weeks of life: is early surgery better? J AAPOS 2003; 7: 81-85.
25. Haargaard B, Ritz C, Oudin A, et al. Risk of glaucoma after pediatric cataract surgery. Invest Ophthalmol Vis Sci 2008; 49: 1791-1796.
26. Koc F, Kargi S, Biglan AW, et al. The aetiology in paediatric aphakic glaucoma. Eye 2006; 20: 1360-1365.
27. Kirwan C, O'Keefe M, Lanigan B, Mahmood U. Ahmed valve drainage implant surgery in the management of paediatric aphakic glaucoma. Br J Ophthalmol 2005; 89: 855-858.
28. Asrani S, Freedman S, Hasselblad V, et al. Does primary intraocular lens implantation prevent "aphakic" glaucoma in children? J AAPOS 2000; 4: 33-39.
29. O'Keefe M, Fenton S, Lanigan B. Visual outcomes and complications of posterior chamber intraocular lens implantation in the first year of life. J Cataract Refract Surg 2001; 27: 2006-2011.
30. Ahmadieh H, Javadi MA. Intra-ocular lens implantation in children. Curr Opin Ophthalmol 2001; 12: 30-34.
31. Beck A, Freedman S, Lynn M, et al. Glaucoma-Related Adverse Events in the Infant Aphakia Treatment Study: 1-Year Results. Arch Ophthalmol 2012; 130: 300-305.
32. Johnson CP, Keech RV. Prevalence of glaucoma after surgery for PHPV and infantile cataracts. J Pediatric Ophthalmol Strabismus 1996; 33: 14-17.
33. Simon J, O'Malley M, Gandham S, et al. Central corneal thickness and glaucoma in aphakic and pseudophakic children. J AAPOS 2005; 9: 326-329.
34. Simsek T, Mutluay AH, Elgin U, et al. Glaucoma and increased central corneal thickness in aphakic and pseudophakic patients after congenital cataract surgery. Br J Ophthalmol 2006; 90: 1103-1106.
35. Tai TY, Mills MD, Beck AD, et al. Central corneal thickness and corneal diameter in patients with childhood glaucoma. J Glaucoma 2006; 15: 524-528.
36. Lim Z, Muir KW, Duncan L, Freedman SF. Acquired central corneal thickness increase following removal of childhood cataracts. Am J Ophthalmol 2011; 151: 434-441.
37. Resende G, Lupinacci A, Árieta C, Costa V. Central corneal thickness and intraocular pressure in children undergoing congenital cataract surgery: a prospective, longitudinal study. Br J Ophthalmol 2012; 96: 1190-1194.
38. Ventura M, Ventura B, Ventura C, et al. Congenital cataract surgery with intracameral triamcinolone: pre- and postoperative central corneal thickness and intraocular pressure. J AAPOS 2012; 16: 441-444.
39. Filous A, Osmera J, Hlozanek M, Mahelkova G. Central corneal thickness in microphthalmic eyes with or without history of congenital cataract surgery. Eur J Ophthalmol 2011; 21: 374-378.
40. Muir KW, Duncan L, Enyedi LB, et al. Central corneal thickness: congenital cataracts and aphakia. Am J Ophthalmol 2007; 144: 502-506.
41. Nilforushan N, Falavarjani KG, Razeghinejad MR, Bakhtiari P. Cataract surgery for congenital cataract: endothelial cell characteristics, corneal thickness, and impact on intraocular pressure. J AAPOS 2007; 11: 159-161.
42. Bhola R, Keech RV, Olson RJ, Petersen DB. Long-term outcome of pediatric aphakic glaucoma. J AAPOS 2006; 10: 243-248.
43. Bothun E, Guo Y, Christiansen S, et al. Outcome of angle surgery in children with aphakic glaucoma. J AAPOS 2010; 14: 235-239.
44. Azuara-Blanco A, Wilson RP, Spaeth GL, et al. Filtration procedures supplemented with mitomycin C in the management of childhood glaucoma. Br J Ophthalmol 1999; 83: 151-156.

45. Beck A, Wilson W, Lynch M, et al. Trabeculectomy with adjunctive mitomycin C in pediatric glaucoma. Am J Ophthalmol 1998; 126: 648-657.
46. Mandal AK, Bagga H, Nutheti R, et al. Trabeculectomy with or without mitomycin-C for paediatric glaucoma in aphakia and pseudophakia following congenital cataract surgery. Eye 2003; 17: 53-62.
47. Beck A, Freedman S, Kammer J, Jin J. Aqueous shunt devices compared with trabeculectomy with mitomycin-C for children in the first two years of life. Am J Ophthalmol 2003; 136: 994-1000.
48. O'Malley Schotthoefer E, Yanovitch TL, Freedman SF. Aqueous drainage device surgery in refractory pediatric glaucomas: I. Long-term outcomes. J AAPOS 2008; 12: 33-39.
49. Chen TC, Bhatia LS, Walton DS. Ahmed valve surgery for refractory pediatric glaucoma: a report of 52 eyes. J Pediatr Ophthalmol Strabismus 2005; 42: 274-283; quiz 304-305.
50. Cunliffe I, Molteno A. Long-term follow-up of Molteno drains used in the treatment of glaucoma presenting in childhood. Eye 1998; 12: 379-385.
51. Pakravan M, Homayoon N, Shahin Y, Ali Reza BR. Trabeculectomy with mitomycin C versus Ahmed glaucoma implant with mitomycin C for treatment of pediatric aphakic glaucoma. J Glaucoma 2007; 16: 631-636.
52. Kirwan J, Shah P, Khaw P. Diode laser cyclophotocoagulation. Ophthalmology 2002; 109: 316-323.
53. Neely D, Plager D. Endocyclophotocoagulation for management of difficult pediatric glaucomas. J AAPOS 2001; 5: 221-229.
54. Carter BC, Plager DA, Neely DE, et al. Endoscopic diode laser cyclophotocoagulation in the management of aphakic and pseudophakic glaucoma in children. J AAPOS 2007; 11: 34-40.
55. Bradford G, Keech R, Scott W. Factors affecting visual outcome after surgery for bilateral congenital cataracts. Am J Ophthalmol 1994; 117: 58-64.
56. Parks M, Johnson D, Reed G. Long-term visual results and complications in children with aphakia. A function of cataract type. Ophthalmology 1993; 100: 826-840.

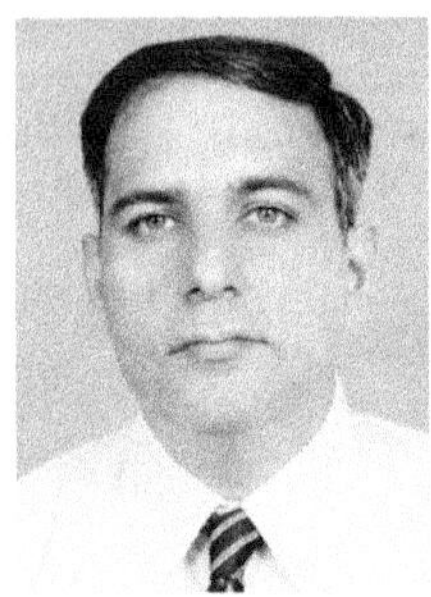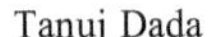

Tanuj Dada

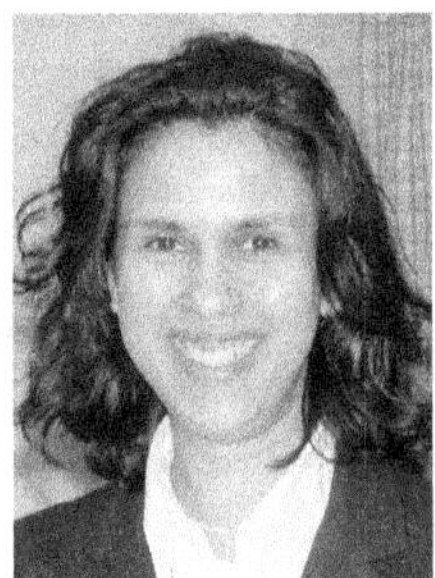

Jugnoo Rahi

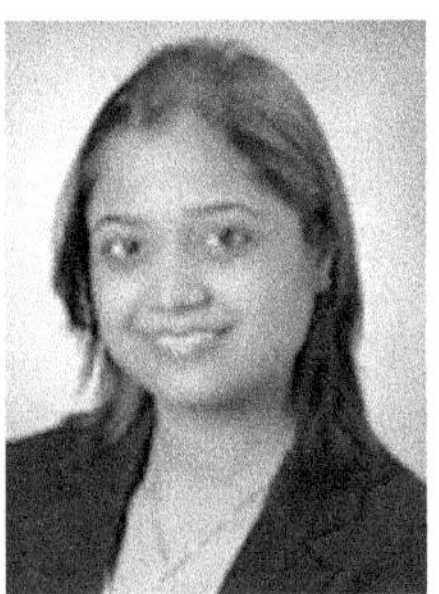

Shveta Jindal Bali

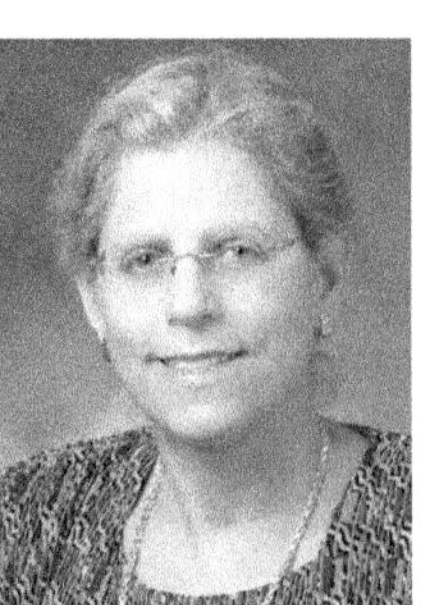

Sharon Freedman

ADDENDUM – PATIENTS, PARENTS AND PROVIDERS AS PARTNERS IN MANAGING CHILDHOOD GLAUCOMA

Tanuj Dada, Jugnoo Rahi, Shveta Jindal Bali, Sharon Freedman

Summary

1. Glaucoma affects the child's health-related quality of life (QoL) and impacts their functioning from early childhood through adolescence and adulthood both at home and school.
2. There is a lack of information on the patient's and parents/caregivers perspective of the impact of glaucoma and its treatment.
3. The emotional and psychological burden of caregivers of patients with childhood glaucoma has been poorly reported, but extrapolation from other visually disability disorders in childhood would suggest that the impact is likely to be considerable.
4. Parent-focused interventions that reduce parental stress and enhance parental confidence, may have a positive effect on the behaviors and outcomes of children with glaucoma.
5. The practitioner and parents/patient should work as partners, developing strategies that give them the best chance to control the child's disease and reduce the physical, psychological, social, and economic consequences of childhood glaucoma.

The worldwide prevalence of childhood blindness ranges from 0.03% in high-income countries to 0.12% in undeveloped countries.[1] The causes of severe visual impairment and blindness are varied and complex. Glaucoma accounts for 4.2 to 5% of blindness in the pediatric population.[2,3] The management of childhood glaucoma requires surgical intervention in almost all cases, while 30%-40% of cases require repeat surgical intervention for the control of intraocular pressure.[4,5] As the prognosis of childhood glaucoma has improved over the years, there has been an increasing emphasis on the impact of the condition and healthcare on the child and its parents/caregivers. Furthermore, patient-led assessment of the impact of disease has developed a high profile in health service planning and policy.

Childhood Glaucoma, pp. 249-254
Edited by Robert N. Weinreb, Alana L. Grajewski, Maria Papadopoulos, John Grigg, and Sharon Freedman
2013 © Kugler Publications, Amsterdam, The Netherlands

Glaucoma affects the child's health-related quality of life (QoL) and impacts their functioning from early childhood through adolescence and adulthood both at home and school.[6] It is known that visual impairment in childhood has a significant and lifelong impact on all aspects of development (physical, social, emotional and cognitive), education, employment opportunities, independence and social integration. In order to understand the psychometric impact of childhood glaucoma, it is vital to have measures/instruments for the evaluation of multidimensional health status that are child and condition specific. Evaluation of methodology in this area[7] and recognition of the importance of the measuring the impact of illness/disability and treatment from the patient's perspective has resulted in development of Patient-Reported Outcome Measures (PROMs) for use in specific scenarios within pediatric ophthalmology, *e.g.*, Cardiff Visual Ability Questionnaire for Children (CVAQC), Impact of Vision Impairment on Children (IVI_C), LV Prasad-Functional Vision Questionnaire Second Version (LVP-FVQII).[8-10] PROMs include outcomes such as 'health-related quality of life', 'activities of daily living' or 'health status'. There is a paucity of vision specific PROMs for use in children for numerous reasons. Firstly, it reflects the lack of defined vision-related constructs to be measured. For example, the 'impact of visual disability' is variably described in the literature as visual function (*e.g.*, visual acuity), functional vision (mobility capacity for a given visual function) and vision related quality of life (how patients living with an eye condition or visual impairment feel about their life). These are conceptually distinct aspects of the impact of vision/eye condition and must be clearly defined and assessed. Secondly there is the challenge of age appropriate methodology and finally the lack of a universally accepted definition of QoL. The consensus is that a person's perception of their quality of life is a subjective psychological impression derived from many aspects of life, for example physical, emotional, social and independence. Instruments should capture the impact of a condition across all QoL areas.

There is a definite need for the development of childhood glaucoma specific instruments that can be self reported and are sensitive to changes over time with respect to natural history and/or treatment.[11] Yet to be assessed and documented in childhood glaucoma is the specific impact to the child regarding: (1) the glaucoma diagnosis – chronic condition with uncertain prognosis, pain, cosmesis; (2) glaucoma-related visual impairment; (3) treatment; and (4) economic consequences. Furthermore, it is essential to include this aspect in the comprehensive management of children with glaucoma, so that the health policies can be shaped in accordance with what matters most to children with glaucoma related visual impairment.[11]

The ophthalmic care for children with glaucoma is potentially complex and a demanding task, with the immediate burden of the disease borne by the caregivers; *i.e.*, parents, siblings, and the family unit as a whole, with assumed high personal opportunity costs. Therefore, the diagnosis affects the child with glaucoma and its caregivers and so management should focus not only on the child, but must also support the needs of the family. However, again there is a lack of Patient Reported

Experience Measures (PREMs) which capture the health service experiences of patients and their families, *e.g.*, the degree to which services meets their needs in relation to information and support in a family centered way.

Caregiver burden has been defined as the type of stress or strain that caregivers experience related to the problems and challenges they face as a result of the status of the patient.[12] Significant caregiver stress has been identified in chronic systemic illnesses.[13,14] A number of studies have reported significant anxiety and depression associated with the demanding task of care giving for patients with chronic systemic ailments such as dementia, stroke, cancer and heart failure.[15-18] Studies have shown that caregivers of children with disabilities suffer greater emotional disturbances and also higher incidence of systemic disorders like back pain, migraine headaches and stomach/intestinal ulcers.[19-21] The parents must coordinate their children's medical, developmental and educational needs while balancing their family and occupational roles.[22] Even when the affected children had a excellent long-term outcome, Mitra *et al.* identified moderate to severe depression in 48% of caregivers to children with nephrotic syndrome. [23] In children with chronic kidney disease, caregiver stress, particularly in mothers, has been noted to lead to behavioral disturbances in children.[24,25]

Limited literature is available on the relationship between care burden and depression in caregivers of visually impaired individuals.[26] There is evidence of significant time-dependent, emotional, existential and physical burden; and depression among individuals caring for legally blind patients.[27] Hours of close supervision and intensity of care-giving have been identified as factors related to the overall burden. In the same study, depression was found to be prevalent in 16%-48% of population caring for legally blind individuals. This is relatively high compared to 6.7% to 15.1% prevalence of major depression in countries like the USA and India, respectively.[28,29]

In a recently published study, Dada *et al.* assessed the magnitude of caregiver burden and depression in primary congenital glaucoma.[30] Of the 55 parents evaluated, nearly 70% of the participants were identified to have significant socioeconomic, emotional, and psychological burden related to their striving to provide eye care and rehabilitation for their visually disabled children. A moderate level of depression was observed in 22% of individuals, and as high as 11% of parents had either severe or very severe depression. This may have greater implications for a developing nation where there is a relative lack of support organizations and specialized care services. The majority of individuals pay for medical expenses out of their pocket due to the lack of medical insurance, which is affordable only to the top 30% of wage earners in the country.[31]

However, it is also important to acknowledge that this rather pessimistic view is balanced by clinical reports and extensive empirical evidence that not all disabled children and their parents are negatively affected by the child's disability, that they adapt to the situation, and that they function well as a family. Hence, the 'disability paradox' – that those with the most severe objectively measured functional limitations report better quality of life than those with less severe impairment – is well described in the childhood disability literature. In a study conducted on family caregivers of persons with dementia, it was reported that care giving was associated with moderate burden and great satisfaction at the same time.[32] In another study of caregivers for children with disabilities, the investigators reported that caring for their children had a positive spiritual impact.[33]

In light of the definite impact on caregivers of visually disabled children, caregiver-focused interventions may have a positive effect on the outcomes of children with glaucoma by reducing caregiver stress and enhancing confidence. In particular 'key worker' services providing information, support and liaison have been shown to be effective in pediatric ophthalmology.[34] Coping mechanisms noted in the literature include – social support (caregiver relationships with extended family and friends), family function (extent to which the family works as a unit) and personal strategies and practices the caregiver utilizes for stress management.[35] Recent studies have suggested a role of yoga and meditation as an effective strategy to reduce stress in caregivers of individuals with dementia.[36-38] Danucalov *et al.* noted that an eight-week session of yoga and meditation significantly reduced stress, anxiety and depression in such caregivers.[36] Reduction in salivary cortisol and increase in telomerase activity was documented as a result of such interventional therapies.[36,37]

In summary, there is an emerging emphasis on the impact of illness and healthcare on both the patient's and caregivers' quality of life. Not only should practitioners be aware of this multifaceted impact, but its evaluation should be an essential part of the holistic approach for management of childhood glaucoma. There is an unmet need for instruments to identify the impact of childhood glaucoma on the patient and caregivers, which requires further research. Evaluation of impact should include the assessment of the process, experience and the outcomes of care. The practitioner, caregivers and patient should work together to develop strategies that provide the best chance not only to control the child's disease, but also to reduce the physical, psychological, social, and economic consequences of childhood glaucoma on the affected individuals as well as the caregivers. Efficient and effective health management for childhood glaucoma demands a team-based approach for the appropriate care of affected individuals as well as their caregivers.

References

1. Kong L, Fry M, Al-Samarraie M, Gilbert C, Steinkuller PG. An update on progress and the changing epidemiology of causes of childhood blindness worldwide. J AAPOS 2012; 16: 501-507.
2. Dandona L, Williams JD, Williams BC, Rao GN. Population-based assessment of childhood blindness in southern India. Arch Ophthalmol 1998; 116: 545-546.
3. Gilbert CE, Rahi JS, Quinn GE. Visual impairment and blindness in children. In: Johnson GJ, Minassian DC, Weale RA, West SK (Eds.), The Epidemiology of Eye Disease, 2nd ed. London: Hodder Arnold 2003, pp. 260-286.

4. Tourame B, Ben Younes N, Guigou S, Denis D. Congenital glaucoma: future of vision and pressure: results of an 11-year study. J Fr Ophtalmol 2009; 32: 335-340.
5. Kargi SH, Koc F, Biglan AW, Davis JS. Visual acuity in children with glaucoma. Ophthalmology 2006; 113: 229-238.
6. Zhang XL, Du SL, Ge J, et al. Quality of life in patients with primary congenital glaucoma following antiglaucoma surgical management. Zhonghua Yan Ke Za Zhi 2009; 45: 514-521.
7. Rahi JS, Tadić V, Keeley S, Lewando-Hundt G. Vision-related Quality of Life Group. Capturing children and young people's perspectives to identify the content for a novel vision-related quality of life instrument. Ophthalmology 2011; 118: 819-824.
8. Khadka J, Ryan B, Margrain TH, Court H, Woodhouse JM. Development of the 25-item Cardiff Visual Ability Questionnaire for Children (CVAQC). Br J Ophthalmol 2010; 94: 730-735.
9. Cochrane GM, Marella M, Keeffe JE, Lamoureux EL. The Impact of Vision Impairment for Children (IVI_C): validation of a vision-specific pediatric quality-of-life questionnaire using Rasch analysis. Invest Ophthalmol Vis Sci 2011; 52: 1632-1640.
10. Gothwal VK, Sumalini R, Bharani S, Reddy SP, Bagga DK. The second version of the L. V. Prasad-functional vision questionnaire.Optom Vis Sci 2012; 89: 1601-1610.
11. Tadic V, Hogan A, Sobti N, Knowles RL, Rahi JS. Patient-reported outcome measures (PROMs) in paediatric ophthalmology: a systematic review. Br J Ophthalmol 2013.
12. Zarit SH, Reever KE, Bach-Peterson J. Relatives of the impaired elderly: correlates of feelings of burden. Gerontologist 1980; 20: 649-655.
13. Rudnick A. Burden of caregivers of mentally ill individuals in Israel: a family participatory study. Int J Psychosocial Rehabil 2004; 9: 147-152.
14. Parks S, Novielli KD. A practical guide to caring for caregivers. Am Fam Physician 2000; 62: 2613-2620, 2621-2622.
15. Rabow MW, Hauser JM, Adams J. Supporting family caregivers at the end of life: "they don't know what they don't know." JAMA 2004; 291: 483-491.
16. Kasuya R, Polgar BP, Takeuchi R. Caregiver burden and burnout: a guide for primary care physicians. Postgrad Med 2000; 108: 1-7.
17. Pochard F, Azoulay E, Chevret S, et al. Symptoms of anxiety and depression in family members of intensive care unit patients: ethical hypothesis regarding decision-making capacity. Crit Care Med 2001; 29: 1893-1897.
18. Cannuscio CC, Jones C, Kawachi I, Colditz GA, Berkman L, Rimm E. Reverberations of family illness: a longitudinal assessment of informal caregiving and mental health status in the Nurses' Health Study. Am J Public Health 2002; 92: 1305-1311.
19. Tong HC, Haig AJ, Nelson VS, Yamakawa KS, Kandala G, Shin KY. Low back pain in adult female caregivers of children with physical disabilities. Archives of Pediatrics and Adolescent Medicine 2003; 157: 1128-1133.
20. Wang KW, Barnard A. Technology-dependent children and their families: a review. J Adv Nursing 2004; 45: 36-46.
21. Brehaut JC, Kohen DE, Raina P, et al. The health of primary caregivers of children with cerebral palsy: how does it compare with that of other Canadian caregivers? Pediatrics 2004; 114: e182-e191.
22. Silver EJ, Westbrook LE, Stein RE. Relationship of parental psychological distress to consequences of chronic health conditions in children. J Pediat Psychol 1998; 23: 5-15.
23. Mitra S, Banerjee S. The impact of pediatric nephrotic syndrome on families. Pediatr Nephrol 2011; 26: 1235-1240.
24. Mehta M, Bagga A, Pande P, Bajaj G, Srivastava RN. Behavior problems in nephrotic syndrome. Indian Pediatr 1995; 32: 1281-1286.
25. Rüth EM, Landolt MA, Neuhaus TJ, Kemper MJ. Health-related quality of life and psychosocial adjustment in steroid sensitive nephrotic syndrome. J Pediatr 2004; 145: 778-783.

26. Hamblion EL, Moore AT, Rahi JS. The health-related quality of life of children with hereditary retinal disorders and the psychosocial impact on their families. Invest Ophthalmol Vis Sci 2011; 52: 7981-7986.

27. Braich PS, Lal V, Hollands S, Almeida DR. Burden and depression in the caregivers of blind patients in India. Ophthalmology 2012; 119: 221-226.

28. Kessler RC, Chiu WT, Demler O, Merikangas KR, Walters EE. Prevalence, severity, and comorbidity of 12-month DSM-IV disorders in the National Comorbidity Survey Replication. Arch Gen Psychiatry 2005; 62: 617-627.

29. Poongothai S, Pradeepa R, Ganesan A, Mohan V. Prevalence of depression in a large urban South Indian population--the Chennai Urban Rural Epidemiology Study (CURES-70). PLoS One 2009; 28; 4:e7185.

30. Dada T, Aggarwal A, Bali SJ, Wadhwani M, Tinwala S, Sagar R. Caregiver burden assessment in primary congenital glaucoma. Eur J Ophthalmol 2013; 23: 324-328.

31. Healthcare in India. Boston, MA: Boston Analytics 2009, pp. 16-19.

32. Andren S, Elmstahl S. Family caregivers' subjective experiences of satisfaction in dementia care: aspects of burden, subjective health and sense of coherence. Scand J of Caring Science 2005; 19:157-168.

33. Marshall ES, Olsen SF, Mandleco BL, Dyches TT, Allred KW, Sansom N. 'This is a Spiritual Experience': perspectives of Latter-Day Saint families living with a child with disabilities. Qualitative Health Research 2003; 13: 57-76.

34. Rahi JS, Manaras I, Tuomainen H, Hundt GL. Meeting the needs of parents around the time of diagnosis of disability among their children: evaluation of a novel program for information, support, and liaison by key workers. Pediatrics 2004; 114: e477-82.

35. Raina P, O'Donnell M, Schwellnus H, et al. Caregiving process and caregiver burden: conceptual models to guide research and practice. BMC Pediatr 2004; 4: 1.

36. Danucalov MA, Kozasa EH, Ribas KT, et al. A yoga and compassion meditation program reduces stress in familial caregivers of Alzheimer's disease patients. Evid Based Complement Alternat Med 2013; 2013: 513149.

37. Lavretsky H, Epel ES, Siddarth P, et al. A pilot study of yogic meditation for family dementia caregivers with depressive symptoms: effects on mental health, cognition, and telomerase activity. Int J Geriatr Psychiatry 2013; 28: 57-65.

38. Oken BS, Fonareva I, Haas M, et al. Pilot controlled trial of mindfulness meditation and education for dementia caregivers. J Altern Complement Med 2010; 16: 1031-1038.

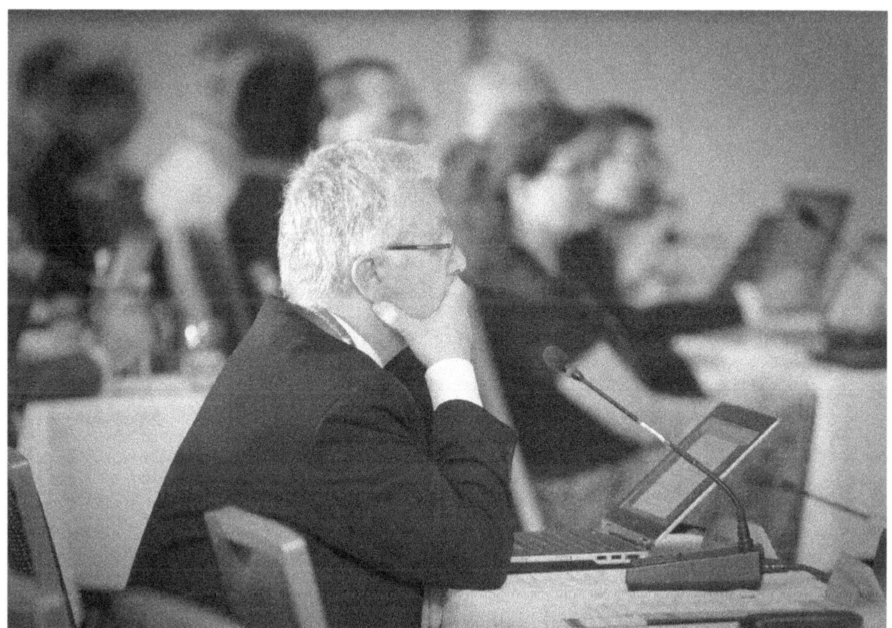

Mohamad S. Jaafar

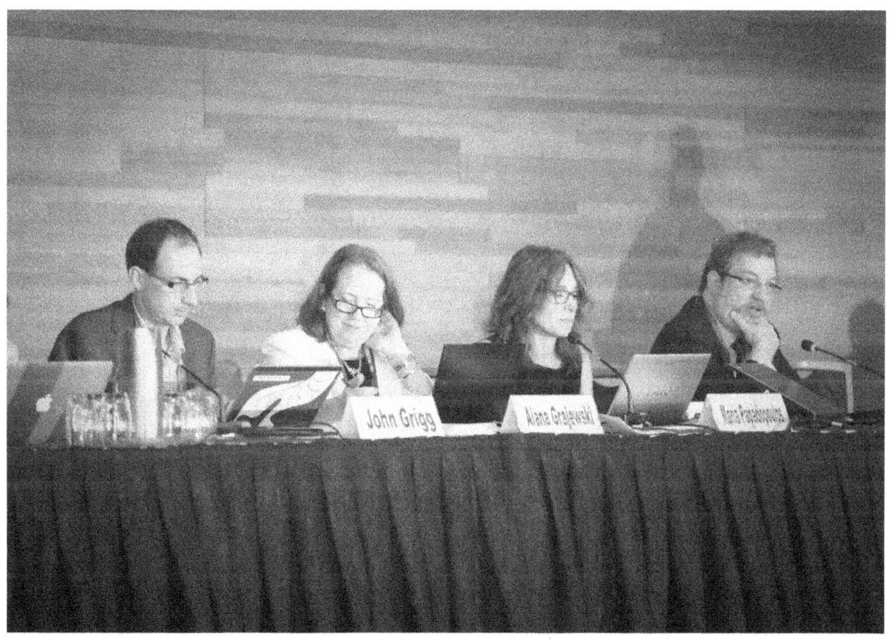

John Grigg, Alana L. Grajewski, Maria Papadopoulos, James D. Brandt (L-R)

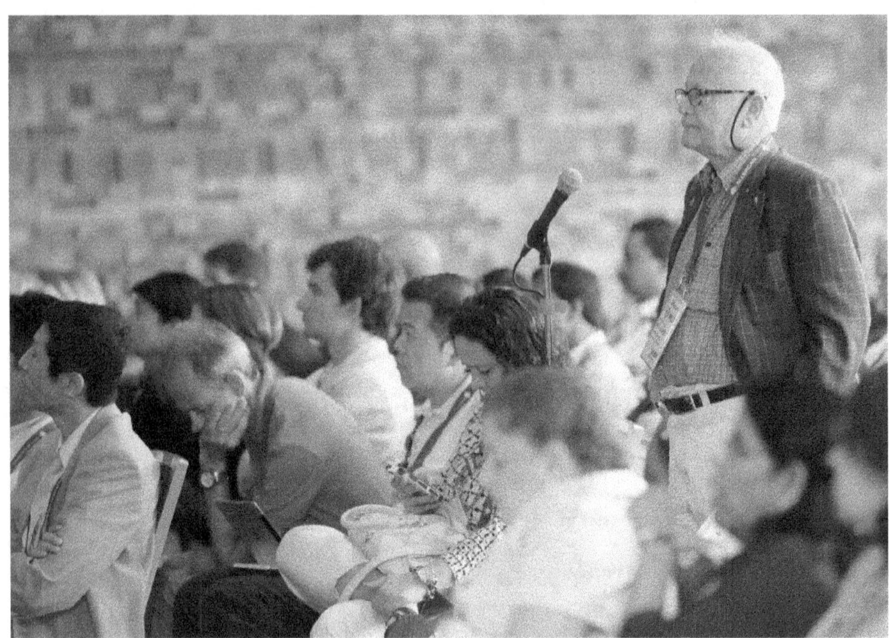

Robert Ritch

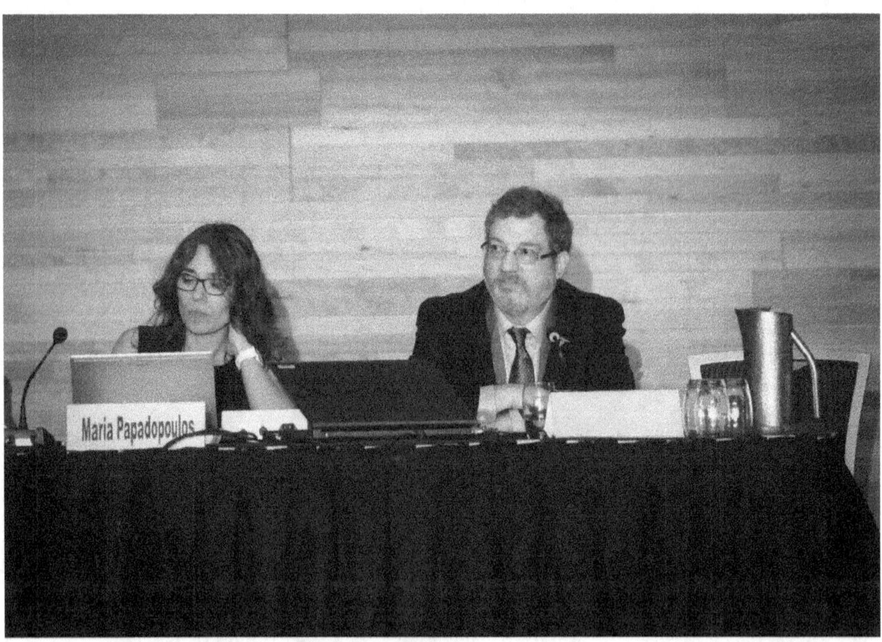

Maria Papadopoulos, James D. Brandt (L-R)

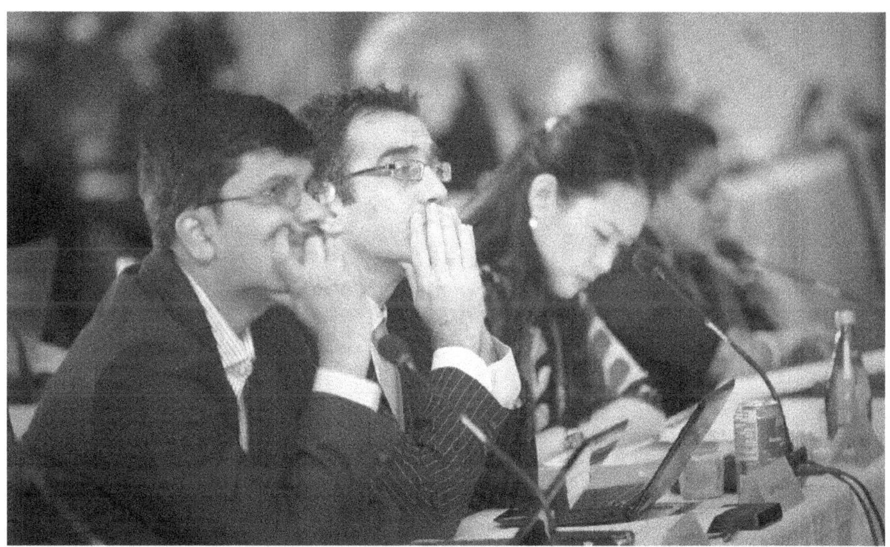

Viney Gupta, Julian Garcia Feijoo, Ching Lin Ho (L-R)

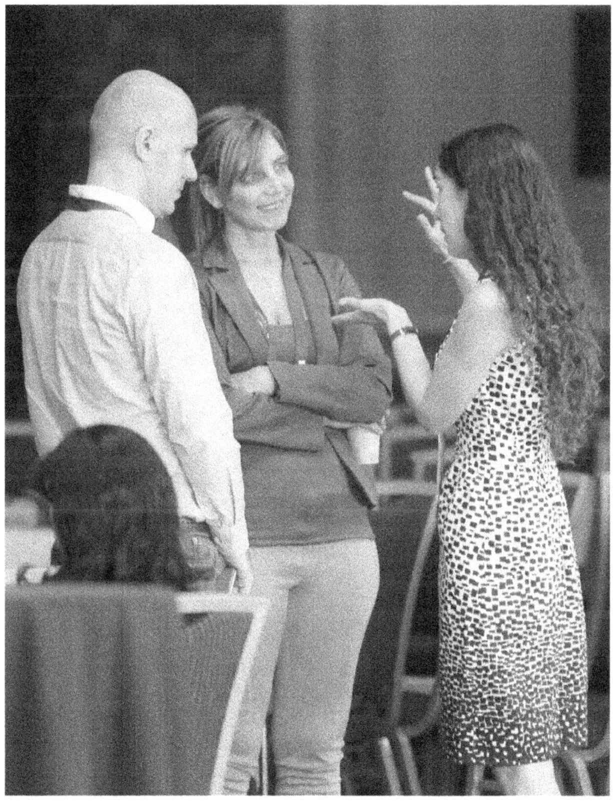

Hector Fontana, María Moussalli, Elena Bitrian (L-R)

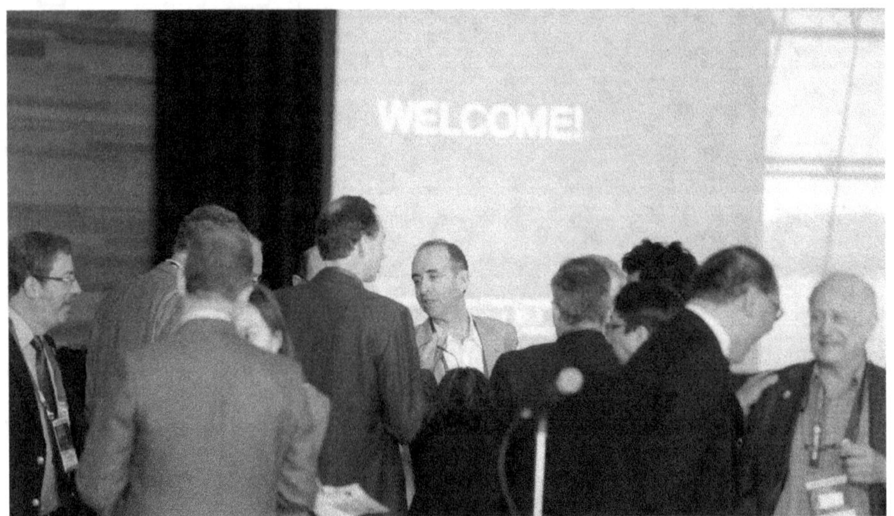

James D. Brandt, John Grigg, Jeffrey M. Liebmann, Peng T. Khaw, Robert Rich (L-R)

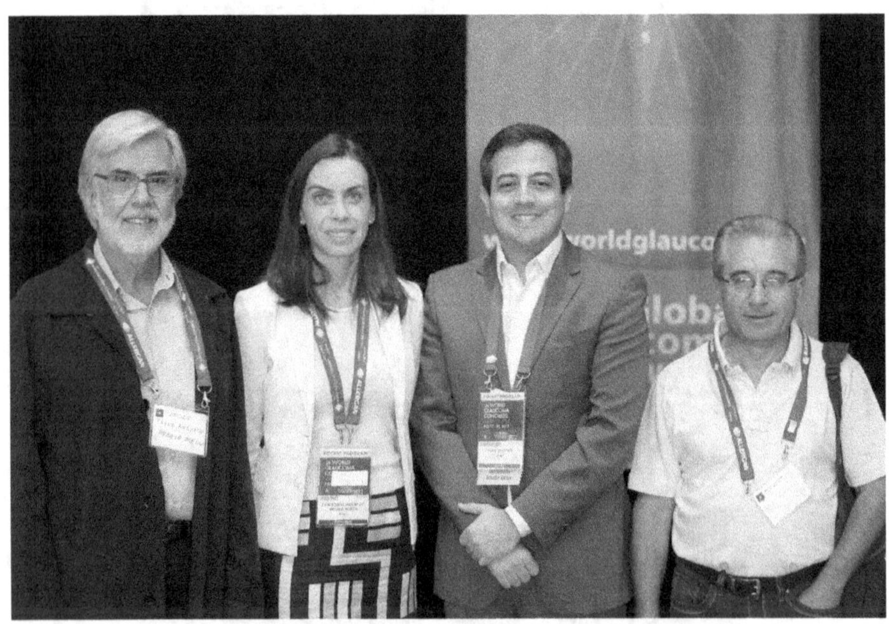

Paulo Augusto Arruda Mello, Christiane Rolim de Moura, Ivan Tavares, Felicio Silva (L-R)

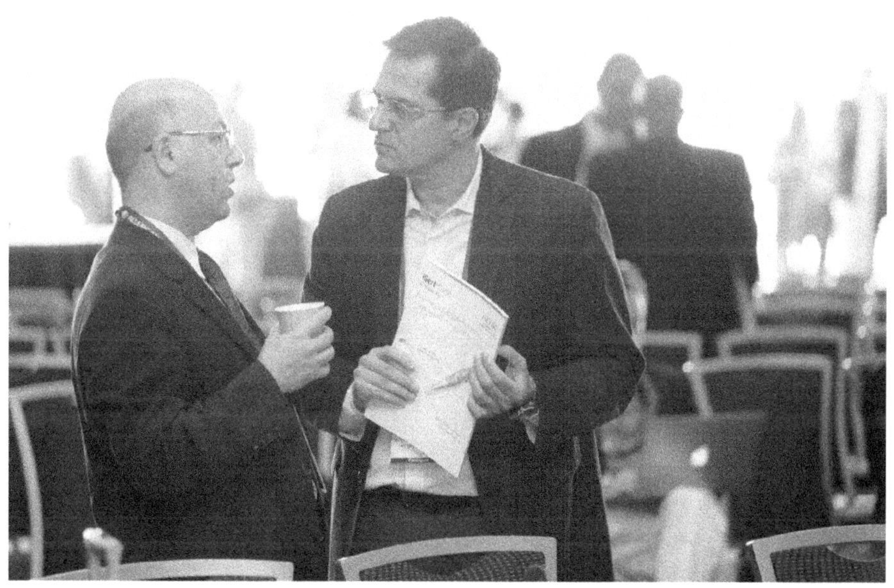

Albert Khouri, Mohammad Pakravan (L-R)

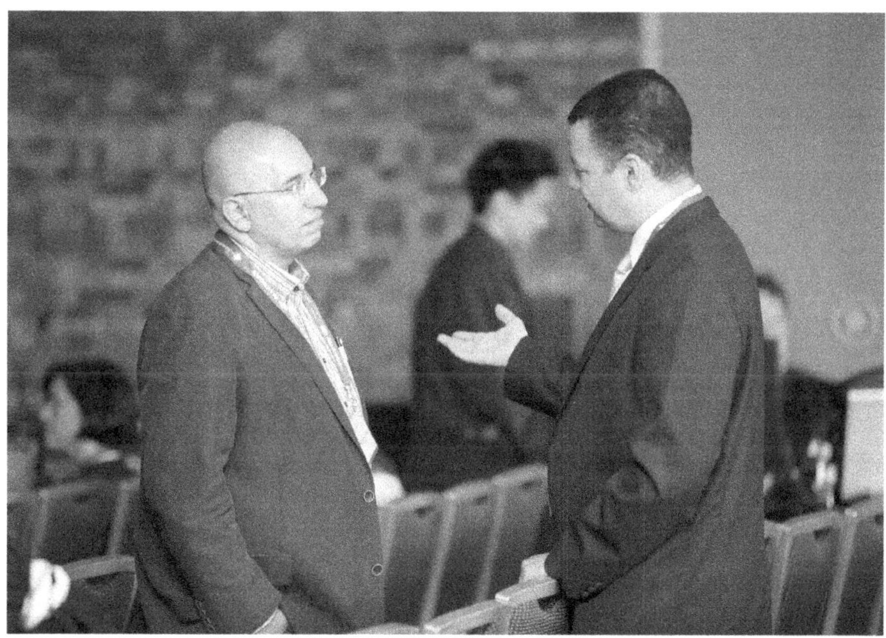

Ahmed Abdelrahman and Oscar Albis-Donado (L-R)

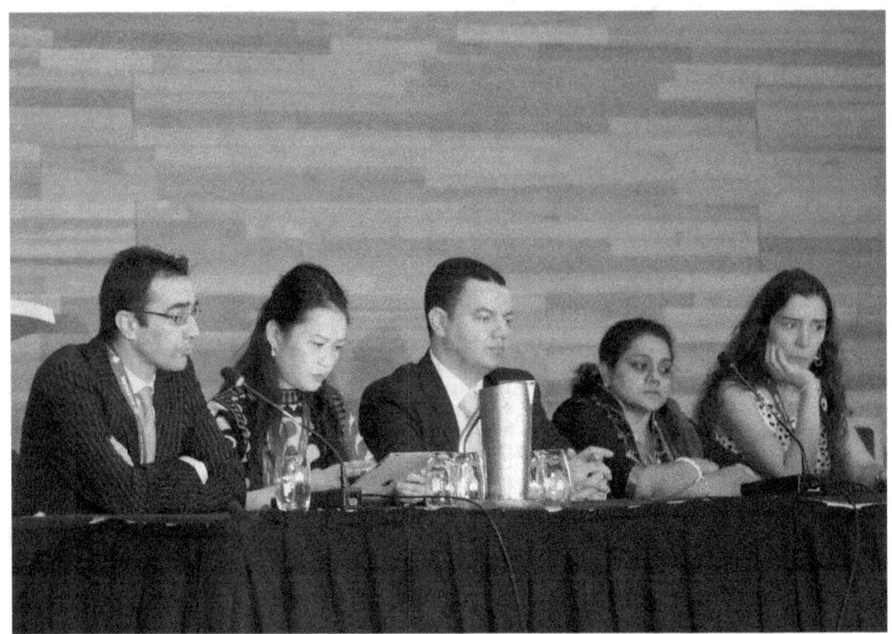

Julian Garcia Feijoo, Ching Lin Ho, Oscar Albis-Donado, Manju Anilkumar, Elena Bitrian (L-R)

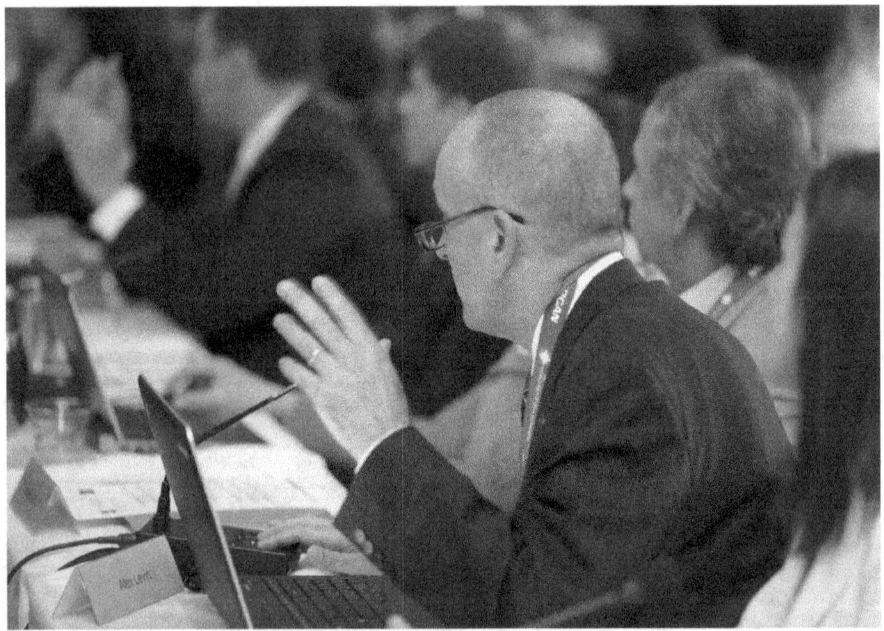

Alex Levin

SUMMARY CONSENSUS POINTS

Section 1 – Definition, classification, differential diagnosis

1. Childhood glaucoma is intraocular pressure (IOP) related damage to the eye.
   Comment: In addition to the IOP, optic disc appearance and visual fields, the definition of glaucoma also reflects the effect of IOP on other ocular structures in infancy.
2. The interpretation of IOP measurement in infants and young children, especially during examination under anesthesia, can potentially be affected by many factors.
   Comment: Other signs of glaucoma in infants and young children, such as ocular enlargement, Haab striae and increased cup-to-disc ratio, may be more important than the IOP value in the assessment.
3. Childhood glaucoma is classified as primary or secondary. Secondary childhood glaucoma is further classified according to whether the condition is acquired after birth or is present at birth (non-acquired). Non-acquired childhood glaucoma is categorized according to whether the signs are mainly ocular or systemic.
   Comment: Terms such as 'developmental', 'congenital' or 'infantile' glaucoma lack clear definition and their use is to be discouraged.
4. A child should not be labeled as having glaucoma or subjected to surgical treatment unless one is reasonably sure of the diagnosis and has excluded other conditions that may mimic glaucoma.

Section 2 – Establishing the diagnosis and determining glaucoma progression

1. Prompt diagnosis of childhood glaucoma and appropriate prompt treatment can minimize the degree of visual impairment.
   Comment: Examination under anesthesia or sedation may be appropriate to make the diagnosis, perform surgery or plan further treatment.
2. A child should not be labeled as having glaucoma or subjected to surgical treatment unless one is reasonably sure of the diagnosis and has excluded other conditions that may mimic glaucoma.
   Comment: If doubt exists about the diagnosis or evidence of progression cannot be determined, then appropriately timed follow-up or examination under anesthesia or sedation is advisable.
   Comment: Children should be encouraged onto the slit lamp for more accurate evaluation [intraocular pressure (IOP) measurement and optic disc assessment] when it appears this may be possible.
3. Glaucoma in children is characterized by the presence of elevated IOP and characteristic optic disc cupping. In addition to these features, glaucoma in infancy is associated with ocular enlargement, *buphthalmos*.

Comment: IOP measurement and optic disc appearance are fundamental features of the examination throughout the life of a child with glaucoma. In an infant whose eye is still vulnerable to other effects of elevated IOP, proxies of persistent elevated IOP (enlarging corneal diameter, increasing axial length and progressive myopia) also need to be taken into consideration and regularly assessed.

Comment: In children, the conclusion with regard to the diagnosis or progression of glaucoma must be based on the overall clinical findings and investigation results.

4. IOP measurement *in infancy and early childhood* can be influenced by many factors so is often unreliable when used in diagnosis and management.

5. IOP response to anesthetic agents is unpredictable. All inhaled agents lower IOP, sometimes rapidly and profoundly.

   Comment: Chloral hydrate, ketamine and midazolam appear not to lower IOP.

   Comment: Use the same anesthetic for serial examinations.

6. Increasing corneal diameter is the hallmark of all forms of glaucoma in infancy and early childhood.

   Comment: Corneal enlargement due to elevated IOP usually occurs before three years of age. Serial corneal diameter measurements are useful in establishing the diagnosis and in the monitoring of progression of glaucoma up to the age of three years.

   Comment: Central corneal thickness (CCT) should not be used to adjust IOP measurements as its role in childhood tonometry remains to be determined.

7. Gonioscopy is crucial in making the correct diagnosis and for planning surgical treatment. It should be performed at least once when possible.

8. Optic disc appearance is an important and sensitive parameter for both diagnosis and determination of progression in childhood glaucoma.

   Comment: Optic nerve size, the cup-disc ratio, focal areas of rim loss, and nerve fiber layer defects should be documented, preferably through a large pupil.

   Comment: A magnified binocular view is preferable, so attempt to examine a child on the slit lamp as soon as they are cooperative.

   Comment: Documenting the appearance of the disc at baseline and follow-up is desirable in determining both diagnosis and response to treatment.

   Comment: Cupping reversal is common in successfully-treated childhood glaucoma.

   Comment: Automated optic nerve imaging (*e.g.*, OCT) is limited by the lack of normative data and portability of the devices.

9. Rapid changes in refractive status and axial length (AL) determination are helpful in both diagnosing the disease and determining response to treatment while the sclera remains vulnerable to the effects of elevated IOP.

   Comment: AL outside normal limits is strongly suggestive of glaucoma.

   Comment: Continued enlargement of AL beyond the normal range suggests inadequately-treated glaucoma.

   Comment: Progressive myopia is additional evidence of glaucoma progression.

10. Assessment of the visual field in children can be useful but is challenging.
    Comment: It may be helpful to use the shortest possible test (*e.g.*, program 24-2
    Sita Fast).
    Comment: Repeat visual fields to confirm deficits. If repeated testing shows
    consistent findings, the measurements are probably valid.
    Comment: Although there is no normative database for children, age correction
    of the mean deviation for standard automated perimetry is small (0.7 db/decade).
    Moreover, useful metrics, such as pattern standard deviation, glaucoma hemi-
    field test and glaucoma change probability, are largely unaffected by age.

Section 3 – Genetics

1. Genetic evaluation of childhood glaucoma is especially important in those types
   of glaucoma when genotype phenotype correlations are known to exist.
   Comment: The results of these tests may be important in counseling, prognosis
   and management.
2. There is a known correlation between primary congenital glaucoma (PCG) and
   mutations in the *CYP1B1* gene.
   Comment: Performing carrier testing for at risk relatives is possible if both
   disease causing alleles of an affected family member have been identified.
3. Families affected by autosomal dominant juvenile open angle glaucoma (JOAG)
   have been found to have mutations in the *MYOC* gene.
   Comment: Genetic screening and genetic counseling could be considered in
   these patients to help diagnose pre-symptomatic cases among first and second-
   degree relatives of these patients.
4. Axenfeld-Rieger anomaly and syndrome have been associated with *PITX2* and
   FOXC1 mutations.
   Comment: *PITX2* mutations are more likely to be associated with systemic findings, while the risk of glaucoma is increased with *FOXC1* duplications and
   PITX2 mutations.
   Comment: Prospective parents may consider genetic counseling for risk calculation.
5. Aniridia is usually inherited in an autosomal-dominant fashion with high penetrance and variable expressivity, and it is almost exclusively caused by *PAX6*
   mutations.
   Comment: A child with sporadic aniridia should have ultrasound surveillance
   for Wilms tumor unless genetic testing rules out a microdeletion involving the
   Wilms tumor gene.
6. The *LTBP2* mutations seem to be involved in complex ocular phenotypes including ectopia lentis, megalocornea (unrelated to elevated intraocular pressure),
   microspherophakia and associated secondary glaucoma.
7. To optimize genetic counseling for families, accurate clinical ophthalmic diagnosis is critical.

Comment: Marked variation in penetrance and expression in primary and secondary childhood glaucomas exist, so parents and siblings of an affected child should be examined to provide maximally accurate phenotypic diagnoses for the clinical geneticist.

8. General pediatric assessment forms an important part of the management for children with glaucoma and can greatly assist in identifying systemic associations and initiating early management.

9. Genetics review plays a number of important roles including confirming or identifying syndromic diagnoses, recurrence risk assessment, genetic diagnosis, interpretation of molecular data, and reproductive counseling where this may be requested by the family after appropriate genetic counseling.

Section 4 – Medications

1. Medications alone rarely show sustained efficacy as primary treatment for glaucoma in infants and young children, especially in primary congenital glaucoma (PCG).
Comment: Medical therapy is frequently needed as temporizing intraocular pressure (IOP) lowering treatment before surgery or as adjuvant therapy after partially successful surgical procedures in childhood glaucoma.
Comment: IOP-reducing medication may help reduce corneal edema prior to surgery for childhood glaucoma.
Comment: Medical therapy should be considered first-line for some cases of childhood glaucoma (*e.g.*, uveitis-related, glaucoma after cataract removal).

2. Childhood glaucomas are heterogeneous in their causation as well as in their responses to different glaucoma medications.

3. Systemic pharmocokinetics for glaucoma medications are different in children than in adults.
Comment: Systemic absorption can be significant and may be reduced by advising parents to close the lids (if possible), remove excess periocular liquid and perform naso-lacrimal occlusion.
Comment: Use minimum frequency and concentration to achieve target IOP.

4. Potentially serious or fatal systemic adverse reactions which are rarely seen in adults may occur in young children after exposure to glaucoma medications.
Comment: Adverse side effects may manifest atypically in children (*e.g.*, nocturnal cough with beta blockers rather than wheeze with reactive airways).
Comment: Brimonidine should be avoided in young children.
Comment: Children are more vulnerable to adverse effects of medications as they may be unable to verbalize symptoms and parents may not readily recognize them.
Comment: Parents must be informed of the potential side effects.

5. Compliance and adherence issues are greater and more complex in children due to their dependence on caregivers or parents, possible lack of cooperation in the

administration of treatment, as well as concurrent medical conditions that may complicate medical therapy.

6. Target pressure must be chosen and reassessed with all available information concerning whether glaucoma is adequately controlled.
   Comment: Limitations on ability to perform structural and functional testing of optic nerve make verification of glaucoma control more difficult in children.

7. Consider surgery when medical treatment fails to control glaucoma.
   Comment: Glaucoma therapy in children has to be individualized, especially in situations where the risk of surgery outweighs the benefits of continuing medical therapy.

Section 5 – Glaucoma surgery in children

1. Surgery is a critical component of the management of childhood glaucoma.
   Comment: It is important to prepare patients and parents or caregivers for lifelong follow-up and possible future surgeries.

2. Glaucoma surgery should preferably be performed by a trained surgeon in centers where there is sufficient volume to ensure surgical experience and skill, and safe anesthesia.
   Comment: A long-term surgical strategy including choice of procedures should be based on training, experience, logistics, and surgeon's preference.
   Comment: The first chance for surgery is often the best chance, and it is important to choose the most appropriate operation.

3. Glaucoma surgery in children is more challenging than in adults with a higher failure and complication rate than in adults.

4. Angle surgery (goniotomy and trabeculotomy – conventional or circumferential) is the procedure of choice for primary congenital glaucoma with the exact choice dictated by corneal clarity and the surgeon's experience and preference.
   Comment: Angle surgery success rates for secondary childhood glaucomas are generally not as good as for primary congenital glaucoma (PCG) with certain exceptions [*e.g.*, glaucoma with acquired condition (uveitis) in juvenile idiopathic arthritis (JIA)].

5. Trabeculectomy, when performed by experienced childhood glaucoma surgeons, can be associated with good outcomes in appropriate cases.
   Comment: Anti-scarring agents and other adjunctive techniques may be beneficial.

6. Glaucoma drainage devices (GDD) may offer the most effective long-term intraocular pressure (IOP) control in many childhood glaucomas especially those that are refractory to other surgical treatment.
   Comment: There is no prospective evidence that anti-scarring agents influence drainage device outcomes.

7. Cyclophotocoagulation with the diode laser has limited long-term success and often requires re-treatment and the continuation of medications.

8. Other glaucoma procedures advocated in children for the treatment of glaucoma have not been widely adopted either because of the technical challenges in buphthalmic eyes or because they are yet to be proven efficacious or safe in children.

9. Concurrent with glaucoma therapy, visual development needs to be evaluated and optimized with ametropic correction and amblyopia therapy.

10. With childhood glaucoma surgery, one needs carefully to consider the risks and benefits of each intervention, especially in refractory cases when the fellow eye is healthier, and in only eyes.

    Comment: Whenever possible, the assent of the child should be sought when making these difficult decisions.

Section 6 – Primary congenital glaucoma and juvenile open-angle glaucoma

1. Primary congenital glaucoma (PCG) is the most common non-sydromic glaucoma in infancy and is classified according to onset of signs. Its worldwide incidence is variable and influenced by consanguinity.

2. PCG is usually inherited in an autosomal recessive manner, with a family history reported in 10-40% of cases and is more common in consanguineous populations.

    Comment: Mutations in the *CYP1B1* gene have been identified and show variable expressivity and phenotypes.

    Comment: Clinical screening of current and future siblings is essential if there is parental consanguinity.

3. The pathogenesis of PCG remains uncertain but the immature angle appearance seen clinically is thought to result from the arrested maturation of tissues derived from cranial neural crest cells.

4. PCG is a surgical condition and the surgical procedure of choice is usually angle surgery (goniotomy or trabeculotomy) with high rates of success reported for both in favorable cases and after multiple procedures.

    Comment: Combined trabeculotomy with trabeculectomy as an initial procedure is suggested by some to be more successful than either procedure performed alone in certain populations. There are no supporting prospective comparisons in the literature.

5. Once angle surgery fails, the next procedure of choice is either trabeculectomy or a glaucoma drainage device.

6. Juvenile open-angle glaucoma (JOAG) is a relatively rare form of childhood glaucoma usually presenting after the age of four years, with a normal angle appearance and no signs of other ocular anomalies or systemic disease.

7. Depending on age, medical therapy is the first-line treatment for JOAG, although surgery is often required.

8. Evidence remains weak for the optimum first-line surgical intervention for JOAG.

Section 7 – Glaucoma associated with non-acquired ocular anomalies

1. Children who have non-acquired ocular anomalies often have systemic conditions that require pediatric evaluation and/or treatment.
2. Many non-acquired ocular anomalies are genetic in nature.
   Comment: Screening of family members in such cases and genetic counseling is indicated.
3. Glaucoma related to non-acquired ocular anomalies may be present at birth or may develop over time, so regular lifelong monitoring is necessary.
4. Before glaucoma develops, one should consider treating elevated intraocular pressure (IOP) associated with non-acquired ocular anomalies (secondary ocular hypertension).
5. Infantile onset of glaucoma related to non-acquired ocular anomalies is associated with buphthalmos and the risk of Descemet membrane breaks.
6. Medical treatment is usually first-line, but surgery is often required early for congenital/infantile presentations and should not be delayed.
   Comment: Angle surgery in infants may be effective although the results are usually not as good as for primary congenital glaucoma (PCG).
   Comment: Often trabeculectomy with anti-scarring agents or primary tube surgery is necessary for IOP control.
   Comment: Cyclodestruction may be considered after failed trabeculectomy or tube surgery.
7. There is considerable phenotypic variability associated with genetic mutations recognized in children with non-acquired ocular anomalies.
8. Axenfeld-Rieger (AR) anomaly is recognized now to represent a spectrum of disease previously referred to as Axenfeld anomaly and Rieger anomaly. Axenfeld-Rieger syndrome includes the ocular findings of Axenfeld-Rieger anomaly with the addition of systemic abnormalities.
   Comment: Examination of family members including gonioscopy is important to determine whether the patient is part of a larger pedigree or a new case.
9. Peters anomaly is usually seen as an isolated ocular disorder but can be associated with systemic abnormalities of neural crest origin and is referred to as Peters plus syndrome.
   Comment: It is important to exclude the presence of systemic involvement and when it is present, to co-manage it with a pediatrician.
   Comment: Assessing for glaucoma can be challenging as typical IOP measurement over the central cornea may be inaccurate and the optic discs may not be visible. Measure the IOP in a clear area of cornea if possible.
10. Aniridia is commonly associated with glaucoma and is due to both open- and closed-angle mechanisms.
    Comment: Children with sporadic aniridia should be screened for Wilms tumor.
11. Management of persistent fetal vasculature can be challenging because of the heterogeneity of clinical presentation.

Comment: Surgical treatment is aimed towards obtaining useful vision and preventing or treating secondary complications such as glaucoma.

Section 8 – Glaucoma associated with non-acquired systemic disease or syndrome

1. Syndromes with system anomalies or systemic diseases that are present at birth can be associated with ocular signs that include glaucoma.
   Comment: Patients should be regularly monitored for glaucoma throughout life and elevated intraocular pressure (IOP) treated, should it occur.
   Comment: Patients also should be assessed for systemic manifestations of their disease.
2. Sturge-Weber syndrome (SWS) is commonly associated with glaucoma.
   Comment: Periocular port-wine marks are associated with ipsilateral glaucoma. Lid involvement and/or episcleral capillary vascular malformation appear to further increase the risk of glaucoma.
   Comment: Choroidal hemangioma increases the risk of serous choroidal effusion and suprachoroidal hemorrhage with surgery, especially if the IOP drops precipitously or hypotony develops. Modifications to the surgical technique must be employed to minimize risk of hypotony.
   Comment: Patients should be assessed, perhaps including neuroimaging, for other manifestations of SWS.
3. Neurofibromatosis (NF1) is uncommonly associated with glaucoma.
   Comment: Optic pathway gliomas affect 12-15% of patients with neurofibromatosis and can present with decreased vision distinct from glaucoma.
4. Ectopia Lentis (EL) can present as an isolated ocular anomaly or be associated with other ocular or systemic findings.
   Comment: Patients with EL are at risk of acute pupillary block.
   Comment: All patients without a proven or obvious cause of EL should be tested for homocystinura by urine analysis and investigated for blood homocyteine levels prior to any anesthesia or sedation because of life-threatening vascular risks.
   Comment: Patients with Marfan syndrome should have echocardiography and cardiology consultation prior to surgery.
5. Maintain close follow-up for infants with known or suspected congenital rubella, since glaucoma signs might be less evident at birth in some cases.
   Comment: Rubella keratitis should be differentiated from corneal findings associated with IOP related corneal edema.

Section 9 – Glaucoma associated with acquired conditions

1. Managing uveitic glaucoma in children is challenging. The control of intraocular inflammation with adequate immunosuppression, topical and/or systemic agents, is a crucial part of management.
   Comment: Hypotony is a particular concern with surgery and modifications to the surgical technique must be employed to minimize its risk.
2. Traumatic glaucoma pathogenesis is multifactorial.
   Comment: Patients with sickle cell disease (not trait) are at higher risk for re-bleed and are likely to develop glaucomatous optic nerve damage, even with only moderately raised intraocular pressure (IOP).
   Comment: Management is aimed at controlling IOP and minimizing damage to the cornea and optic nerve. Consider surgical intervention with sustained elevated IOP > 30 mmHg unresponsive to maximum medical therapy or if corneal staining is present.
3. Steroid-induced elevated IOP is not uncommon and may be severe in children treated with ocular and systemic corticosteroids.
   Comment: Consider discontinuing the corticosteroid if possible or switching to a steroid sparing agent to ensure underlying disease control, which takes priority.
   Comment: IOP elevation may persist for months, years or even become permanent, requiring medical or surgical intervention.
4. Glaucoma secondary to intraocular tumors in children is a relatively rare event.
   Comment: Patients can be symptomatic with acute glaucoma due to the fast growth of the tumor, or symptom free in the case of a progressive, slow growing tumor.
   Comment: In cases of unexplained glaucoma, the possibility of an intraocular tumor should be considered, especially when a child presents with a severe chronic uveitis associated with high IOP.
   Comment: Incisional surgical intervention to lower IOP is contra-indicated for glaucoma secondary to malignant ocular lesions.
5. The causes of retinopathy of prematurity (ROP) induced glaucoma are multifactorial in nature but largely due to secondary angle closure.
   Comment: Glaucoma may develop years or decades later in patients with treated or untreated Stage-4 or -5 ROP, so long-term surveillance is warranted.
   Comment: IOP elevation may follow laser therapy for threshold ROP.

Section 10 – Glaucoma following cataract surgery

1. Glaucoma following cataract surgery is that which occurs after pediatric cataract removal of either congenital idiopathic cataract, cataract associated with ocular or systemic syndromes and acquired cataract.
2. Glaucoma can occur in aphakic and pseudophakic eyes.

3. Young age at the time of cataract surgery and microcornea increase the risk of glaucoma.
4. Glaucoma usually occurs in eyes with open angles but angle closure can occur, and it is important to elucidate the underlying mechanism when possible (*e.g.*, by gonioscopy).
5. The risk of glaucoma following cataract surgery in children is lifelong, so regular monitoring is necessary.
6. Medical intraocular pressure (IOP) lowering therapy is usually first line treatment for glaucoma following cataract surgery. When medical therapy fails, surgical therapy is indicated but there is no consensus on the preferred approach.

INDEX OF AUTHORS